PsychoPolitics

'One of the most prolific, versatile and scholarly of this country's socialist writers.'
—*The Times*

'A unique voice, politically committed but always balanced, urgent but always laced with humour.'
—*New Statesman*

PsychoPolitics

Peter Sedgwick

New Introduction by Tad Tietze

PLUTO PRESS

First published 1982; this edition published 2022 by Pluto Press
New Wing, Somerset House, Strand, London WC2R 1LA

www.plutobooks.com

British Library Cataloguing in Publication Data
A catalogue record for this book is available from the British Library

ISBN 978 0 7453 4725 7 Hardback
ISBN 978 0 7453 4722 6 Paperback
ISBN 978 0 7453 4724 0 PDF
ISBN 978 0 7453 4723 3 EPUB

This book is printed on paper suitable for recycling and made from fully managed and sustained forest sources. Logging, pulping and manufacturing processes are expected to conform to the environmental standards of the country of origin.

Typeset by Riverside Publishing Solutions, Salisbury, England

Simultaneously printed in the United Kingdom and United States of America

Contents

Introduction to the New Edition

MENTAL HEALTH POLITICS, 40 YEARS LATER

When *PsychoPolitics* first came out in 1982, the year before Peter Sedgwick took his own life, the politics of mental illness and the wider political world were in a very different place to where they are now. Sedgwick, who had identified with revolutionary marxism, working-class struggle, and the radical left for most of his adult life, was swimming against two interconnected tides when the book was assembled.

The first of these tides was the rise of a new biomedical psychiatry as embodied in the publication of the *Diagnostic and Statistical Manual of Mental Disorders*, 3rd Edition (*DSM-III*) in 1980. This was generally seen as a 'paradigm shift' ushering in a new, more rational and rigorous, approach to mental disorders, one which rebutted accusations that psychiatry was an anti-scientific enterprise whose true purpose was the coercive control of behaviours deemed deviant by society.

The second tide Sedgwick swam against was the impasse of the social and political movements that had swept the West, including his native Britain, from the late 1960s. These movements had, as one of their consequences, inspired activism and experimentation around issues of mental health and illness. When they went into decline, not only was the door opened to political reaction – in Britain exemplified by Thatcherism – but to defensiveness and retreat by those involved in radical mental health politics. Nevertheless, in 1982 their residue still hung in the air, leaving open the prospect of future clashes between a resurgent biomedical psychiatry and its anti-psychiatric critics.

Forty years later, neither of these conditions obtains.

Biomedical psychiatry has foundered on its own contradictions, after the attempt to unite around a new neuroscientific paradigm with the *DSM*-5 provoked theoretical divisions, professional turf wars and criticism from leaders of the earlier DSM-III revolution.[1] The new manual – finally released amid fierce public controversy in 2013 – was seen as little different from its predecessors. And psychiatric research has stagnated, eschewing aspirations of further far-reaching innovation and instead focusing on tinkering at the edges of existing theories and treatments.[2]

Meanwhile, political struggles and theoretical perspectives critical of psychiatry have also waned, paralleling the decline of working-class and social movement activity and a concomitant retreat and fragmentation of the left. Socially transformative demands around mental health have given way to narrower questions of 'consumer participation', 'rights', 'lived experience', 'identity' and 'trauma' that have largely been incorporated by mainstream, bureaucratic healthcare systems.

This double impasse of mainstream psychiatry and its militant critics has created a fitting moment for the republication of *PsychoPolitics*. This is because Sedgwick developed his ground-breaking critique of modern psychiatry via a concurrent critique of anti-psychiatric thinkers and movements. His key move in this respect was to broaden the scope of his inquiry to the concepts of health and illness *in general* – physical as well as mental – thereby opening up new and different ways of tackling the debates swirling at the time rather than forcing them into mutually hostile, pro- and anti-psychiatry, camps.

My own engagement with Sedgwick's ideas started when I read *PsychoPolitics* for the first time soon before I completed my psychiatric training. Sedgwick had an unusual ability – even among marxists – to interrogate a wide range of critical concepts without once allowing them to become disconnected from their basis in material social relations and the political economy of healthcare. Thus grounded, the polarisation between psychiatry and its detractors became more apparent as *Sturm und Drang* that obscured real power structures more than it exposed or challenged them.

What's more, having been a generalist doctor for a decade before commencing postgraduate training, I was struck by Sedgwick's refusal to single psychiatry out as qualitatively different to (and worse than) the rest of medicine. This was not only a clearsighted riposte to the dualism that shapes perceptions of both, but one thoroughly supported by the medical realities I'd experienced. Sedgwick was by no means letting the mad doctors off the hook; rather, he was exposing their physical health counterparts to much-deserved scrutiny at a time their authority was still near its historical peak.

WHAT IS ILLNESS?

The dual nature of Sedgwick's critique also helps explain why his arguments have been taken seriously by activists and writers generally inclined to be sharply critical of psychiatry, as well as within the psychiatric profession itself as it grappled with its own upheavals in the 1970s and 1980s.[3] Today they can help us comprehend the exhaustion of mainstream psychiatry and its anti-psychiatric opponents, and what alternatives to this state of affairs might be possible.

The first part of *PsychoPolitics* is dominated by richly detailed critical analyses of the ideas of prominent thinkers associated with anti-psychiatric movements of the late 1960s and early 1970s, in particular the American sociologist Erving Goffman, the Scottish psychiatrist R.D. Laing, the libertarian Hungarian-American psychiatrist Thomas Szasz, and the French philosopher Michel Foucault. These theorists, as well as more mainstream authors, provide the counterpoints against which Sedgwick's theoretical innovations are elaborated and refracted.

Although 'anti-psychiatry' refers to a heterogeneous and at times contradictory range of ideas, politics and activities, common themes emerge: that psychiatry relies on low-quality or absent 'scientific' evidence when compared with physical healthcare professions; that mainstream mental healthcare is basically repressive, structured around detention and forced treatment; and that psychiatric diagnosis is fundamentally value-laden, labelling certain types of social deviancy as 'mental illness'.[4]

Sedgwick congratulated anti-psychiatric thinkers for expressing 'a consistent and convergent *tendency of opposition* directed against *positivist method* in the study of abnormal human behaviour'. Positivism was defined in the medical context as 'an approach towards the investigation of human pathology which, modelling itself upon antecedents it believes to be characteristic of the natural sciences, (a) postulates a radical separation between "facts" and "values" (declaring only the former to be the subject matter of the professional investigator) and (b) suppresses the interactive relationship between the investigator and the "facts" on which she or he works'.[5]

For all their scrutiny of psychiatry's positivist claims about mental disorder, the profession's critics smuggled positivism back in when they came to contrast psychiatry with physical medicine, which they tended to treat as an area of human activity that could indeed proceed on 'objective', value-free scientific lines. Thus, 'Anti-psychiatry can only operate by positing a mechanical and inaccurate model of physical illness and its medical diagnosis'.[6]

This contradiction emerged from what Sedgwick saw as the anti-psychiatrists' failure to interrogate not just *mental* illness but the logically prior and more inclusive concept of *illness* in general.

> [I]t appears to me that none of these thinkers have begun by asking the question: What is *illness*? Only in the light of an answer to *this* question could we determine our answer to the question: Is mental illness really illness in the 'medical' sense?[7]

Sedgwick drew on medical epidemiologist René Dubos's descriptions of how social and political measures had produced the vast bulk of effective responses to ill-health in human history and how modern medicine – focused on the biotechnical treatment of sick individuals – was only a small part of the story. Medicine was just one way that humans had tried to explain and manage ill-health within historically specific circumstances. The medical enterprise is, on this view, 'from its inception value-loaded; it is not simply an applied biology, but a biology applied in accordance with the dictates of social interest'.[8]

From this came Sedgwick's radical conclusion about the status of all health and illness:

> If we examine the logical structure of our judgements of illness (whether 'physical' or 'mental') it may prove possible to reduce the distance between psychiatry and other streams of medicine… not by annexing psychopathology to the technical instrumentation of the natural sciences but by revealing the character of all illness and disease, health and treatment, as social constructions. For social constructions they most certainly are.[9]

Sedgwick contended that 'Outside the significances that we voluntarily attach to certain conditions, *there are no illnesses or diseases in nature*'.[10] By this he did not mean that there are no biological or other material correlates of what humans refer to as illness, but that it is a human – indeed *social* – decision as to what is defined and treated as 'illness'.

Understood this way, 'all sickness is essentially deviancy' from social norms, because 'no attribution of sickness to any being can be made without the expectation of some alternative state of affairs [i.e. health] which is considered more desirable'.[11] By this Sedgwick did not mean that all social deviancies will be labelled illnesses and therefore fall within the remit of healthcare processes. To understand why such attributions are made – why some problems and not others are treated as forms of sickness or disease – requires a concrete analysis of the interests and conflicts at play within a given society at a given time. The same is true of situations in which there are unresolved disputes over whether a particular social problem should fall within a health/illness framework; for example, over whether the diagnosis of 'psychopathy' or 'antisocial personality disorder' should be grounds for diminished criminal responsibility.

Post-traumatic stress disorder (PTSD) provides a striking example of a psychiatric diagnosis 'invented' due to the assertion of certain social interests. Emerging from a campaign by American Vietnam War veterans and their health worker allies to have their wartime suffering officially recognised rather than written off as personal failing, the diagnosis was effectively a product of anti-war radicalisation.[12] Over time, however, it has become integral to the rise of 'trauma' as a professional and lay concept explaining why people suffer emotional distress and dysfunction after exposure to certain types of triggering events, with a resulting expansion of PTSD diagnoses. The rise of PTSD has thus come to fit with the interests not only of people who have had such experiences and health professionals who want to provide them with help, but such disparate groups as insurers needing clear guidelines for reimbursement, bosses wanting to deal with their employees' reactions to work stress, and activists pursuing recognition of past wrongs within a medicalised framework.[13]

Sedgwick also deployed this approach to explain the devaluation of mental when compared to physical illness in modern times. Because the concept of illness had grown up in close association with the social practice of treatment, as therapies became more technologically based, so too did concepts of illness become more tied up with biotechnical models, alienated from the social relationships in which they had originated. Mental disorder, less amenable to biotechnical explanations and interventions, became ever more open to the accusation that it was not a true illness, putting pressure on psychiatrists to adhere to a positivist biomedical frame.[14]

INDIVIDUALISING, PRIVATISING AND ATOMISING

Identifying the implicit acceptance of a positivist, narrowly biotechnological view of physical health and illness among both psychiatry's defenders and critics, Sedgwick transcended that dualism to forge a critique of modern medicine *in toto*, which could evaluate the common features of physical and mental healthcare.

For example, in a 1974 article on 'medical individualism' Sedgwick took aim at its 'consistent bias towards individualizing, privatizing, and atomizing concepts and practices in treatment which ought to be interpreted and produced socially, collectively, and integrally', by examining how these tendencies undermine care in the very different medical specialties of surgery and psychiatry. The real-world failures of individualist and contractual forms of healthcare lead inexorably to the bureaucratic state stepping in to provide a mass-produced and institutional alternative, but with the result that the two forms come to be in permanent competition with each other without a true 'socialisation' of care, let alone its rational integration into collective human action.[15]

Physical medicine has repeatedly displayed flaws akin to those that psychiatry's critics have often implied are specific to mental healthcare. For example, all of medicine (and not just psychiatry) has been wracked by scandals exposing the corrupting influence of the pharmaceutical industry, leading to the popular impression that the profession can't be trusted to do what is best for patients.[16] Alongside this have been revelations that many doctors were prescribing ineffective or dangerous treatments despite there being no evidence supporting their use, resulting in embarrassing 'medical reversals' in which therapies had to be withdrawn.[17]

Even if we put aside such improprieties, a major 2012 statistical comparison of psychiatric versus general medicine drugs showed that, apart from a few exceptions, many of the most commonly used medications for physical illnesses had effect sizes little different from their psychiatric counterparts. While this data was used by some defenders of mainstream psychiatry to extol the virtues of psychotropic medications, in fact what the study revealed was the relatively limited effectiveness of medicines for physical illness, very far from their portrayal as miracles of modern science.[18]

It is similarly untenable to see psychiatry as qualitatively different from physical medicine because its determinations of health and illness are directly bound up with its role in coercive treatment. As I have written elsewhere, such a perspective ignores how the vast majority of psychiatric treatment today occurs on a voluntary basis in private or public outpatient settings, as well as eliding how many practices in contractually based physical medicine involve elements of coercion certified by doctors' value judgements:

> From the impossibility of 'informed consent' when there are large asymmetries of knowledge and power between doctors and patients, to the informally non-consensual treatment of severely ill patients in emergency and acute medical settings, to the use of various legal instruments such as 'guardianship' orders to impose treatment and control on patients found to lack decision-making 'capacity', the individual freedom of patients being treated by physicians and surgeons is often only apparent and partial.[19]

Most strikingly, the governments of liberal democracies around the world have just spent two years imposing extraordinary restrictions on their citizens' lives, justified on the basis of expert medical consensus that deemed these measures necessary to combat the COVID-19 pandemic. Medical authority was mobilised by governments, with many health experts rising to prominence arguing the official line, in order to justify unprecedented state coercion, often on the basis of terrifying modelling projections of health system collapse and mass death – most of which turned out to be wildly inaccurate[20] – if the public didn't obey.

It's hard to imagine a cruder application of a narrow, positivist medical rationality on the panoply of divergent (and often competing) interests that make up modern societies. Moreover, many of the restrictions represented a sudden reversal of previous expert consensus contained in pandemic planning documents, one that cannot be explained by the emergence of new scientific evidence.[21]

Yet if it was an unsustainable proposition that politicians were merely 'following the science' in imposing lockdowns, border closures and other controls, such measures were made possible – as was the marginalisation of dissenting voices arguing for a more holistic view of their social impacts – precisely because most of the public had voluntarily withdrawn to the presumed safety of an atomised private sphere. This retreat gave a material weight to government-imposed restrictions that would have been considered intolerable just months earlier. Perversely, this was often justified in terms of saving health systems from having to deal with too many sick patients, a logic accepted even by many of those on the left who had previously campaigned for more and better healthcare.

The almost unimaginably costly suppression of large swathes of economic and social life was in effect prioritised over mobilising society's resources towards better care and protection of those most vulnerable to the virus's ravages. Rather than simply accepting the hegemonic narrative that all this was scientifically grounded and socially necessary, Sedgwick's approach encourages us to inquire which actors were acting in whose interests, as well as considering the effects of such unprecedented actions not just on select COVID-19-related health outcomes but on the wider social fabric in which health and illness are embedded.

THE CENTRAL PROBLEM OF THE ASYLUM

PsychoPolitics also helps us comprehend how struggles over diagnosis and treatment are themselves embedded in social relations and can express (even if in distorted form) conflicts between determinate social interests. Sedgwick's critique historicises these issues and forces us to think about the problems with modern healthcare in general, and the society that spawns it, rather than to focus on the problems of psychiatry in isolation.

This conception of illness (including that of mental illness) was, for him, essential to placing demands on health services. Moreover, because questions of health and illness are based in and inseparable from real social relations and struggles, 'Mental illness, like mental health, is a fundamentally *critical* concept: or can be made into one provided that those who use it are prepared to place demands and pressures on the existing organisation of society'.[22] Such demands should not be limited to the reallocation of resources to overcome disparities in access to healthcare but should also posit what type of care would be needed. As Mark Cresswell and Helen Spandler have noted, this goes beyond the bounds of narrow biotechnical conceptions of treatment:

> Sedgwick is pro-medicine precisely to the extent that he envisages a *radically socialized* medicine applicable equally to physical and mental health. Such examples of socialized medicine include, '[t]he insertion of windows into working-class houses' and 'the provision of a pure water supply and an efficient sewage disposal'.[23]

This is very far from calls for 'parity' or 'parity of esteem' between mental and physical health. These concepts emerged in the United States in the 1990s and have more recently been taken up in Britain as a way of shining a light on gross deficits in healthcare access and outcomes suffered by people with mental illness. They rest on the notion that a health system dominated by profit-motivated insurers and/or government bean-counters should apply the same accounting rules to 'value' both varieties of problems equally. While they might represent a step forward in terms of funding, such measures also further imbricate care in cold cost-benefit calculations and systems of rationing. Because parity doesn't eliminate the separate status of mental and physical disorders, solutions tend to be posed in terms of competition over limited healthcare resources rather than provision according to patients' needs.

Also conspicuous over the last 40 years has been the incorporation of much of even the most radical mental health activism into channels that leave existing healthcare hierarchies intact. This is not only a result of the decline of social struggles that previously gave energy to militancy around mental health. Activists' one-sided opposition to the entire enterprise of psychiatry allowed many of them to be assimilated by existing power structures and used as a cudgel to manage health systems. In an address to the Royal College of Psychiatrists soon before his death, Sedgwick presciently warned how the 'libertarian' critique of psychiatric authority emanating from sections of the ascendant Thatcherite right – criticisms that strongly overlapped with anti-psychiatric attacks – would underpin assaults on 'collective' government provision of care without challenging the repressive power of the state.[24]

Concepts and practices drawn from activist and reform demands – such as 'consumer participation', 'human rights', 'trauma-informed care', and 'patient-centred care' as well as a place within systems for the 'lived experience' of consumer representatives and peer workers – have not been an uncomplicated boon. Rather, for all the ways they formally recognise patients' needs, existing hierarchies also use them to performance-manage clinicians, bureaucratically restructure workplaces, and cut costs by replacing highly trained clinical care with lower-paid, ex-patient staff.[25] Meanwhile, changes to mental health law purported to enshrine greater patient rights have increased the legal-bureaucratic pressures on clinicians while doing little to arrest upward trends in involuntary treatment – or have had the perverse but predictable effect of extruding patients out of psychiatric care and into custodial settings.

In the second part of *PsychoPolitics*, Sedgwick surveys activism, political demands, and radical therapeutic experimentation around mental health. His sobering conclusion is that such struggles have had minimal impact on the institutions that deliver psychiatric care, and that they have often created as many problems for people suffering from mental disability as they intended to solve:

> The civil-libertarian stance, the corporate trade-union response, the hyper-politicised annexation of anti-psychiatry by the far left, the 'alternative therapies' which cater only for the milder and the acuter forms of distress all stand as glib, guilt-discharging displacements of the central problem of the asylum: how to create the economic means of employment, the material apparatus of housing, the ethical structures of fellowship and solidarity, for those who through various forms of mental disability cannot purchase these benefits as commodities in the market-place. It will not suffice to reverse the long historical process of hospitalising the mentally disabled by despatching them back to their families.[26]

The politicisation of medical goals must not, therefore, be limited to the reform (or replacement) of psychiatry or the hospital carried out in isolation from more fundamental social change. The embryonic efforts by patients, their supporters, clinicians, and other social forces to expand, improve and transform mental healthcare can only properly unite and come to fruition in the context of society revolutionising itself. Sedgwick's was a deeply humanist orientation, one that demanded the greatest possible care for the suffering individual, indissolubly tied to a profoundly critical social practice.

THE FUTURE BELONGS TO ILLNESS

Sedgwick predicted that while some conditions might be shifted from the ledger of illness to that of another category of social deviancy – or even to be considered 'normal' – the rapid expansion of medical technology and its ability to control various aspects of the natural world meant it was more likely that, '*The future belongs to illness*: we just are going to get more and more diseases, since our expectations of health are going to become more expansive and sophisticated'.[27] The massive growth over the last 40 years of diagnoses, as well as of conditions (for example, baldness in men) whose status is not that of illness but which are seen as amenable to medical treatment, have confirmed his forecast to the point that it would not be an exaggeration to speak of 'the medicalisation of society'.[28]

Despite the expansion of its involvement in social life, the medical profession has not been immune from experiencing a version of the kind of crisis of authority that has bedevilled multiple social and political institutions in recent decades. These difficulties have intensified with the growing involvement of medical experts in political advocacy, perhaps most prominently seen during the pandemic, further weakening their claim to be standing above society and dispensing objective scientific advice. The more that society is medicalised, the more the purveyors of medicine are expected to resolve (social) problems well beyond their control, with disappointment and resentment inevitably following close behind.

The current moment is fertile for the intervention of movements seeking to transform how mental disorder is treated by societies and the individuals who constitute them. What have so far been absent are the wider social foment and resistance that Sedgwick tended to see as an indispensable precondition for the emergence of such movements, and which can unite patients, clinicians, and others around common interests. Because it draws on the experiences and lessons of past periods of radicalism, when such movements do erupt, *PsychoPolitics* will come into its own not just as acutely perceptive critique but as an essential guide to effective social action.

About the Author

Peter Sedgwick was the youngest of four children. In June 1934 at three months old he was separated from his siblings and adopted by his uncle and aunt in Liverpool (his elder siblings were told that he was dead). On their mother's death, a year later, they were taken into care in Southampton.

In contrast to his siblings, Peter's material circumstances were comfortable. Together with his adoptive brothers, he lived in a large house, where his adoptive father ran a dental practice in Anfield. Peter developed curvature of the spine, however, and he was forbidden to play outdoors.

Pressed by his adoptive mother to study, Peter gained a place at the Liverpool Collegiate. There, teachers and fellow pupils applauded not only his achievements – his results were the highest ever attained at the school – but his jocularity and wit. In 1952 Peter won a scholarship to read Classics at Balliol College, Oxford. As he wrote in his introduction to the first edition of this book, 'a series of catastrophic events in my family home' impelled him to break from his linguistic and literary studies and turn to a biologically-based science.

During his early student days Peter was a devout Christian and his ambition was to become Archbishop of Canterbury. Even after his friend Raphael Samuel converted him to Communism, Peter retained his faith: he prayed for the Rosenbergs on their execution for espionage in the United States in 1953.

Repulsed by the Soviet Union's crushing of the Hungary Uprising in 1956, Peter and Raphael left the Communist Party. Together with other socialist historians such as Edward Thompson, and the cultural critic Stuart Hall, they founded the New Left. From the mid-1950s, Peter's articles spanned a spectrum of concerns, from mental health – in 1955 his piece 'Psychopolitics' appeared in *The Oxford Clarion*, the journal of the Oxford University Labour Club – to the struggles of African colonies for independence.

In 1955, Peter had met another seminal Balliol student, Michael Kidron. Drawn to Kidron's luminosity and economic critique of, inter alia the Soviet Union as 'state capitalist', and the debates underway in the Socialist Review Group, Peter moved away from the 'old New Left' (his term). As a founder member of the International Socialism group (predecessor to the Socialist Workers Party, which he never joined) he threw himself into activism in the 'new New Left'.

To support his young family in Liverpool – after Liverpool University sacked him for publishing an article demanding an end to the London Rubber Company's monopoly of Durex – he found work with children, first as a school teacher and then as a child guidance psychologist. Terrified by the escalating arms race, Peter and his wife, Edie, were absorbed in the anti-nuclear movement (his prescient words, from 1959, were cited by Thompson in his 'Notes on Exterminism', *New Left Review* May–June 1980, when both were active in the campaign for European Nuclear Disarmament).

By the 1960s, Peter's scholarly focus was Victor Serge: he edited and translated his *Memoirs of a Revolutionary*, published in 1963 (*Year One of the Russian Revolution* came out in 1972). Peter then moved to Grendon prison, as tutor-organiser, before returning to Oxford for research into head injuries.

By spring 1968, Peter had obtained a post as lecturer in politics at York University. Ever sceptical of fads, his scholarly attention was diverted in the early 1970s to the theses of R.D. Laing, as well as progressives' embrace of anti-psychiatry. In addition to insisting that 'mental illness is illness', Peter's critical review of Ken Loach's film *Family Life* (a remake of David Mercer's play *In Two Minds* about a young woman with schizophrenia), published in the weekly *Socialist Worker*, provoked the most letters of complaint to the editor ever received by the paper. It almost provoked a near riot among the comrades at one of IS's annual educational rallies at Skegness, where he, with Tirril Harris, defended his position against a hostile audience.

In 1970, Peter had been commissioned to write a rapid pot-boiler on R.D. Laing for the newly-founded Pluto Press, by the press's founder, Richard Kuper. The six-week deadline receded and various draft chapters of what was becoming a much larger project appeared in the journal *Salmagundi*. The book itself, substantially transformed, was to be published over a decade later, in 1982, as *Psycho Politics*, now including a significant second part on mental health movements and issues.

In the years preceding this, after his split from Edie, Peter funded himself and his family by teaching at York and Leeds universities and by writing reviews. As the sociologist Hilary Rose suggested after Peter's death in September 1983 – not only was his brilliance luminous, but that his writing was born of personal pain was palpable.

That notwithstanding, in his work with the Alzheimer's Disease Society (now the Alzheimer's Society) and the National Schizophrenia Fellowship (now Rethink) – in the latter asserting the therapeutic benefits of work – Peter campaigned tirelessly for good psychiatric care for the mentally ill, and for proper support to the families of sufferers.

Acknowledgements

The preparation of this book has been considerably assisted by the following people who read drafts of the different chapters: Tom Arie, Arthur Bowen, Anthony Clare, Alan Dabbs, Michael Fears, David Goldberg, Tirril Harris, Ann Howard, Ursula Huws, Alec Jenner, John Pringle, Colin Pritchard, Jonathan Rée, Geoff Richman, Naomi Richman and Andrew Scull. I have not always followed their suggestions and am entirely responsible for error and mis-statements that remain. Liz Jakab offered consistent encouragement and sympathy from the New York side of this publishing endeavour. Robert Boyers, editor of *Salmagundi*, has been an indefatigable reader, critic and promoter of a number of draft chapters of this book. Richard Kuper has proven a most invaluable editor. Particular thanks must go to the indexer, Sheila Hartley.

The completion of this book has not been assisted by any grants from academic departments, learned institutions or private or other foundations: indeed, when one such private source expressed an interest in funding my work on Laing, the offer was immediately withdrawn (by Alfred Sherman, now an ideological adviser to Margaret Thatcher) as soon as the content of my argument was perused. But it should be emphasised that most of the learning I underwent in order to complete this book was undertaken with the help of a large number of therapeutic and educational collectives in Britain and the United States.

Peter Sedgwick

Part One:
Anti-Psychiatry

1. Anti-Psychiatry, Illness and the Mentally Ill

The arc of argument within the politics of psychiatry which is traversed by the ideological celebrities discussed in these chapters extends over a lengthy epoch of debate and action: from the later fifties, with their burden of post-war reconstruction and health-service planning, through the more exuberant (and also more tormented) sixties and seventies, into our own anxious and regressive decade. And my own involvement in psychiatry and its various counter movements or challenges has covered an almost exactly similar span. For it was in the mid-fifties, when the enlargement of the in-patient population of the mental hospitals of Britain was reaching its all-time maximum, that I broke from the predominantly literary and linguistic studies which had occupied me since earlier years, and began an avocation towards a scientific training in experimental and social psychology. The immediate occasion which impelled me towards the systematic study of what is still (in however social its aspects) a biologically-based science was a series of catastrophic events in my family home in which, finally, a close relative of mine was admitted, in a condition of extreme dementia, into the charge of a crowded and custodial local mental hospital, in which she quite shortly afterwards died. Today that hospital still stands, less crowded perhaps, but still locked and, for masses of its chronic patients, lacking in many of the elements of a humane care.

My studies in the psychological sciences, and my subsequent work as a psychologist and educator in various fields of paramedical treatment, left me with very little knowledge either of the reasons which lay behind my particular family disaster (and, doubtless, behind countless similar family tragedies) or of the practical remedies, whether in individual person-to-person treatment or in a wider social provision, which could at least minimise and possibly even prevent the worst of the devastations which attend the communicative breakdown known as psychosis or madness. As an active partisan of many left-wing causes and movements, I was amazed (as the expansion of radical or revolutionary groupings gathered force in the late sixties and the seventies) to discover that on the left the most popular attitude towards the mental illnesses was to deny their very existence.

The problems of practice in the healing and care of the mentally ill were, among the circles where I usually felt the broadest ideological and personal sympathy, dissolved neatly into two categories.

Firstly, there were bad practices, which were the result of capitalism's tendency to label various deviants and dissidents as 'mentally ill' as a prelude to lobotomising, electro-shocking, sedating or incarcerating these valiant unfortunates. Secondly, there were (or there were about to be, or there ultimately *would be* under the aegis of a socialist state, when the more urgent priority of overthrowing the capitalist order had at last been achieved) some good practices towards the mentally deviant. These included leaving them well alone to become the good healthy rebels that they undoubtedly ought to be, or inducting them into any one of a range of genuinely radical and genuinely therapeutic milieux (of the sort being pioneered by R.D. Laing, David Cooper or a number of clinicians on the West Coast of the United States). A more militant perspective included aiding them to mount collective actions of opposition against psychiatrists, psychologists, neuro-surgeons, drug companies and hospital institutions, as well as more individual actions of protest against their relatives or other do-gooders who were nothing less than co-conspirators in the manoeuvrings directed by the macro-structure of capitalism against the innocent insane.

The books that propagated this vision of psychiatry as modern capitalism's (or modern bureaucracy's) ultimate weapon of social control against dissidence were commonly best-sellers, available widely in frequently reprinted cheap editions to mass audiences both on and away from univeristy campuses. Their utility as a provocation for a wider social critique, outside the strict realm of public policy in mental health, is still manifest even for those of us who disagree with their implications for psychiatry's future direction. Their weaknesses will be discussed in the chapters that follow. But nobody situated now, at the fagend of a century that has seen the coming and passing of innumerable avant-gardes of critical promise, should underrate the importance of this cohort of anti-psychiatric writers and thinkers. Erving Goffman, for example, won an immediate and thoroughly deserved recognition with the publication in 1961 of his *Asylums: Essays on the Social Situation of Mental Patients and other Inmates*. This was a powerful and compelling study – based largely on Goffman's first-hand anthropological fieldwork as a participant-observer on a traditional mental ward – of the moulding of 'psychiatric' symptoms and of the typical 'chronic' patient's career through the de-humanising repressiveness of the pyschiatric hospital's customary regulations. When in the early seventies I taught in a New York City University with a mass intake of introductory sociology students, Goffman's *Asylums* was the prime text listed as required reading for sophomore undergraduates by teacher after teacher in classes and lectures offering a first orientation to the general discipline of sociology. Although the direct influence of Goffman both on general sociology and on the sociology of mental health has abated since the early seventies, workers in the kindred field of what is usually called 'labelling theory' have continued to create a credible and persuasive imagery of the construction of psychiatric deviancies through enforced pressures by medical and social agencies. Among academic (and often publicised) contributors we may mention Thomas Scheff, author of the 1966 book *Being Mentally Ill: A Sociological Identity*, and D.L. Rosenhan, whose 1973 paper 'On Being Sane in Insane Places', published in the prestigious review *Science*, kindled an instant furore through its report that psychologically normal investigators, who presented themselves at a mental hospital's admission desk with a claim to one single (and entirely fabricated) psychotic symptom, were promptly committed to in-patient care for periods of between seven and 52 days even though they never subsequently provided their medical assessors with either that particular sign or with any other evidence of a deluded psychopathology. Other innovative work in what may loosely be called a Goffmanesque vein has come from anti-psychiatric writers in film, the theatre and the novel. Ken Kesey's fiction (and later film-script) *One Flew Over the Cuckoo's Nest*, and David Mercer's account of the precipitate hospitalisation of a schizophrenic, *In Two Minds* (for British television) and *Family Life* (as a film for the cinema), both perhaps belong in the literary-anthropological tradition of *Asylums*, although all the anti-psychiatric contributions to the wider media in the last couple of decades also bear the impress of R.D. Laing's notoriety.

Goffman may need some introduction to a lay readership in the eighties; Laing, even at this distance from the peak of his reputation, will need little or none. During my earlier involvement with the socialist-humanist New Left of Britain I found (towards the very end of the fifties) that his work on the inner rationality of schizophrenic behaviour was becoming the focus of some sympathetic attention on the intellectual left; but I did not see or hear Laing until 1964 (and then only at a distance, as a member of a respectful audience at a social psychiatry conference) when he delivered what was to become a key paper in the establishment of his best-known position, soon to be printed in an updated version as the chapter on 'The Schizophrenic Experience' in his book *The Politics of Experience and the Bird of Paradise* (1967). I was very, very sceptical as to the value of Laing's inferences on the supposedly normal and life-enhancing qualities of the schizophrenic frenzy; by the time I had developed these reservations in some draft talks and articles expressing the position outlined in this book, virtually the entire left and an enormous proportion of the liberal-arts and social-studies reading public was convinced that R.D. Laing and his band of colleagues had produced novel and essentially accurate renderings of what psychotic experience truly signified. Seldom can a vanguard minority of researchers, opposed to the main orthodoxies of a dominant applied science, have achieved in so short a span of years a cultural and even political dominance of their own among progressive circles of the public with a pretension to discrimination in the matter of ideas.

The thrust of Laingian theorising accords so well with the loose romanticism and libertarianism implicit in a number of contemporary creeds and moods that it can easily generate support and acquire plausibility. It is only four years since I walked into a gathering of 30 or 40 postgraduate trainees in social work, to introduce them to two parents of schizophrenic children, both of them activists with me in a local pressure group for the welfare of schizophrenia sufferers. Much to the surprise of the parents and myself, this audience of social-work trainees directed a barrage of hostile questions and comments at us. Was not psychiatric diagnosis just a matter of labelling awkward people, just like in Russia? How could we be sure that we were talking about a real illness, and not something that was the product of faulty family handling? Faced with these attacks, which might have been quite uncomfortable for the morale of ordinary parents outside the gamut of the doubts and guilts that afflict the families of the handicapped, the three of us from the support group became increasingly more defensive, conventional and lame in our replies. We left an audience that had been sympathetic to Laing before we entered the room and was now more Laingian than Laing himself: for had they not witnessed the evasiveness and inauthenticity of a repressive and authoritarian parenthood left in charge of an innocent deviancy? Musing on the experience afterwards, one of the parents, a robust and good-humoured mother who had to look after her seriously ill black adolescent son in a suburban neighbourhood not distinguished for its racial tolerance (and still less for its mental-health liberalism), remarked that she could quite understand the reactions of our interrogators. 'We must have looked very conservative and square; and besides, only a few years ago, I read Laing and accepted his story completely – before we had any knowledge at home of what these things were really like.'

It is only two years since the publication, following a series of widely-hailed performances, of the play *Mary Barnes*, dealing with the most celebrated case-study from the Laingian school, written at a high pitch of dramatic excitement by one of Britain's most brilliant tragedians, David Edgar. For those who know a little about schizophrenic illnesses, and can read behind the lines of the published accounts of the Kingsley Hall settlement where Laing and his associate enthusiasts conducted their experiments in permissive therapy, there is something distinctly incongruous in presenting the Barnes life-history as some kind of vindication for Laing's methods with schizophrenia. For one thing, this patient's demeanour is more obviously hysterical than schizophrenic;[1] for another, the primary account of the treatment (on which the play is based) is related by a therapist from Kingsley Hall who despite his considerable charm and intelligence is obviously possessed of a strongly partisan zeal, invoking in his presentation neither any alternative suggestions of what might be going on nor any checks on the account from more objective witnesses. Nevertheless, the publicity for the book of the play describes it as: 'based on a true story – the story of Mary Barnes's journey through madness and her emergence from it' via the Laingian therapeutic method. The drama critic of the *Daily Telegraph* found the author's approach 'meticulous' and his 'study' of the case 'absorbing': the *Guardian's* theatre critic saw it as a 'specific, well-documented account of one treatment that worked'.

The play *Mary Barnes* will doubtless continue to enjoy repeat performances, deservedly, for it is indeed a very strong piece, with ample scope for the bravura of talented lead-acting. On stage or as a printed text, it will therefore continue to indoctrinate further audiences, and perhaps even a few more critics, in the validity of Laing's theories of schizophrenia and in the efficacy of the techniques – a combination of charisma in the therapist (most suitably male) and infantilism in the patient (predictably female) – which have been canvassed by him and his following for the cure of this complex and exacting condition. It is because of the potential tenacity of Laing's influence upon future generations of the credulous – or of those unwilling for other reasons to confront the great seriousness and specificity of the dementing illnesses which can strike at any home, including the private addresses of social workers, theatrical habitués and political militants of various progressive causes – that I have devoted special attention in this book to the scientific and logical evaluation of Laingian concepts of psychosis and its treatment.

Few introductory comments are required to explain the appearance in these pages of Michel Foucault and Thomas Szasz, as the work of these authors touches on questions of public provision in the care of the mentally ill. I have learnt a great deal both from Szasz and from Foucault as general intellectual innovators. Szasz's early game-playing analysis of neurotic behaviour remains of considerable use (though it has been taken much further, and far more fruitfully, by later 'transactional' analysts such as Eric Berne and Claude Steiner). However, the game-playing approach to mental illness needs to be used in conjunction with another, more material model of mental pathology which I shall outline below.

The reader will not find here any attempt at a general summing-up of the intellectual endeavours of that polemical polymath of our time, Michel Foucault. Several such overviews have recently been published in English, although with the exception of the vivacious and lucid introductory volume offered by his main translator (Alan Sheridan, *Michel Foucault: The Will to Truth*, 1980) they tend to be composed in a flat and ponderous prose unlike Foucault's own glittering style. Some of these expositions have their own worth as paraphrases or glosses on a writer who can at times be wilfully tantalizing; some of the criticisms of Foucault from a more marxist perspective (such as those furnished by Nicos Poulantzas in his final theoretical testament, *State, Power, Socialism,* published in 1978) do focus on a number of his crucial flaws, such as his inability to pose the central questions of power raised in the exploitative extraction of a surplus from those who toil, or in the concentration of authority which still lies, whatever the force of more miniaturised and mundane components of coercion, within the grand and obdurate apparatus of the centralised state itself. But all of these commentaries on Foucault, whether they be sympathetic or adversary, still take for granted the substance of his many statements of fact, i.e. of apparent or alleged fact, which season the main course of his argument and indeed form a staple ingredient of its piquant impact on the present-day consumer. As a researcher on historical themes, Foucault can be quite careless and even licentious in the handling of evidence. He does not steep himself in an abundance of primary sources before pronouncing on the direction of an important historical trend. Indeed, at the rate of his current production of titles claiming to discern the ultimate logic (never previously fathomed) of psychiatry, government, physiology, criminology, natural-scientific method and – most recently – sexual desire, one can hardly expect a very deep familiarity with the primary source material in any one field – although it should be clear that, in the treatment of particular core-sources for the cultural outlook of a given age, his mode of analysis can be (and very often is) not only penetrating but positively riveting.

The chapter I have assigned to the status of Michel Foucault as a psychiatric historian is based not on any first-hand source work of my own but on the compilation of the best available materials produced by a growing collective of scholars in the field of psychohistorical research. It is a particularly sad paradox that those structuralist and post-structuralist writers who, like Foucault, have staked their entire venture upon the evacuation of the individual 'subject' from any rational account of human action should also be those who in the public consciousness have done most to confirm the stereotype of the individual genius, the single-handed author of germinal ideas, the *maître penseur* of the cogito working – as Foucault almost always does – without a single research colleague and without any other human being to acknowledge as a contributory influence, except some predecessor – *maîtres* who (like his old supervisor Georges Cangouilhem) passed on the torch of individual authorship-authority. It is my own belief (and one, moreover, not original to me, but stemming from a number of vanguard communist thinkers from Kropotkin to the radicals of the Chinese Cultural Revolution) that serious work in the arts and the sciences is above all a collective production. In my chapter of historical reportage I wish above all to pay tribute to a commune of savants who will never be picked up in the literary pages of prestige magazines or have their names on the front covers of best-selling paperbacks, but who are taking on, thoroughly and with insight, the exploration of a small part of a very large, important and treacherous terrain.

Let me conclude these prefatory comments with an aside about my lengthy treatment of an author already referred to, Thomas S. Szasz. I began looking at Szasz's politico-psychiatric ideology in the course of the seventies, before the arrival in governmental power of the laissez-fairist and right-libertarian philosophies of welfare (or rather of the running-down of what has been hitherto accepted as welfare) now predominant in Britain and the United States. When I drafted these sections, my demonstration of the coincidence between Szasz's philosophy of neglect for psychiatric disability and the nineteenth-century philosopher Herbert Spencer's advocacy of 'negative beneficence' (i.e. letting the weak go to the wall) might have appeared as an idle antiquarian exercise. Surely no political thinker or practitioner of the modern age would conceive of reviving these brutal and long-discarded notions of an unfeeling Victorian industrialism? Yet Social Darwinism is alive and quite well today; Herbert Spencer walks the corridors of power denied to him even in his own miserly and flint-hearted epoch. The Spencerians and the Szaszians of the modern party system win hearts and minds: and, for a short while at the very least, even win elections.

The criticisms of the various anti-psychiatric founding figures which I have sketched above, and which will be developed fully later, are of a disparate and divergent quality. This is not surprising since the figures themselves have very different cases to argue. There is, however, a central issue which unites them in a common framework of assumption and inference, and upon which my own disagreement with their position takes the shape of a single, integral and co-ordinated polemic, directed against what I take to be their shared error. All the modern 'revisionists' of the psychiatric enterprise who are discussed in this book take as their starting point a sociological, indeed socially deterministic, orientation on the nature of mental illness. It will be necessary to offer some remarks on this sociological project of the re-definition of mental illness. But it appears that none of these thinkers have begun by posing a prior question of definition: What is *illness*? Only in the light of an answer to *this* question, surely, can we determine our answer to the question: Is mental illness really illness in the 'medical' sense?[2]

The attempt by so many sensitive modern theorists to find the root-meaning of the idea of illness in the wilder scrublands of sociology rather than in the neatly planted park of the medical sciences should occasion no surprise or demurral. Any inspection of the current state of discussion in the medical press about the real nature of illness and disease will undermine any confidence the reader may have had that our doctors have the faintest idea of what it is, in the most general sense, that they are trying to cure, treat or palliate. Dr F. Kräupl Taylor, to take one recent example, has suggested the coining of an attribute to be known as 'morbidity' to characterise the class of 'persons who are ill organically, psychologically or otherwise'. Morbidity is to be conceived as the overlap of two further attributes: 'abnormality (a statistically significant deviation of an attribute from a norm)' and 'therapeutic concern for a person felt by the person himself and/or his social environment'.[3] To be ill, therefore, is to be a statistical oddity and, at the same time, a candidate (perhaps through self-referral) for the attention of anyone who sets up a business as a therapist. It is a definition of the sick state which admirably reflects the two major obvious concerns of the contemporary medicine man: an attachment to quantitative criteria for classification (heaven help a patient of Dr Kräupl Taylor who appears at the surgery with a deviation that falls below statistical significance), and an awareness that nobody can be ill nowadays without joining the great and growing class of 'possible patients', the mellifluous term with which Dr Taylor describes those who are at some point in the queue for his profession's standing invitation to open their mouths and say 'Aaah!' or else to drop their trousers and cough.

Both of these criteria for the definition of what it means to be ill – the statistical and the diagnostic – suffer from obvious implausibilities. Although probabilistic concepts of what counts as a biological abnormality have an ancestral appeal, extending back to the first attempts by nineteenth-century French pioneers of science to place notions of 'pathology' on a firm objective footing,[4] very few modern classifiers of the abnormal regard the criterion of statistical infrequency as anything other than an aberration. The deviation constituted by disease or illness is not necessarily an infrequent sort of event, as witness the common cold and infants' colic: rare attributes are not necessarily diseases, as witness the ability to talk to sad-looking strangers at bus-stops, the willingness to strike in support of sacked colleagues, the capacity to write a warm letter to a friend who really needs to hear from you, and other attributes of uncommon saintly virtue. Kräupl Taylor's attempt to evolve a definition of illness as the propensity to behave like a patient is also confusing; in the words of one of the doctors in the debate:

> Equating illness with a complaint allows the individual to be the sole arbiter of whether he is ill or not, and is unsatisfactory because some people who should be complaining don't do so, and others who do so repeatedly don't seem to have adequate reasons for doing so.[5]

This breath of common sense is, unfortunately, not maintained in the later portions of Professor Bob Kendell's counterargument to the cruder medical model of disease. His own position relies heavily on an influential suggestion made by J.G. Scadding in the *Lancet* for 1967. According to Scadding's proposal, diseased living organisms have to possess

> a specified common characteristic or set of characteristics by which they differ from the norm for their species in such a way as to place them at a biological disadvantage.[6]

Kendell's gloss on Scadding's criterion of 'biological disadvantage' emphasises, for illnesses in human beings, the increased risk for mortality and the reduction in fertility prospects which an adequately defined disease must be held to confer. This refined Scadding definition is offered on the grounds that it encompasses a conception of disease founded on the consequences of illness rather than of its alleged antecedents – which are often unclear or contentious. Further, 'the concept of "biological disadvantage"' is, compared with other accounts of illness based on consequence, 'more fundamental, less obviously an epiphenomenon, and… immune to the idiosyncratic personal judgments, of patients or doctors, that had proved the undoing of its predecessors.'

Kendell's development of the Scadding criterion for illness does (as he immediately admits) have the consequence that those human complaints such as psoriasis and post-herpetic neuralgia which neither reduce the patients' fertility nor shorten their lifespan cannot be regarded as illnesses, though they may have for a long time been the subject of specialised and even effective medical attention. On the other hand, various mental illnesses such as schizophrenia, and also (though the argument is here less compelling) manic-depressive psychosis, neurosis and psychopathy, can be unambiguously defined as disease conditions since the patients who bear these diagnostic labels are often found to display a child-producing capacity which is well below average. At times, Kendell seems slightly oblivious to the possibility that the reduced fertility associated with some diagnostic categories may be due to the lack of sexual opportunities conferred on them by institutionalisation (or by the shortage of cash for a social life) rather than to factors more directly attributable to a disease-state. His sympathetic reporting of 'suggestions that the fertility of criminal psychopaths is below that of the general population' thus has about it a somewhat unsophisticated ring.

The main difficulty with the Scadding-Kendell case, however, is that it imposes a compulsory common definition of health on all citizens. Nobody is allowed to be both healthy and infertile: a puzzling requirement, since even though a certain level of reproductiveness is undoubtedly required by a society in order to keep it going, very few cultures have actually demanded in practice that all their members should have parenting as their major preoccupation. At one point Kendell appears to withdraw from the perspective of an unremitting baby boom as the index of society's biological well-being: 'in an era of explosive population growth,' he concedes, 'it might be beneficial to a community to have its fertility reduced.' But the notion that, in whatever epoch of national fertility pressures, it might be beneficial for some individuals to rear families and for others to abstain from parenting appears to be a difficult one to entertain within this all-embracing concept of healthiness.

A particular test case for Kendell's view of health as fertility is the part played in society by gay men and women. He oscillates between an insistence that 'in simple biological terms their lack of interest in sexual activity capable of resulting in conception puts homosexuals… at a quite daunting negative selection advantage' and a recognition that 'it might be positively advantageous to a community to have a proportion of homosexual members' if the latter should possess 'valuable aptitudes which others lacked.' In a personal letter to me, replying to my complaint of an anti-homosexual bias in his original paper, Kendell has made the interesting remark that:

> I think it should be stressed that it is not homosexuality per se that is to be regarded as an illness but rather the inability to maintain a heterosexual relationship and the associated male/female pair bonding necessary for the successful rearing of offspring. In other words there is, or should be, a crucial distinction between medical and social attitudes to homosexuality. It is what homosexuals and other sexual deviants *do* that generates strong feelings and social attitudes; it is what they *cannot* do that matters to medicine.[7]

But the split being advocated here between 'medical' and 'social' determinations of the homosexual's status simply reinforces the value-loadedness of the supposedly biological element being canvassed in the total appraisal. Why should the presence of gay men and women in a community be seen as a counter-biological, socially conferred benefit only if homosexuals can be seen to possess some extra virtues which are relatively scarce in the straight citizenry? Why is the capacity for parenthood, even in a narrow biological perspective aiming towards the reproduction of the species, presented here as a norm to which every human being should aim on pain of being branded as 'ill' if he or she proves to be childless? Why cannot a loving and committed parenthood be offered as a conscious, voluntary option for those who wish seriously to assume its burdens – which do tend to be part of the package wrapped up with its benefits?

If I have dwelt in some detail on what I take to be logical and political shortcomings in the arguments of Kräupl Taylor and Kendell, it is not because these two authors suffer from any special partiality towards error. They merely illustrate the pitfalls of a biologistic approach towards the definition of health: an approach which, in attempting to eradicate social and personal value-judgments, may smuggle them back in through unexplored assumptions which are highly contentious.

When one disagrees with the verdict of one's doctor, it is well to seek the second opinion of a further physician. When the disagreement is a more general, theoretical one involving a dissent from doctoring itself as an endeavour applicable to one whole class of client or patient, the second opinion can only be sought outside medicine and within another discipline of human enquiry. The part of this alternative theoretical voice which counters and contradicts the medical enterprise is usually played by sociology. 'Revisionism' in the mental-health field, of the kind that radically challenges the validity of psychiatry, is unthinkable without the long and serious contribution of a critical sociology to the appraisal of psychiatric concepts.

Of course not all sociologists working in mental-health problems are revisers and some of the key 'revisers' of mental health are not sociologists at all. The highly suggestive and consequential work of Thomas Szasz, Professer of Psychiatry in the State University of New York, rarely depends on any material from the deviancy experts of the sociological profession (although it is braced by many striking allusions drawn from political science, law, economics, creative fiction and the medical and psychoanalytic literature). Michel Foucault has long pioneered the study of cultural relativism in psychiatric categories; his book *Madness and Civilisation*, published in English in 1965, has become deservedly famous among sociologists and sociologically inclined historians who have followed in the same track. But Foucault has never been classifiable as a sociologist: he is a historical and philosophical analyst of ideas in the social and natural sciences who has worked in complete independence from the academic specialism of sociology as defined in either its American or European branches.

On the other hand, the bulk of medical-sociological writing in the sphere of psychiatry merely represents a parallel with the developed science of 'epidemiology' in the prevalence and incidence of physical disease by different social classes, age ranges, cultures and other social variables. These researches take it for granted that 'mental illnesses' exist as facts of life (to be correlated with other, social facts) and do not discuss the logical status or the social nature of either diagnosis or therapy in the psychopathological field. Even the more advanced and closely focused studies of 'family process' or 'psychiatrically induced mental disorder' which are characteristic of the best work in British and American social psychiatry begin their analysis at a very late stage of the *total possible analysis* of mental illness. Chronic mental patients deteriorate, we are told, through spending long years in overcrowded locked wards: but what, pray, is a 'mental patient'? How does such a person come to exist, in terms of his own definition 'I am a mental patient', the definitions of others to the same effect, and the relations between these ascribed and self-ascribed identities? Family pressures, according to the American schizophrenia researchers, impel susceptible people into severe breakdowns which necessitate their treatment in a suitably equipped clinical institution. The problem is to discover how the illness began, so that once again our very notion of a mental illness is never posed as constituting any kind of problem. That trend in the sociology of psychiatric classification and treatment which, on the contrary, takes 'mental illness' and its 'treatment' as problematic, to be analysed as value-laden *social constructions*, is an unpopular trend in psychological medicine – though it dominates the teaching of deviancy-sociology in many American colleges. We have a constrast, in brief, between what might be called an *exterior* sociology of mental illness and an *immanent* (or indwelling) sociology of 'mental-illness-as-a-social-construct'. The same contrast, as a matter of fact, is visible in the sociological treatment of several social problem areas outside the aetiology of madness: prostitution, homosexuality, drug addiction and criminal delinquency are all topics which can be discussed in the literature either via an external sociology analysing pathological 'givens' or from an immanent, critical perspective which sees the official counts and categories of deviancy as mere projections of society's formal or informal control process, and performs an imaginative entry into the deviant's own actions, viewing these as an attempt to manufacture significance for his or her life within and against a rejecting, 'labelling' world.[8]

Immanent theorists of mental illness, whether in sociology or outside it, have usually had to begin by denying the validity of a natural science perspective on psychological abnormalities. Thus we have Szasz, Leifer and Goffman drawing a sharp distinction between the natural-scientific, value-free language of physical medicine and the socially and politically loaded language of psychiatry. Szasz believes that, in physical illnesses, 'the notion of a bodily symptom is tied to an *anatomical* and *genetic* context' as distinct from the social or ethical context which informs psychiatric judgments. Our description of the norm of physical health (a deviation from which constitutes a physical illness or disease) is just a description, which 'can be stated in anatomical and physiological terms'.[9]

Indeed, according to Szasz, even a corpse can have a disease, since a bodily symptom can occur just as much in a dead body as in a living one: 'Every "ordinary" illness that persons have, cadavers also have. A cadaver may thus be said to "have" cancer, pneumonia, or myocardial infarction.'[10] Szasz's disciple, Ronald Leifer, while paying due tribute to the social grounding of medicine as a profession, still insists that in physical diagnosis and treatment 'the term "disease" refers to phenomena that are not regulated by social custom, morality and law, namely bodily structure and function'; psychiatric concepts of disease refer, on the contrary, to 'behaviour, which is subject to the regulation of custom, morality and law'.[11]

Erving Goffman, the most influential sociological theorist in the anti-psychiatry tradition, offers in different works a number of quite distinct approaches in the demarcation of physical from psychiatric disorders. One of his most readable books, *Stigma*, applies a careful phenomenological and interpersonal analysis to the victims of physical handicap and disfigurement, with a method very similar to that adopted in his celebrated study of 'The Moral Career of the Mental Patient'.[12]

Goffman would appear to be using a unitary schema in which the division of the patients' case-files into 'psychiatric' versus 'physical' categories would contribute nothing to our further understanding of the difficulties experienced by the subject in various social settings and encounters. Elsewhere in Goffman's work, a more definite distinction between physical and psychiatric symptom construction is propounded. At one point, the 'political' vested interests surrounding the procedures of mental medicine are contrasted with the presumably apolitical practices of ordinary doctoring: thus, decisions concerning behavioural (psychiatric) pathology 'tend to be political, in the sense of expressing the interest of some particular faction or person rather than interests that can be said to be above the concerns of any particular grouping as in the case of physical pathology'.[13] There is an assumption here that the language of body pathology works within a unanimously common culture, rising above the historically evolved social formations whose notorious diversity has been an important traditional beginning point of sociological investigation. We shall have occasion later to question this assumption and to provide a few examples of wide cultural variation within conceptions of physical illness. Even in the strange sense of 'political' whereby politics means only open dissent among factions (so that, e.g. there could be no such thing as the 'politics' of a successfully manipulated consensus), it is extremely sweeping of Goffman to announce that decisions about physical pathology never involve conflicting interests between different parties to the situation. It is perhaps not surprising that, in a subsequent exposition of the difference between 'mental' and 'medical' symptom patterns,[14] Goffman falls back on an unsophisticated Szasz-type contrast between the purely biological, value-free substrate of medical classifications and the socially determined character of judgements about mental symptoms.

> Signs and symptoms in a *medical* disorder presumably refer to underlying pathologies in the individual organism, and these constitute deviations from biological norms maintained by the homeostatic functioning of the human machine. The system of reference here is plainly [*sic*] the individual organism, and the term 'norm' ideally at least, has no moral or social connotation… biological and social norms are quite different things.[15]

The position of the Laing School is different again. Unlike Szasz and Leifer, Laing does not give a general endorsement to face-to-face psychoanalysis as the method *par excellence* for dealing with disturbed patients in an ethically acceptable (because non-medical) framework, but instead devotes much effort to the critique of psychoanalytic and psychological explanations of human pathology, on the grounds that they do not, with the exception of his own perspective, do justice to the actual experience of persons.[16] The argument is extended by David Cooper in a distinction between 'two types of rationality' within the range of scientific knowledge. The study of humankind is to be conducted through a *dialectical rationality* which uses a historical-biographical method modelled on Sartre's interpretation of Jean Genet's life. *Analytic rationality* is the method of the natural sciences, which works for 'inert' data in physics, biology etc., but is inapplicable to the study of people.[17] It is not clear where this leaves the role of medical science. Cooper concurs with Szasz and Goffman in assigning physiological descriptions of human bodily states to a sphere that lies outside the proper understanding of people. Physiological explanation amounts to a 'reductive analysis', the misuse of analytic rationality in an area (the science of persons) for which it is inappropriate. But learning theory and psychoanalysis, at any rate in the Freudian form, are equally 'reductive analyses', and just as bad as physiology. However, the Laingian classification of the sciences still has room for the medical role in the treatment of patients. Laing refers to himself as a physician and a psychiatrist,[18] and Cooper offers similar identifiers, complaining only that other doctors should deal with the physical ailments of schizophrenics and that non-medical administrators should attend to the procedural paraphernalia that are at present left to hospital psychiatrists.[19]

To sum up these rather complex alignments of position: it looks as though Laingians deny the applicability of a natural science method to human investigations but claim that psychiatry (or else anti-psychiatry – which must be 'anti' only in the sense that the Anti-Popes were rivalling the Popes) can still be scientifically based within a suitable Sartrean methodology. There is no special division between the study of bodily states and the study of people: wrong forms of people-study are on one side of the divide, along with the psychiatric misuse of physiology and body science generally, while the other brighter shore is occupied by a Laingian 'science of persons' which is admittedly still being developed. Szaszians, in contrast, allocate the natural sciences to an area dealing with medically reputable complaints (those referring to diseased organs of the body) and then set up another, non-medical, autonomous zone for what is at present called psychiatry; concepts and methods are admitted rather eclectically to this liberated territory, on the sole proviso that psychiatric practitioners must see themselves as consultants responsible to their clients rather than as social agents programming the mentally ill. The 'scientific' status of Free Psychiatry is left indeterminate: Szasz writes at one point as if it had a descriptive, empirical foundation, but elsewhere he has celebrated the 'moral science' of a liberated psychiatry which refuses any classification of persons – including (one may take it) a classification in terms of their level of social development.[20]

The position of the philosopher-historian Michel Foucault is hard to compare with any of the above theoreticians of present-day psychiatry. In an important early text, *Maladie mentale et psychologie* (1962),[21] Foucault appears concerned not so much to destroy the concepts of psychiatric diagnosis and treatment as to point out carefully that each sequence of civilisation, from the medieval period to modern times, has had its own view of madness which closely reflects the general social and logical preoccupations of the time. Psychopathology is not independent of social history, for each age has drawn the split between madness and reason at a different point and in a fundamentally different fashion. Still it is permissible to seek a psychodynamic or a genetic or an existential account of an individual patient's behaviour, so long as we do not 'make these aspects of the illness into ontological forms', real essences which then require 'a mythological explanation like the evolution of psychic structure, or the theory of instincts, or an existential anthropology' to support them.[22]

Psychological descriptions of insanity 'are not to be suppressed by some explanatory or reductive principle which is exterior to them', but simply situated within the forgotten social-historical framework which has given them birth. It is possible, for example, to speak of the psychological state of 'regression' (i.e. of a resumption of infantile patterns) only in a society which has separated infancy as a pre-adult refuge: 'neuroses of regression do not display the neurotic character of childhood, but incriminate the archaic nature of the institutions which are concerned with children.' Thus, unlike the sociological and other re-definers of mental illness, Foucault does not *eliminate* the psychological and the medical enterprises: instead he brackets them, and shows the text of other human meanings which lies just outside the thin bounds of the parenthesis. And, while for other critics the present world may have room for a liberated region of psychiatry – Szasz's 'moral science' for neurotic life-problems or Laing's existential therapy for schizophrenia – which will be immune from the deceits and compulsions of the orthodox medical tradition, there is no such sanctuary in Foucault's psychiatric universe. The moral tyranny and cultural bondage of the Reasonable Human's superior confrontation with Unreason are just as manifest in the psychoanalyst's consulting room as in the locked wards of the asylum: they are no less implicit in our social attitudes towards neurosis than in our dismissal of the mad person's rantings. The images of psychoanalysis, with their percipient charting of defense shields, traumas, anxieties and other embodiments of conflict, do not (as the analysts imagine) reveal the true workings of an inner psychic machinery, but rather reflect 'how mankind has made mankind into a contradiction-laden experience', ridden by the theme of 'competition, exploitation, group-rivalry and class struggle'. Normal social structure is always the hidden truth of the psychology of the abnormal: so that if we may believe that one day, perhaps a genuine communion between Reason and Unreason can be restored, it will be within a new form of society which will see, as one of its natural consequences, the liberation of human thought from psychology.[23] In the here and now, we are left with no hope for a reformed or even radicalised psychology of madness, and no choice, in working with patients, except to use the psychologised descriptions which have been bequeathed to us as the deposit and the disguise of social classifications made by previous centuries.

The various 'immanent' theorists of mental illness thus diverge, radically in theory and drastically for practice, in the same breath that they converge, as criticism and as negation, upon the established doctrines of psychiatric medicine. Immamentist theory does not present itself as a solid, cumulative mass of concepts which can be wielded as a single heavy weapon against the institutions of psychiatry. The prickled barbs of its various critiques project and tend in so many opposed directions that any attempt to grasp them for use as a unitary whole will wound the critic to the bone of his or her own logic. It is quite erroneous to speak, as one journalistic enthusiast did in the 1960s (in a manner which would be applauded by many other devotees), of a 'school of thought' including Szasz, Goffman, Bateson, Cooper and Laing, 'which offers this radical reformulation in our ideas about the true nature of mental illness, with its corresponding subversive critique of the established society and culture.'[24] Not all of these theorists have expressed beliefs about 'the true nature of mental illness'. The views of Laing and Cooper (and Bateson) are confined to schizophrenia alone, and Goffman's theory of mental illness comes from quite a different 'school of thought' from that of Szasz. Neither Goffman nor Szasz offers any 'subversive critique' of larger social institutions, and indeed it appears that these two authors offer an explicitly conservative vision of societal process, founded in Goffman's case on a total immobilism of micro-structures and a total indifference to macro-structures, and in Szasz on the glorification of private medical practice at the expense of social welfare and on an anti-collective individualism which savours far more of America's 'radical-libertarian' right wing than of any revolutionary social philosophy. Foucault's 'critique of the established society and culture' has changed very considerably from the association he allowed to develop after the events of May 1968 between his name and the revolutionary political current of *gauchisme* to the present undivided concentration he now applies to the analysis of the 'capillary' effect of power in micro-arenas of social life: an analysis which necessarily excludes any confrontation with capital or the state. Other 'immanentist' writers like Thomas Scheff or Edwin Lemert (who for reasons of space are not discussed in this book) are quite silent on the general nature of American (or of capitalist) society, being content to apply, within the special field of mental illness, the theoretical constructs of 'labelling' that have been developed by their sociological tendency for many types and settings of social deviancy.

We have not got here a colony of 'subversives', or even the theoretical base for an 'anti-psychiatry' which would be able to agree on some working alternatives – conceptual or tactical – to the current dominant framework of psychiatric treatment. What we do have is a consistent and convergent *tendency of opposition* directed against *positivist method* in the study of abnormal human behaviour. 'Positivism', for the present discussion, may be taken to refer to an approach towards the investigation of human pathology which, modelling itself upon antecedents it believes to be characteristic of the natural sciences, (a) postulates a radical separation between 'facts' and 'values' (declaring only the former to be the subject matter of the professional investigator) and (b) suppresses the interactive relationship between the investigator and the 'facts' on which she or he works.[25] The psychiatric labels which are catalogued in textbooks of medicine and clinical psychology are, on a positivist account, terms which represent, or at least approximate towards, existent processes inhabiting an objective structure within the individual. The structure may be the psyche, the autonomic nervous system, perhaps even in the last resort the brain, but it stands towards the investigator as the ultimate object of reference towards which hypotheses, empirical techniques and standards of validation all tend. To be sure, we may remain suitably guarded in the finality or the completeness of the claims we may make for our disease categories. The judgements of psychiatrists on individual patients are notoriously prone to discordance:

a fact which, in one variant of the positivist school, has stimulated the search for more accurate 'measurements' of the deeper dimensions on which personality characteristics may be said to lie. Or it may be pointed out that we are working, at best, with hypothetical constructs of our own devising: a confession that offers little in the way of modest disavowal, since on the positivist account all scientific concepts whatsoever – from atomic particles to the Germ Theory of Disease, from chemical valencies to the mechanics of blood coagulation – are equally the inventive constructions of the mind, provisional models which may be more firmly based in empirical evidence and theoretical elegance than, say, the Hippocratic humours or the nineteenth-century Ether, but are still artifacts of human production. The stance of the scientific investigator before the categories of psychopathology differs, on the positivist case, in no essential way from her or his relationship to the categories of biological disease, to the molecular arrangements of the elements, or to the orderings of animal species suggested by evolutionary theory. Our conceptual units for the subdivision and understanding of the natural world are, if you like, solid; or, if you like, tenuous; but in any case of a muchness. The chair in which the psychiatrist sits and the motions she or he engages in to sign a certificate exist and function at different levels of the organisation of matter; their existence and functioning may be understood in different departments of the organisation of theory. And the categories of human disorders which the psychiatrist employs in making professional decisions about patients come from yet another area of the natural sciences, clouded (it is true) by greater complexities of error and uncertainty; they refer to yet another, higher level of the organisation of reality, to the precise inspection of which our instruments have not yet advanced.

Even the most advanced areas of clinical psychiatry bear, in their most basic terminology, the impress of this positivist tradition. We have the thriving discipline of 'the epidemiology of mental disorders', which has repeatedly displayed the considerable social variation, across classes and communities, in the incidence of the major psychological illnesses; yet it achieves this social insight by regarding the contours of the boxes into which its numerations fall as uncontroversial, objective boundaries, analogous to the physical disease categories that are studied in other branches of the same discipline. ('Epidemiology' means originally, after all, the study of epidemics, that is to say of infectiously transmitted diseases like cholera and tuberculosis, and if the concept of an epidemic is nowadays commonly extended to the germless plagues of heart disease, heroin addiction or schizophrenia, it is still supposed to mark the occurrence of morbid conditions as distinct and unambiguous as those produced by actual bacilli.) Similarly, in the application of statistical techniques for the fresh classification of mental disorders (in an attempt to reach groupings of symptoms which will be more systematic than those drawn from clinical experience), we find a reliance on the method of a 'numerical taxonomy' which was originally devised for the sorting of microbes according to the clustering of their objective characteristics.[26] The judgemental, valuational element in psychiatric assessments, in other words their *social* and cultural quality, is simply ignored in these taxonomic investigations. And the same can be said of the manifold drug trials, behaviour therapy studies, reports on hospital ward reform, symptom questionnaires and the like, which comprise the bulk of the serious journals of present-day clinical psychology and psychiatry.[27]

It is to the permanent credit of the immanentist critics of psychiatry that they have exposed the inadequacy of this positivist framework for the understanding of mental illness. Whatever exaggerations the more radical anti-psychiatrists and labelling-theory sociologists have engaged in, they have shown convincingly that both diagnoses and treatment measures in psychiatry are founded on ethical judgements and social demands whose content is sometimes reactionary, often controversial and nearly always left unstated. Mental illness is a social construction; psychiatry is a social institution, incorporating the values and demands of its surrounding society. These conclusions, and their supporting arguments, deserve to be placed in the forefront of all teaching material aimed towards those who seek guidance on the problems of mental illness. Foucault and Laing, Goffman and Szasz, Scheff and Lemert, should be made part of the curriculum for all aspirant therapists, nurses and social workers in this field. Never again should it be possible for a lecturer to instruct students, or the public, that 'mental illnesses may be caused by heredity, the environment, or a combination of both', or that 'outcome in psychopathology depends on a combination of exterior stress and the inner predisposition of the patient'. For such dicta, however seemingly authoritative and 'scientifically grounded', simply obscure a number of central features of mental illness and its associated agencies of treatment and care. To say that somebody is mentally ill, or to announce oneself as mentally ill, is to attach complex social meanings to acts and behaviours that in other societies, or in different contingencies within our own society, would be interpreted in the light of quite different concepts. The accidents of heredity and the blows of environment do not add up or multiply into the social position and personal identity of being 'mentally ill', any more than in bygone years they combined sufficiently to form the status of being 'a witch', or of being 'possessed by spirits', or of being 'under the influence of black bile' (to name a few of the alternative significations that have been attached to the behaviours nowadays classified in the light of 'mental illness' concepts). 'Stress' and 'predisposition' are valuable categories for the understanding of organisms and their malfunctioning; but we are concerned, in the understanding of human beings, with the impact of stressful meanings as these affect the predisposition of individuals to screen and consolidate these meanings into their established images of self and society. Trauma and resistance to trauma can, in the human case, be understood not on the analogy of a physical force striking a more or less brittle object, nor on the lines of the invasion of an organism by hostile bacteria, but only through the transformation of elements in a person's identity and capacity to relate to other persons and social collectives. And what positivist accounts of mental illness most flagrantly omit is the serious 'stress' (of socially charged meanings, and not of physical or biological influences) imposed on the subject-patient by the acts of diagnosis, classification, hospitalisation and even, in many cases, 'treatment'. As Marx criticised the utopian socialists for arriving at a position that involved dividing society into two parts of which one (themselves) was seen as 'superior to society', so must the clinical positivism of 'psychopathology' stand condemned for its stance of cultural smugness, its erection of a local, twentieth-century style of assessment into a timeless biological universal, its failure to take stock of its own social role. The utopians, Marx observed, were so busy trying to educate society into socialism that they forgot that 'the educator must himself be educated'. The clinical positivists are so involved in uncovering the factual, objective basis of psychopathology that they have forgotten the subjective valuations which impregnate their whole enterprise. Sooner or later, for good or ill, the valuators must themselves be valued, and their judgements judged.

But the immanentist critique of clinical positivism (and of the latter's ally, the purely exterior 'medical sociology') has begun the task of this evaluation at a somewhat odd starting point. In seizing on the value-laden, subjective, 'political' elements of psychiatric diagnosis and treatment, they have implicitly – and sometimes, indeed, explicitly – conceded the value-free, apolitical and 'objective' character of medicine-in-general: their dismissal of positivism in psychiatry is founded on a contrast with non-psychiatric medicine which actually depends on the acceptance of positivism as a possible method in vital areas of human decision-making. The split between fact and value is reinstated at a superordinate, strategic level precisely in order to attack it in the tactical onslaught against the particular medical specialism of psychiatry. Physical medicine belongs to the world of Fact, of the natural sciences, of anatomy and physiology, of objectively ascertainable disturbed conditions of the body or its 'functioning'; and psychiatry belongs to the world of Value, of ethical judgements on behaviour, of factional coalitions against the unhappy victim, or covert and malignant social and political control. The immanentists of anti-psychiatry *have accomplished the feat of criticising the concept of mental illness without ever examining the (surely more inclusive, and logically prior) concept of illness*. They have focused a merciless lens on psychiatric treatment, detailing its foibles, its fallacies, and its destructiveness towards human self-respect, while at the same time maintaining a posture of reverent myopia towards the chemical, surgical and other therapeutic procedures that are directed by doctors against the many targets of the human organism that lie outside the grey and white matter of the cerebrum.

The evidence of selective myopia among the anti-psychiatric assayers of human pathology is quite overwhelming. As Robert Dingwall observes in an exhaustive study of the literature on critical concepts of physical and mental health, 'this debate (about the applicability of illness-concepts to psychiatry) has almost invariably presupposed a split between mind and body, between physical and psychiatric illness'.[28] Neither early critical appraisals of the medical role such as Shaw's play *The Doctor's Dilemma* (which, along with its searching Preface to the printed edition, remains a classical locus in the overdue debate on health) nor such recent polemics against medical expansionism as Thomas McKeown's momentous *The Role of Medicine* (published by the Nuffield Provincial Hospitals Trust in 1976) have made the slightest impact on the endless re-editions and repetitions of Laingian and Szaszian theorising. If we take into further consideration the current state of anthropological study dealing with medical practice across different cultures, the literature on folk-medicine in relation to physical ailments is small indeed beside the huge bulk of reports on 'ethnopsychiatry' in the less developed societies of the world. As Dingwall comments again, 'the study of folk medicine, with a few exceptions, *is* the study of folk psychiatry'.[29] Among critical philosophers, to take another possible methodology of enquiry, scarcely a single book and hardly more than a handful of articles have treated physical maladies with the same seriousness that has been granted to, for example, Freudian psychopathology. The philosophers of 'ordinary language' in the post-Wittgenstein tradition have singularly refrained from any logical analysis of what it means to be ill or to seek treatment.

The classic phenomenological and linguistic-philosophical discussions of the notions of pain, or of the body, always take place in a curiously non-medical context, in the logician's proverbial armchair rather than on the hard seat of the waiting room or the casualty department's stretcher. Doubtless there exist substantial reasons for this chronically repetitive suspension of the critical faculty in the face of general medicine. Physical medicine and surgery have achieved, after all, extraordinary advances, to the blessing of countless millions. Who wants to pick a quarrel with success, particularly with the success of a miraculous technology projected in the service of universally acclaimed ideals? Yet the problem remains: We cannot review the social institutions of mental illness independently of, or prior to, the institutions and constructions that society has elaborated for the case of plain illness.[30]

What, then, is 'illness'? It will be recalled that critical theory in psychiatry has tended to postulate a fundamental separation between mental illnesses and the general run of human ailments: the former are the expression of social norms, the latter proceed from ascertainable bodily states which have an 'objective' existence within the individual. One critic of psychopathological concepts, Barbara Wootton, has suggested that the expurgation of normative references from psychiatry is at least a theoretical ideal, though one immensely difficult to achieve:

> anti-social behaviour is the precipitating factor that leads to mental treatment. But at the same time the fact of the illness is itself inferred from the behavior... But any disease, the morbidity of which is established only by the social failure that it involves, must rank as fundamentally different from those of which the symptoms are independent of the social norms... long indeed is the road to be travelled before we can hope to reach a definition of mental-cum-physical health which is objective, scientific and wholly free of social value judgements and before we shall be able, consistently and without qualification, to treat mental and physical disorders on exactly the same footing.[31]

Wootton's view has stimulated at least one attempt to begin the task of purging all cultural norms – with their inconvenient variability from one society to another – from the diagnosis of mental illness: Dr Joseph Zubin has reported some work on 'culture-free' assessments of schizophrenia which involve the analysis of reaction times, responses to electrical stimulation, and the like, among schizophrenic patients.[32] It would be fair to say that research in the refinement of psychiatric categories has been mounted with a similar perspective in mind, straining towards the physical medicine ideal of a set of symptom descriptions 'independent of the social norms'. Value judgements and cultural stereotypes are seen as one form of 'error' coming between the investigator and the desired data; and the ultimate standard sought in the description of illness is to be taken to be a sociologically inert, culturally sterile specification of facts and processes which are grounded in bacteriology, biochemistry, physiology or perhaps some variety of cybernetic systems theory.

But this enterprise, tending constantly towards the microscopic and molecular analysis of the 'objective' substrate of behaviour, forms only one of the ways in which we might begin to place mental and physical illnesses 'on exactly the same footing'. If we examine the logical structure of our judgements of illness (whether 'physical' or 'mental') it may prove possible to reduce the distance between psychiatry and other streams of medicine by working in the reverse direction to Wootton: not by annexing psychopathology to the technical instrumentation of the natural sciences but by revealing the character of all illness and disease, health and treatment, as social constructions. For social constructions they most certainly are.

All departments of nature, below the level of mankind are exempt both from disease and from treatment – until people intervene with their own human classifications of disease and treatment. The blight that strikes at corn or at potatoes is a *human invention*, for if we wished to cultivate parasites (rather than potatoes or corn) there would be no 'blight', but simply the necessary foddering of the parasite crop. Animals do not have diseases either, prior to the presence of humans in a meaningful relation with them. A tiger may experience pain or feebleness from a variety of causes (we do not intend to build our case on the supposition that animals, especially higher animals, cannot have experiences or feelings). It may be infected by a germ, trodden by an elephant, scratched by another tiger, or subjected to the ageing processes of its own cells. It does not present itself as being *ill* (though it may present itself to another animal as being highly distressed or uncomfortable) except in the eyes of a human observer who can discriminate illness from other sources of pain or enfeeblement.

Outside the significances that we voluntarily attach to certain conditions, *there are no illnesses or diseases in nature.* We are nowadays so heavily indoctrinated with concepts deriving from the technical medical discoveries of the last century-and-a-half that we are tempted to think that nature does contain diseases. Just as the sophisticated Parisian or New Yorker classes the excrement of dogs and cats as one more form of 'pollution' ruining the pre-established harmony of pavements and gardens, so do modern technologised folk perceive nature to be mined and infested with all kinds of specifically morbid entities and agencies. What, they will protest, are there no diseases in nature? Are there not infectious and contagious bacilli? Are there not definite and objective lesions in the cellular structures of the human body? Are there not fractures of bones, the fatal ruptures of tissues, the malignant multiplications of tumorous growths? Are not these, surely, events of nature? Yet these, as natural events, do not constitute illnesses, sicknesses or diseases prior to the human social meanings we attach to them. The fracture of a septuagenarian's femur has, within the world of nature, no more significance than the snapping of an autumn leaf from its twig: and the invasion of a human organism by cholera germs carries with it no more than the stamp of 'illness' than does the souring of milk by other forms of bacteria.[32] Human beings, like all other naturally occurring structures, are characterised by a variety of inbuilt limitations or liabilities, any of which may (given the presence of further stressful circumstances) lead to the weakening or the collapse of the organism. Mountains as well as moles, stars as well as shrubs, protozoa no less than persons have their dates of expiry set in advance, over a time span which varies greatly over different classes of structure but which is usually at least roughly predictable. Out of anthropocentric self-interest, we have chosen to consider as 'illnesses' or 'diseases' those natural circumstances which precipitate the death (or the failure to function according to certain values) of a limited number of biological species: ourselves, our pets and other cherished livestock, and the plant varieties we cultivate for gain or pleasure. Around these select areas of structural failure we create, in proportion to the progress of our technology, specialised combat institutions for the control and cure of 'disease': the different branches of the medical and nursing profession, veterinary doctors, and the botanical specialists in plant disease. Despite their common concern with disease, and their common use of experimental natural science, these institutions operate according to very different criteria and codes. The use of euthanasia by vets, and of ruthless eugenic policies by plant pathologists, departs from most current medical practice with human patients. All the same, the fact that these specialisms share the categories of disease and illness indicates the selective quality of our perceptions in this field. Children and cattle may fall ill, have diseases and seem as sick, but who has ever imagined that spiders or lizards can be sick or diseased? Plant diseases may strike at tulips, turnips or such prized features of the natural landscape as elm trees, but if some plant species in which we had no interest (a desert grass, let us say) were to be attacked by a fungus or parasite, we should speak not of a disease, but merely of the competition between two species. The medical enterprise is from its inception value-loaded; it is not simply an applied biology, but a biology applied in accordance with the dictates of social interest.

It could be argued that our discussion of animal and plant pathology deals in cases that are too marginal to our central concepts of health and illness to form a satisfactory basis for analysis. Such marginal instances are of course frequently used by logicians in the analysis of concepts since their peripheral character often usefully tests the limits within which our ideas can be seen to be applicable or inapplicable. However, a careful examination of the concept of illness in the human species will reveal the same value-impregnation, the same dependency of apparently descriptive, natural-scientific notions upon our norms of what is desirable. To complain of illness, or to ascribe illness to another person, is not to make a descriptive statement about physiology or anatomy. Concepts of illness were in use among people for centuries before the advent of any reliable knowledge of the human body, and are still employed today within societies which favour a non-physiological (magical or religious) account of the nature of human maladies. Our own classification and explanation of specific illnesses or diseases is of course tremendously different from the categories that are current in earlier ages or in contemporary tribal societies; but it is implausible to suppose that the state of illness itself has no common logical features over different types of society. Homer's sick warriors were tended by magical incantations as well as by herbs and other primitive technical remedies,[34] but the avowal and ascription of illness in Homer does not set up a distance between his characters and ourselves but rather (like his descriptions of bereavement or of sexual attraction) a powerful resonance across the ages. Similarly, the meaning of illness among primitive peoples is usually sufficiently close to our own to enable them to take advantage of modern medical facilities when these are made accessible within their territories. Tribesmen and peasants do not have to be indoctrinated into Western physiological concepts before they can accept help from physicians and nurses trained in advanced societies. Sickness and disease may be conceptualised, in different cultures, as originating within bodily states, or within perturbations of the spirit, or as a mixture of both. Yet there appear to be common features in the declaration or attribution of the sick state, regardless of the causal explanation that is invoked.

All sickness is essentially deviancy. That is to say, no attribution of sickness to any being can be made without the expectation of some alternative state of affairs which is considered more desirable. In the absence of this normative alternative, the presence of a particular bodily or subjective state will not in itself lead to an attribution of illness. Thus, where an entire community is by Western standards 'ill', because it has been infected for generations by parasites which diminish energy, illness will not be recognised in any individual except by outsiders.[35] The Rockefeller Sanitary Commission on Hookworm found in 1911 that this disease was regarded as part of normal health in some areas of North Africa.[36] And in one South American Indian tribe the disease of dyschromic spirochetosis, which is marked by the appearance of coloured spots on the skin, was so 'normal' that those who did not have them were regarded as pathological and excluded from marriage.[37] Even within modern urbanised nations we cannot assume that aches, pains and other discomforts are uniformly categorised as signs of illness among all sections of the community. Although little work has been done on social class variations in the construction of what constitutes 'health' and 'sickness',[38] the example of tooth decay is suggestive: among millions of British working-class families, it is taken for granted that children will lose their teeth and require artificial dentures. The process of tooth loss is not seen as a disease but as something like an act of fate. Among dentists, on the other hand, and in those more educated sections of the community who are socialised into dental ideology, the loss of teeth arises through a definite disease process known as caries, whose aetiology is established.[39] Social and cultural norms also plainly govern the varying perception, either as essentially 'normal', or as essentially 'pathological', of such characteristic as baldness, obesity, infestation by lice, venereal infection, and the presence of tonsils and foreskins among children.

Once again it can be argued that these cultural variations apply only to marginal cases of sickness and health, that there are some physical or psychological conditions which are *ipso facto* symptomatic of illness, whether among Bushmen or Brobdignagians, duchesses or dockworkers. But there is no reason to believe that the 'standardised' varieties of human pathology operate according to a different logic from the 'culturally dependent' varieties. The existence of common or even universal illnesses testifies, not to the absence of a normative framework for judging pathology, but to the presence of very widespread norms. To be ill, after all, is not the same thing as to feel pain, or to experience weakness, or to fail to manifest this or that kind of behaviour. Rather it is to experience discomfort (or to manifest behavioural failure) in a context of a particular kind. Consider the following imaginary conversations between physician and client:

(a) *Client* Doctor, I want you to examine me, I keep feeling terrible pains in my right shoulder.
Doctor Really? What are they like?
Client Stabbing and intense.
Doctor How often do they happen?

Client Every evening after I get home from work.
Doctor Always in the same spot?
Client Yes, just in the place where my husband hits me with the rolling-pin.

(b) *Client* (telephoning doctor) Doctor, I haven't consulted you before but things are getting desperate. I'm feeling so weak, I can't lift anything heavy.
Doctor Goodness, when does this come on you?
Client Every time I try to lift something or make an effort. I have to walk quite slowly up the stairs and last night when I was packing the big suitcase I found I couldn't lift it off the bed.
Doctor Well, let's have some details about you before you come in. Name?
Client John Smith.
Doctor Age?
Client Ninety-two last February.

In the first example, the 'patient's' pain is not an illness because we expect pain as a normal response to being hit in tender places; indeed, *not* feeling pain when hit or prodded would be taken as a sign of some disease involving nerve degeneration. In the second example, the 'patient's' infirmity would usually be ascribed not to the category of 'illness' but to that of 'ageing'. (If he had given his age as 'twenty-two' the case would be different.) In our culture we expect old people to find difficulty in lifting heavy weights, although it is easy to conceive of a culture in which mass rejuvenation among the aged had been perfected (perhaps by the injection of hormones, vitamins or other pep pills into the water supply) and where, in consequence, a dialogue of the type recounted would lead to a perfectly ordinary referral for medical treatment. The attribution of illness always proceeds from the computation of a gap between presented behaviour (or feeling) and some social norm. In practice of course we take the norm for granted, so that the broken arm or the elevated temperature is seen alone as the illness. But the broken arm would be no more of an illness than a broken fingernail unless it stopped us from achieving certain socially constructed goals; just as, if we could all function according to approved social requirements within any range of body temperature, thermometers would disappear from the household medical kit.

This is not to say that illness amounts to any deviancy whatsoever from social expectations about how we should function. Some deviancies are regarded as instances not of sickness but of criminality, wickedness, poor upbringing or bad manners (though not all cultures do in fact draw a firm line between illness and these other deviations, e.g. primitive societies for which illness is also a moral flaw and modern liberal circles for which drug addiction is categorised in medical as well as moral terms). Looking over the very wide range of folk concepts and technical ideas about illness which exist in the history of human societies, it is difficult to discern a common structural element which distinguishes the notion of illness from other attributions of social failure. Provisionally, it is possible to suggest that illness is set apart from other deviances insofar as the description (or, at a deeper level, the explanation) of the sick state is located within a relatively restricted set of causal factors operating within the boundaries of the individual human being. One may become ill as the result of being infected by germs, or through being entered by evil demons, or visited by a curse from the Almighty. Each culturally specific account of illness must involve a theory of the person, of the boundaries between the person and the world 'outside', and of the ways in which adverse influences can trespass over these limits and besiege or grip the individual. If the current theory of the person is positivistic and physical, the agencies of illness will be seen as arising from factors within (or at the boundaries of) the body; in cultures with an animistic tradition, the invasion will be one of the spirit or soul. But, however variously the nature of illness is specified from culture to culture, the attribution of illness appears to include a *quest for explanation*, or at least the descriptive delimiting of certain types of causal factor, as well as the normative component outlined above.

It is indeed likely that the concept of illness has arisen in close parallel with the social practice of therapy, i.e. with the development of techniques to control those human afflictions which can be controlled at the boundaries of the individual person. It is hard to see how the category of illness, as a distinct construction separate from other kinds of misfortune, could have arisen without the discovery that some varieties of pain and affliction could be succoured through individual specialised attention to the afflicted person. In traditional societies, of course, the institution of medicine is not crystallised out as an applied branch of natural science: 'Therapy' for the Greeks was simply the word used for looking after or tending somebody, and, in ancient Greece as well as elsewhere nowadays, a great deal of therapy goes on either in the patient's household or in conjunction with religious and magical specialisms. A specifically 'medical' framework of treatment is not necessary to provide the link between illness and practical action.

Practice and concept continue their mutual modification over the ages. In a society where the treatment of the sick is still conducted through religious ritual, the notion of illness will not be entirely distinct from the notion of sinfulness or pollution. Correspondingly, with the growth of progressively more technical and more autonomous specialisms of therapy, the concepts of disease and illness themselves become more technical, and thereby more alienated from their implicit normative background. Thus we reach the position of the present day where any characterisation of an 'illness' which is not amenable to a diagnosis drawn from physiology or to a therapy based on chemical, electrical or surgical technique becomes suspect as not constituting, perhaps, an illness at all. Such has been the fate of mental illness in our own epoch. It has been much easier for societies with an animistic theory of the person (and of his or her boundaries and susceptibilities to influence) to view mental disturbances on a par with bodily ailments. Ceremonies of ritual purgation and demon expulsion, along with primitive 'medical' methods of a herbal or surgical type, are used indifferently by traditional healers on patients with a mental or with a bodily dysfunction. Fever and madness, the broken limb or the broken spirit are situated within the same normative frame, within the same explanatory and therapeutic system.

Even the development of a technical-physiological specialism of medicine, such as emerged with the Hippocratic tradition which runs in fits and starts from antiquity to modern times, does not impair the possibility of a unitary perspective on physical and mental illness, *so long as a common structure of valuation and explanation applies over the whole range of disorders of the person*. The medicine of the seventeenth and eighteenth centuries in Western Europe, for instance, was able to interpret our present-day 'mental' disorders as a group of illnesses inhabiting the embodied person on much the same plane as other sorts of malady. The insane or the emotionally disturbed patient was suffering from a fault of 'the vapours', 'the nerves', 'the fluids', 'the animal spirits', 'the spleen', 'the humours', 'the head', or the forces and qualities of the body.[40] This unitary integration of human illnesses was of course only achieved at the cost of a stupendously inaccurate and speculative physiology. But an integrated theory of illness, whether achieved within a unitary-animistic or a unitary-physicalistic doctrine of the person, has one singular advantage over more fragmentary perspective: it is not beset by the kind of crisis we now have in psychopathology and psychiatry, whose conceptual and moral foundation has been exploded now that 'illness' has acquired a technical-physical definition excluding disorders of the whole person from its purview. Animistic and unitary-physicalistic accounts of illness both dealt in the whole embodied individual; but the medical technology of the nineteenth century and onwards has succeeded in classifying illnesses as particular states of the body only.

Hence, indeed, the growing popularity of those therapies in 'alternative medicine', such as acupuncture and the unitary-materialist systems of healing stemming from India, which have refused to split the therapeutic enterprise into a collection of specialisms dealing in different body parts and further segments allocated to the mind and the emotions. After this complicated and prestigious process of segmentation and objectification, so typical of modern medicine, psychiatry is left with two seeming alternatives: either to concur with the view that personal, psychological and emotional disorders are really states of the body, objective features of the brain tissue, the genes, the organism-under-stress, or what have you; or else to deny that disorders of the psyche are illnesses at all. If the latter, then the way is open to treat mental illnesses as the expression of social value judgements about the patient, and psychiatry's role will not belong to the disciplines of objective, body-state medicine. Instead, it will be analogous to the value-laden and non-medical disciplines of moral education, police interrogation, criminal punishment or religion (depending on how low or how lofty a view one takes of the values inherent in psychiatric practice).

This dilemma will perhaps seem somewhat to dissolve if we recapitulate what was previously said about the nature of illness as a social construction. *All* illness, whether conceived in localised bodily terms or within a larger view of human functioning, expresses both a social value judgement (contrasting a person's condition with certain understood and accepted norms) and an attempt at explanation (with a view to controlling the disvalued condition). The physicalistic psychiatrists are wrong in their belief that they can find objective disease-entities representing the psychopathological analogues to diabetes, tuberculosis and post-syphilitic paresis. Quite correctly, the anti-psychiatrists have pointed out that psychopathological categories refer to value judgements and that mental illness is deviancy. On the other hand, the anti-psychiatric critics themselves are wrong when they imagine physical medicine to be essentially different in its logic from psychiatry. A diagnosis of diabetes, or paresis, includes the recognition of norms or values. Anti-psychiatry can only operate by positing a mechanical and inaccurate model of physical illness and its medical diagnosis. It follows, therefore, from the above train of argument that mental illnesses can be conceptualised within the disease framework just as easily as physical maladies such as lumbago or TB.

There are several misunderstandings that might arise (have, indeed, already arisen) out of a declaration of this position. In the first place, it does not follow from the position as stated that the existing 'official' categories of mental illness are the most useful or truthful ones that we can reach. The label of 'psychopathy', for example, probably represents no more than an attempt at pseudo-medical mislabelling, for control purposes, by psychiatrists working in tandem with the judicial authorities. It is likely, also, that 'schizophrenia' is a rudimentary dustbin category for a variety of psychic ills which may have little logically or biologically in common with one another. Equally, though, I have no doubt that many current diagnostic categories in physical medicine will disappear in the next century or so, and be replaced by others apparently (and provisionally) more adequate. I can see that, for example, by the year 2081 nobody will be classed as having diabetes or asthma, though they will undergo feelings of discomfort similar to those experienced by present-day diabetics and asthmatics. In the future development of our species, we can anticipate *either* that some conditions now classified as illnesses will be re-allocated to a different framework of deviancy (or, more drastically, become regarded as essentially normal and non-deviant); *or* that, on the contrary, conditions which are nowadays viewed in a non-illness category of deviancy (as sins, perhaps, or as consequences of ageing or excessive effort) will be re-grouped into the range of the illnesses or diseases. The latter prospect – the progressive annexation of not-illness into illness – seems at the moment much more likely to happen than the former, especially since the stupendous achievements of medical technology make it more and more difficult for doctors to sign death certificates under the rubric 'died of natural causes'. The natural causes of death are becoming, more and more, causes that we can control: so that the terminally ill and their relatives will be putting strong pressures on the medical profession to redefine the natural (and inevitable) causes of fatality, rendering them into medical (and hence controllable) pathologies which require the services of a doctor rather than of a mortician. *The future belongs to illness*: we are just going to get more and more diseases, since our expectations of health are going to become more expansive and sophisticated. Maybe one day there will be a backlash, perhaps at the point when everybody has become so luxuriantly ill, physically or mentally, that there will be poster-parades of protest outside medical conventions with slogans like 'Illness Is Not So Bad, You Know?' or 'Disease Is The Highest Form of Health'. But for the moment, it seems that illness is going to be 'in': a rising tide of really chronic sickness. Even despite the Canutes of deviancy-sociology.

Secondly and much more importantly, nothing in my argument confirms the technologising of illness; the specialised medical model of illness is not the only possible one, as I have already indicated.

As René Dubos points out in his fundamental work *The Mirage of Health*, the greatest advances in the control of disease have often come about through non-medical measures, and in particular through social and political change. The insertion of windows into working-class houses (with the consequent beneficial influx of sunlight), or the provision of a pure water supply and an efficient sewage disposal, did more to clear up the plagues of modern epidemic infection than did the identification of particular microbes or the synthesis of 'medical discoveries' like the various antibiotics and antitoxins.

There are some authorities, notably Miriam Siegler and Humphrey Osmond,[41] who argue that, since the category of illness is infinitely preferable, from the standpoint of the mentally deranged, to any other variety of deviancy, we have to concentrate entirely on a narrow medical model for explaining diseases and curing them. In their view, social explanations for the onset of illnesses like schizophrenia and drug addiction are incompatible with any illness model, and so should be ruthlessly jettisoned But we do not need to technologise illness beyond the point at which we decide that it is helpful to do so. Even with physical illness, the concept of a 'social disease' is indispensable in the understanding and treatment of, for example, tuberculosis. Preventive medicine and public medicine are bound to invoke social explanations and social measures, to occupy a space which occurs, in short, at the intersection of medicine and politics. My case points, not to the technologising of illness, to the medicalisation of moral values (so obvious in the practice of psychiatry that it needs no fresh rehearsal here), but, on the contrary, to the politicisation of medical goals, I am arguing that, without the concept of illness – including that of mental illness since to exclude it would constitute the crudest dualism – we shall be unable to *make demands* on the health service facilities of the society we live in.

Those labelling theorists who like to yearn for the Lost Territories of deviancy now occupied by the invading armies of medical diagnosis, are committing a *sociological irredentism* quite as offensive as the better known bogey of Psychiatric Imperialism. Assemblies of deviancy experts remind me of nothing so much as the sad, moral boosting reunions of Sudeten Germans in the Federal Republic: they appear dangerous to the Czechs, but basically such gatherings are those of the devotees of a lost cause, joining in old songs and refurbished regional accents in order to maintain a losing identity against the harsh world that offers many rival opportunities for re-socialisation. The 'demands' of the Sudeten Germans are, in 1981, a ritual, even if they were not so in 1938. The demands of the sociological revisionists of mental illness are not very obvious even as ritual; they appear to want more money for their own research, and one or two of their allies want to be left undisturbed to carry on rewarding private psychoanalytic practices. But theirs is a passive irredentism; after all, the sociologists never actually lived in the territories that the psychiatric colonisers have now taken over, so there cannot be very much energy in their grumbles.

This very passivity is, however, highly dangerous in the present historical period when the amount of public money available for investment in the health services is so grossly inadequate. The voice of labelling sociology, including a good many of the 'immanentist' theoreticians, chimes in with the cautious, restrictive tones of the cheese-paring politician who is out to deny the priority of resource allocation for the public psychiatric services (at the same time budgeting lavishly for the military and police). Public psychiatry, as the result of the onslaughts of Szasz, Goffman and Laing and – to a smaller extent – of the academic 'anti-psychiatrists', has become thoroughly unpopular with the general reading public. And since this middle-class public forms the great reservoir of candidates from which the officer class of possible pressure groups gets selected, the unpopularity of public health psychiatry is an important factor which prevents the crystallisation of a vocal and determined lobby for the provision of intensive psychiatric facilities on a mass scale. Mental illness, like mental health, is a fundamentally *critical* concept: or can be made into one provided that those who use it are prepared to place demands and pressures on the existing organisation of society. In trying to remove and reduce the concept of mental illness, the revisionist theorists have made it that bit harder for a powerful campaign of reform in the mental-health services to get off the ground. The revisionists have thought themselves, and their public, into a state of complete inertia. They can expose the hypocrisies and annotate the tragedies of official psychiatry, but the concepts which they have developed enable them to engage in no public action grander than that of wringing their hands. Of course they do it beautifully. But the tragic stance of labelling theory and anti-psychiatric sociology cannot be taken seriously as a posture which is 'above the battle' for the priorities of spending within our bureaucratised and militarised capitalism. It is *in* the battle, on the wrong side: the side of those who want to close down intensive psychiatric units and throw the victims of mental illness on to the streets, with the occasional shot of tranquilliser injected in them to assure the public that something medical is still happening.

Cynics are, quite simply, people who have no hope, and therefore have no capacity to express any demands for the future. The sociological critics of the 'mental illness' concept are, as ideologues, deeply cynical: if they do have hope, or any possibility of formulating demands in the mental-health field, such hope is not made manifest through the ideas contained in their books and articles. And the cynic cannot really be a critic; the radical who is only a radical nihilist, or a radical tragedian, is for practical purposes the most adamant of conservatives.

I have caught, in some discussions of a draft of this paper, a certain pervasive anxiety among my audience, an anxiety which is afraid lest psychiatry may, in the service of our abominable social and economic order, succeed in 'adjusting' the mentally ill to its goals. It is as though people believe that there is only a finite pool of grievances and maladjustments available in this society for radicals to work with. The fear is that psychiatry, with its tranquillisers, hospitals and whatnot, may succeed in mopping up this limited supply of miseries, discharging its patients into the hell of the factory and the purgatory of the home as permanently 'cured' and adjusted robots. Once again, if capitalism could really 'adjust' people, through psychiatry or any other technology, who would want to quarrel with it? I myself am perfectly happy to see as many mentally-ill persons as possible treated, fully and effectively, in this society: for no matter how many maladjustments may become adjusted through expert techniques, the workings of capitalism will ever create newer and larger discontents, infinitely more dangerous to the system than any number of individual neuroses or manias. Some people in this audience have seemed to me to be wanting to hoard the existing supply of neuroses and insanities, by leaving them untreated as long as possible, in the conviction that these are the best grievances we have got, and once they have gone, where will we get any more? I can suggest plenty more alternative sources of maladjustment, within our present-day society. But I forbear from doing so; for there is no arguing with people who will not read the newspapers.

2. Psycho-Medical Dualism: The Case of Erving Goffman

The thinkers and writers to be discussed in the remaining chapters of Part One have usually attained a distinct celebrity outside the narrow scholarly world. Laing, Szasz, Foucault are irremediably public figures, each leaving a different trail of impressions and impacts behind him in the liberal-intellectual media or even within certain mass publics. My discussion of these innovators will be addressed, therefore, partly to the texts they have written, and partly also to the widespread public influences, in the realm of psychiatric ideology and practice, which they have done so much to create. But our analysis of modern anti-psychiatric thought has to begin with a figure who, despite his tremendous prestige with two or three intellectual generations of sociologists and social psychologists, never moved into the limelight of the wider non-academic media. In this chapter I shall not provide a general survey of Goffman's intellectual history or recount his dealings (which in any case are sparse in number) with the institutions that govern psychiatric policy. Instead, I will try to clarify and extend my argument from the previous chapter by criticising his exposition of the 'psycho-medical dualism' (the view that mental illnesses and physical ailments have a distinct and separate logic) which has been a leading preoccupation of this book so far.

As I suggested in the last chapter, Goffman takes physical medicine more or less for granted. In his analysis, physical disease has essentially nothing to do with the personal, social world of values and meanings; such disease is not the attribute of a 'person' but of the 'organism': 'The most disruptive thing a well organism can do is to acquire deadly contagious disease. The most disruptive thing a person can do is to fail to keep a place that others feel can't be changed for him,'[1] i.e. by acquiring psychiatric symptoms of the acting-out kind. True, the effect of a physical disease-state may be to bring into question the afflicted person's credentials of self-presentation within the world of social encounters: this is the burden of Goffman's treatment of disfiguring physical affliction in the essay *Stigma*. But this is still to keep the nature of the physical disease-condition itself – as distinct from its more disruptively visible effects – bracketed or reserved for the asocial domain of organic pathology, which (as Goffman puts it) remains 'above the concerns of any particular grouping' in society.[2]

In the light of our discussion in the previous chapter, it is possible to dissolve the contrast so plausibly established by Goffman. If we render explicit and obvious the social and valuational context of physical-medicine judgements, it will become clear that there are relatively few basic differences between them and judgements of the psychiatric type. We may begin by noting the strain in Goffman's term 'a well organism'. An organism cannot be well or ill: in the conflict between two organisms, we would not know which one represented the 'disease' and which the 'victim of disease' until we had decided which of the two had our sympathies, i.e. the one whose survival we were committed to. Only persons (or other species in whose survival we have an interest) can be ill or well; in order to examine the physical/psychiatric contrast fully we shall confine our attention to human beings since the absence of language from all other species has ensured that any psychiatric framework for discussing the behaviour of e.g. dogs or chimpanzees could only be very rudimentary.

Goffman argues that mental symptoms are distinct from the physical variety in that the identification of the former depends on a specific social context. Thus, in mental hospitals (see *Asylums*) many of the bizarre forms of behaviour displayed by patients are not the 'signs' of a mental disease-process but rather deliberate self-defensive moves used by the victims of an all-engulfing total institution which is trying to destroy them. This, the most well-known of Goffman's arguments, is actually his mildest: it would be accepted by many psychiatrists and medical adminstrators who are quite prepared to admit that mental institutions tend to make people more peculiar than they were when they went in. Goffman's more radical argument about psychiatric symptoms[3] insists that the identification of a piece of 'mentally abnormal' behaviour is based, not on any difference between it and the general range of 'normal behaviour' but on the context of social demands within face-to-face situation encompassing the putative 'patient' and other people. When forms of behaviour which may be perfectly acceptable within other contexts disrupt the 'public order' of interchange among persons, an assignation of categories like 'psychotic', 'mentally disturbed' or 'crazy' is made by relatives or doctors in order to enclose the perceived disruption by placing it 'within' the personality or character of the offending partner. The ascription of a psychiatric pathology to what are no more than 'situational improprieties' enables society to punish (or in Goffman's term 'sanction') these lapses of 'decorum and demeanour' by passing the offender over to the authorised medical agencies. It is not the hallucination, the depression, the vocal rumination, the manic excitement, the mentioning of the unmentionable (or at least of the inappropriate) or the withdrawal from social contact that, in Goffman's view, constitute the symptom, but rather the occurrences of these and kindred behaviours in a setting where other people's sense of etiquette is outraged. 'I know of no psychotic misconduct which cannot be matched precisely in everyday life by the conduct of persons who are not psychologically ill nor considered to be so!'[4] It is all right to be 'out of contact' if you are a young woman who ignores suggestive remarks from men as you walk along the street; it is all right (or at least it is no concern for a psychiatrist) if you hear supernatural voices in the course of a Pentecostal meeting; you may take off your clothes and dance at a hippie festival of joy and music, you may hector and dominate in a classroom or parade ground, you may refuse attention to onlookers if you are fishing, writing a PhD or meditating on St John of the Cross: but if you try these things at home, in the wrong kind of public place or on the observation ward of a mental institution, heaven help you because you are then 'mad', 'mental' or eligible for some more technical diagnosis! 'The deepest nature of an individual is only skin-deep – the deepness of others' "skin"':[5] scratch those others' skins too hard or too often and they will re-define what your nature is.

According to Goffman, then, the central distinction between the medical disease-symptoms and the 'mental symptoms' lies in the latter's disruption of a person's social posture, i.e. of his agreed placing within the compass of others' expectations. Even severely diseased patients suffering from physical disabilities can know and keep their 'place', by playing the sick roles of cheerful invalid or stoical amputee. No such predictable role-playing can be seen as forthcoming from the disturbed 'mental patient': and indeed such an individual is characterised as 'mental' precisely because he or she cannot and will not play the required games. Such is Goffman's position, which has met with virtually unanimous acclamation among his wide readership of academics and students.

But Goffman's radical case on mental illness stands or falls with the sharpness of the distinction that can be made between the socially neutral or negotiable physical illness and the socially disruptive, context-bound psychiatric disorder. In several ways we can see that the distinction is actually much less sharp than Goffman would like. For physical symptoms also demand a context and a set of values before they can be seen as examples of illness. Our imaginary conversations between doctor and 'physically ill' patient in the previous chapter can be precisely paralleled by similar scenarios between psychiatrist and patient:

Client Doctor, I feel so numb and withdrawn, I can't concentrate, I don't feel like going to work, everything round the house seems empty and useless, I can't get my thoughts together on anything except the past: I just think about me and I feel terrible.
Psychiatrist Anything happened to you lately?
Client Well, now that you ask – my wife dropped dead in the kitchen yesterday.[6]

As Goffman says, we can 'match' psychiatric symptoms by instancing virtually identical behaviours that occur within a socially 'normal' context: but the same holds good for at least a very wide range of physical ill-symptoms. Illness in general is, as we have argued, deviancy of some sort, so it should not surprise us that mental illness is also deviancy, unspecifiable as a set of particular acts, specifiable only when context and norm are attached to highlight the act. And, just as with physical illness, the mere identification of the 'sick' behaviour as being socially deviant does not invalidate the judgement that this is indeed illness. Judgements of illness, we have argued, comprise both a normative judgement and an attempt at rational control through explanation. 'He has a high temperature because he has cholera' exhibits the same logic as 'he is withdrawn because he is in a psychotic depression.' The fact that we could match the symptom of high temperature from a context where it would be considered 'normal' (e.g. if the subject's physiology became adapted to prolonged work near a blast-furnace) does not destroy the judgement that, in the present context, his high temperature can be usefully explained by involving the category of cholera infection. Similarly, the fact that withdrawn social behaviour is, in some social contexts, acceptably 'normal', i.e. not to be regarded as a form of 'illness', cannot be taken in evidence for the inapplicability of the illness category to the same withdrawn behaviour in quite different social contexts.

In the case of both physical and mental illness, the subject's 'breach of decorum' may be legitimately taken to be the outward and visible sign of a pathological inner process; thus, by a series of inferences, the inability of an office-worker to get up in time for the train, to concentrate on the files, or to do the more humdrum chores at home or at work may be traced back either to a psychological illness (e.g. depression) or to a physiological disease (e.g. kidney inflammation). The situational impropriety (or other discrepancy from normal expectation) forms the starting point, the pretext, for the diagnostic quest. If we can reach another satisfactory explanation of the deviancy, then a medical explanation may be seen as unnecessary or even as 'ideological', i.e. as an attempt to undermine the rationality of the subject's actions. Thus, it is inconceivable to psychiatrists in the service of the Russian state bureaucracy that political dissent could arise on rational grounds; these improprieties are therefore labelled as illnesses, to be treated by compulsory confinement in an institution. For anybody who *can* accept that political disagreement is rational, the psychiatric 'labelling' of opposition is bound to appear implausible, a barefaced attempt by the state to silence protesting voices. But the Russian bureaucrat-psychiatrists are incriminated not because they single out or identify improprieties of conduct, but because they attach a dismissive and irrationalist explanation to these malefactions. We cannot say that the appearance of a recognised impropriety is sufficient in itself to disbar an explanation in terms of some inward pathological process: if Goffman were right in supposing this, then Freud's analysis of verbal slips and other lapses of performance, as related to the overspill from unconscious conflicts, would be disqualified from the start. But there is nothing absurd or contradictory in Freud's attempt, even though a psycho-analytic explanation may not be the one we would find acceptable in understanding someone's verbal *faux pas*.

To sum up this point: if we are right in assuming that an attribution of illness is necessarily both an expression of deviancy-perception and an attempt at one or more of several varieties of explanation (medical, magical, psychoanalytic, etc.) in terms of the bounded person, then we can challenge someone's diagnosis of illness in two ways. We can either say that the conduct concerned is not deviant (because we ourselves have different norms and values) or else conclude that the explanation in terms of illness is unfounded. We cannot, as Goffman does, simply conclude that the perception of deviancy is incompatible with an illness-explanation, and thus expel deviant acts or manifestations by *fiat* from the purview of the medical.

Goffman's whole argument turns on the proposition (never argued out or justified)[6] that there are two distinct classes of illness: the 'medical' and the 'mental'. Mental symptoms are socially offensive acts, 'wilful situational improprieties'[7] in which the patient's failure to keep a proper station extends even to a refusal to play the game of being a well-behaved patient. On the other hand, 'the interesting thing about medical symptoms is how utterly nice, how utterly plucky the patient can be in managing them'.[8] Physically ill patients can dissociate themselves from their condition, retain some core of personal identity around which they can manage the presentation of their symptoms; mental patients are unable to make this kind of compromise, and their condition is seen by others as intrinsically bound up with their them-ness, their personality.

It has been pointed out by one critic (answering Szasz rather than Goffman, though on lines that are equally relevant against the latter's case) that mental illness and physical illness are in practice quite difficult to separate at all sharply.[9] Not only do many physical illnesses have important consequences in abnormal personality functioning: a great many psychological illnesses are characterised by some form of serious somatic or behavioural disturbance. Asthma, ulcers, insomnia, obesity, facial tension, chain-smoking: the catalogue of psychosomatic maladjustments can be extended liberally, so liberally indeed that it is a serious hazard nowadays for the physically ill to consult a psychiatrically-minded family doctor who will prescribe tranquillisers or insight-therapy for conditions where speedier relief might be brought by aspirins, antibiotics or even a properly placed splint. The concept of the 'situational impropriety' in any case forms an inept designation for the psychosomatic illnesses, some of which (like nervous tics and the postural rigidities of Wilhelm Reich's 'character-armour') may be situationally disquieting while others, such as migraine or cardiac weaknesses,[10] may flow into the socially acceptable 'sick role'.

The dualism of 'mental' versus 'medical' symptomatology becomes especially insane when one considers how a similar set of symptoms may be produced either through the subject's psychological reactions to social stresses or as the outcome of a determinate, physiologically based disease. A striking example is that of dwarfism. The meagre dimensions of human dwarves are usually explained, with considerable plausibility, by the various biochemical or genetic factors which may programme a somewhat miniaturised circuit for the limits of the individual's growth. However, one form of pituitary dwarfism, with an attendant mental as well as physical retardation, has recently been recognised as a product of 'emotional deprivation and neurotic manipulation' by intensely dominant older relatives: 'released from their parent(s), such children may grow more than an inch a month, their schoolwork improve at similar rate, and their behaviour change dramatically' from withdrawnness and quaintness into normal sociability.[11] Epilepsy, to take a better-known instance, would doubtless be located at the 'medical' rather than the 'mental' pole of the dualist world of illnesses yet it may be associated either with distinct cerebral lesions (especially in the temporal lobes) or, in the so-called 'psychomotor' variety, with a socially comprehensible, subjectively experienced stress. There are of course many abnormal psychiatric states, ranging from memory loss to personality derangement of the 'acting-out' type, which can be convincingly attached to an 'organic' diagnosis of cerebral damage. Often only extensive neurological testing, combined with the taking of the patient's history to determine whether the brain has suffered definite insult, can determine whether an 'organic' or a 'functional' psychosis is present; yet, even prior to the results of this detailed testing, it would be agreed by all observers that the patient was indeed mentally disturbed. Goffman at one point tries to face the difficulties raised for his position by the case when 'a brain-damaged and a functionally ill person manifest similar misconduct'. But, far from accepting this as evidence that 'conduct can be a medically symptomatic thing [*sic*], whether the illness is organic or functional', Goffman asks us to take it that 'it is the organic patient's behaviour that mimics a socially structured delict… and it is the functional patient who manifests withdrawal from contact in its fuller and original form.'[12]

It should be obvious from this little quotation that Goffman's argument at this crucial point is lame. For centuries, after all, in epochs when the modern distinction between 'organic' and 'functional' psychosis was but poorly developed and even when conditions now regarded as 'functional' in origin had a crudely 'organic' explanation attached to them – e.g. the notorious 'masturbatory insanity' of Victorian psychiatry, or the various perturbations of bodily fluids which accounted for madness within the Hippocratic tradition – men and women were seen as manifesting public misconduct which amounted, in the common view of their day, to insanity, or lunacy, or craziness, or psychosis, or whatever term was in current use as a superlative for the display of individual irrationality. Yet Goffman asks us to believe that the category of 'functional mental patient', a modern and sophisticated diagnostic label (and one whose meaning is by no means clear, despite its apparent sophistication) represents the 'fuller' and '*original*' manifestation of psychiatric disorder. We are supposed to acquire the concept of a mental disorder from cases whose aetiology is nowadays satisfactorily determined as non-organic or 'functional'; then, having evolved the notion of mental illnesses or symptoms, we can treat the behaviour displayed in senile or alcoholic brain-syndromes as something analogous to our primary concept of a 'functional' and 'original' psychiatric abnormality. Goffman's logic simply inverts the whole history of psychiatric diagnosis, which, as we have pointed out, was able to certify the insane long before it could separate gross brain damage from other varieties of insult to the personality. 'Conduct', including that whole range of deficiencies and inelegancies in face-to-face encounters which is charted, in descriptive terms, so expertly by Goffman, has from time immemorial been considered by doctors as a clue in the diagnosis of conditions with a distinctly physical or biological explanation. And in the commonsense, everyday diagnostics of the lay public, the conduct of the patient is again taken as part of the evidence for the delivering of a verdict of 'crazy', 'loopy', 'ga-ga', 'nutty', 'round the bend' or any of the several homely classifications which by-pass the technical medical distinction between the neurologist's cases of 'brain-damage' and the psychiatrist's cases of neurosis or functional psychosis. The principal Spanish folkword for the mentally ill, *loco*, can be applied to a schizophrenic, an alcoholic, a retarded imbecile, or indeed a dog with rabies. If Goffman's method of dissolving behavioural disorders into their situational context were to be pursued at all rigorously, we would have to conclude that the dog who is impounded and destroyed after it has rushed around biting several people and alarming the public with its foaming jaws actually has no microbe-caused abnormality which can properly be called 'rabies'. All it has done, after all, is to commit some situational improprieties, violating the rituals of dog-to-person interaction which society has decreed. The medical diagnosis of rabies is simply the means by which hired professionals respond to the public demand by giving the dog a bad name.[13]

Goffman is of course not usually as crude as this. Indeed, his dualistic schema of illnesses is wholly unnecessary for the statement of the insights into mental disorder (vis-à-vis the 'order' at work in small groups) which he has so painstakingly annotated. For once it is conceded that mental illness is not a straightforwardly normative category, but rather – like all illness – occurs at the intersection of two indispensable social imperatives – the urge to identify or 'label' the painful and the urge to explain it (with a view to reducing it by the swiftest and most rational means possible): then no amount of detailing of the social norms governing diagnosis and treatment can impugn the technical rationale of medicine. It is impossible, in short, to define the nature of the 'mental', the psychiatric, by restricting the definition of the 'medical', the therapeutic.

Goffman's description of the special havoc of mental illness in 'The Insanity of Place' – that it destroys the individual's control over any possible acceptable 'sick role' – may be a powerfully accurate account of what goes on in some psychopathological conditions. But we cannot use this as a defining characteristic of mental illnesses to distinguish the latter from 'medical' illnesses. Some mentally sick people make extremely bad patients, refusing to keep their 'place' in the family's or hospital's designated slot. But not all are like this, and perhaps not even most. There are many mental disorders in which the sick person is extremely competent at 'front' and 'face' management. A solitary depressive, for example, living without kin or close friends, may weep in desperation to himself or herself and maintain a brilliantly cheerful face before work-colleagues, shopkeepers and other publics. There are a great many suicides whose death is an occasion for the surprise of all who knew them (and suicide is arguably the severest form of mental illness, since the person who commits it has no inner defences left, not even the hallucinated bulwarks of the psychotic). And there are some patients, with chronic diagnostic labels conferred on them by psychiatrists, who regard their schizophrenia or depression as 'another bad spell', requiring medical attention till the trouble passes, just as an epileptic or rheumatic sufferer does. Indeed, one salient feature of many mental disorders is their *fluctuating* quality: the bad spells come and go, rendering a relatively detached adaptation possible, in keeping with the traditional good patient's role as portrayed by Goffman. Many physical illnesses do not fluctuate but keep on in incessant pain or deteriorating. There is a limit to the agony which most people can endure, and still maintain their 'place' or their 'face'. My own earliest memory of another's severe illness is that of a little boy of nine, in the next bed to my own during the Liverpool diphtheria epidemic of the war-years, who screamed and sobbed all night about his need to use the bedpan, using baby-like expressions quite unbecoming to his age (and mine): a solecism on which I promptly made a jest to my friend who occupied the bed on my other side. I still feel guilty that I drew public attention to this 'situational impropriety', because my young weeping neighbour had been in a high fever, and was taken away dead on the following day. Beside such poignant losses of composure among the physically ill – and in Goffman's passages on physical sickness one feels a great lack of contact compared with his close observation of mental patients – the catatonic might almost be said to be keeping a stiff upper lip.

We have hitherto argued that Goffman, even as a microscopic observer of small-scale pathological behaviour, is seriously inaccurate both in his description of what can be observed and in the comparisons he makes between his observed material and the data that lie outside his microscope's bright disc of viewing. But these errors can be seen to proceed from a much more fundamental flaw in his social philosophy. Quite simply, *Goffman has no room for any sense of the historical contingencies of social institutions*. This deficiency makes it absolutely impossible for him to use his insights, either into particular local 'settings' or into the general quality of everyday life, in any way which is *critical*: i.e. which issues in a demand for change in a definite direction. In Goffman's theatre of action among persons, the possibility of innovation in the staging, in a transformation of structures which would also transform the meaning of the action both for participants and for audience, is fundamentally excluded. I shall press the theatrical metaphor no further: it is already a tired one, though less in Goffman's hands than among his reviewers. But the material in, for instance, Goffman's most compassionate work, his *Stigma: Notes on the Management of Spoiled Identity*, is perfectly capable of provoking a number of serious and searching questions addressed not simply to the torments and embarrassments endured by the handicapped (the overt theme of the book) but to the standards of public acceptability by which those bearing 'stigma' are judged and condemned. *It is assumed*, as a natural fact whose logic is writ by inexorable decree, that society has to adopt some kind of standard about the shape or fitness of the human body, or about proper sexual performance, in virtue of which those who fail to live up to this norm may become discredited if they inform the world of their failure. In other words, Goffman takes it for granted that certain important personal qualities of human beings, which they cannot help having (such as their physique or their state of health), should be fed into a *system of comparisons*, a competitive examination which by definition not everybody can pass. Without the competitive style of comparison, without an excellence to be 'achieved', there would be no failures, and therefore no stigma. Goffman's work in this intimate area thus provides us with a casebook and an etiquette book for existing social practice. But think of the questions that could have been posed, and were not. Do we have to have 'beauty', or even 'presentableness' in facial and other physical characteristics? Could we construct another type of society in which the romantic projections and exaggerations that cluster around physique (in a person of the opposite sex or of the same sex) become at any rate much more muted? Why should the disclosure of an infirmity be any more traumatic, or present any greater problem of tact, than the revealing of any personal matter to another of whose sympathy one is not yet sure: in other words, is not the special pain of a 'discreditableness' hidden within a private space – with its attendant fear of disgrace if the linings of privacy are breached – somewhat reducible, in other possible forms of society, to the general dialectic between privacy and communion, attachment and solitude? We all have to have cupboards but do we have to keep skeletons in them? The 'stigmata' documented by Goffman are the wounds of inner and outer crucifixion inflicted on the vanquished Christs of the sex race, the race race, the money race and the class race by the centurions of a neurotically competitive and mercenary society.

Goffman is of course entitled to despair of the possibility that society's standards might be changed. But the trouble with despair is that it insists on spreading. The hopeless person is not content to drown alone, but must pull others in too: their hope is a threat to his or her bleakness, their vital movement a denial of the frozen fixed state which he or she has elected. In particular, intellectuals without hope are necessarily driven to generalise their own condition by means of a theory which attacks the theories of the hopeful. (And among those of us who personally are hopeful, it must be that we live in a parallel necessity to search and destroy the theories of no-hope.) In the last chapter of *Stigma*, Goffman turns his face towards the phenomenon of political radicalism – the only occasion in his writings when he has acknowledged the existence of the organised left – and adjudges it to be one of the more marginal examples of something he calls 'social deviancy'.[14] The social deviants, who comprise a lengthy gamut of disaffiliated subcultures from hobos to homosexuals, beach dwellers to the urban poor, 'are considered to be engaged in some collective denial of the social order' because of their disrespectful and impious life-style. Group-based political radicals can be considered as 'peripheral instances' of this 'core of social deviancy', along with the travelling rich, the metropolitan unmarried and drifting, the permanent expatriates and so on. And that is all that Goffman has to say about the political left: it is no more than a margin to a margin at the border of his schema of deviancies. The ideology of political radicals – the fact that they in general hold *beliefs* about the structure of society, whether couched in marxist or in populist terms, which start at least on an intellectual par with Goffman's own ideas – is beneath consideration or even condescension. The Vietnam anti-war movement, the socialist traditions of labour radicalism, the organisations for civil rights and black freedom, the theoretical work of critical scholars indebted to Wright Mills or to Karl Marx, the analytic content of thousands of articles in left-wing political journals were all available when Goffman was writing. All can be safely sealed off. They do not have to be looked at, or read. It is enough to 'place' them, permitting the speculation that even these rebellious deviants might have some stabilising social function, though to be sure we cannot quite know this: 'In theory, a deviant community could come to perform for society at large something of the same functions performed by an in-group deviant for his group, but while this is thinkable, no one yet seems to have demonstrated the case.'[15] Goffman here flirts with the well-known conservative position that social conflict is all right after all because it is 'functional', but will not commit himself thus far. More usually for Goffman, political 'deviancy', i.e. opposition and struggle, seems to constitute one more of the precious little spaces within which one finds room to stretch the muscles of personal selfhood, while leaving the dominant institutions of the society unchallenged. The concluding paragraphs of his older essay, 'The Underlife of a Public Institution',[16] rehearse this political subservience very lucidly. There the individual is defined,

> for sociological purposes as a stance-taking entity, a something that takes up a position somewhere between identification with an organisation and opposition to it, and is ready at the slightest pressure to regain its balance by shifting its involvement in either direction. It is thus *against something* that the self can emerge.

The 'inner exile' practised by impotent liberals under totalitarian regimes and the puckish routines of 'secondary adjustment' lived out by the cautious inmates of jails and chronic wards are seen by Goffman as offering a model for the maintenance of selfhood in what, without apparent irony, he terms 'free society', i.e. the macro-structure of advanced capitalism. The existing dominant bourgeois and bureaucratic institutions are necessary, because 'without something to belong to, we have no stable self.' Yet something private and personal must be withheld from these powerful blocs of belongingness, lest we become engulfed and (doubtless) mortified. And so 'the little ways in which we resist the pull' become all-important in asserting individuality. Macro-conservatism may exist in more-or-less peaceful coexistence with a constant mini-anarchism: 'Our status is backed by the solid buildings of the world, while our sense of personal identity often resides in the cracks.'

Goffman's general politics are therefore quite clear. The ruling classes and their managerial hierarchies are to be left firmly in charge of 'the solid buildings of the world': such ruling-class dominion is indeed necessary, for it gives us, importantly, 'our status', and the radical alternative to the pursuit of status – namely, social liberation – is nowhere envisioned in Goffman. Only 'the cracks' are left for us to expand in, the licensed loopholes of idiosyncrasy, to whose sympathetic cataloguing, across innumerable crannies of private integrity (along with their negotiated exits and entrances), Goffman has dedicated an entire moral career of his own.

We must of course recall the historical climate of American academic ideology which prevailed over the period when Goffman wrote and published his masterworks. With the exception of C. Wright Mills's solitary voice – a literary witness of radicalism rather than a participant in a collective radical endeavour (whose very feasibility, outside the brave circles of a small intelligentsia, Mills refused to the last to entertain – the sociological and political science of the United States was the intellectual servitor of the dominant social order. A 'radical sociology', a 'critical sociology', even a determined and principled liberal sociology lay quite outside the frame of academic conceits during those years of the international High Cold War and the domestic capitulation before McCarthyism. Sociology's solid buildings were then inhabited, in the main, by the devotees of a 'functional' social theory which was dumb in any language of opposition or contradiction. As functionalism's lease upon the discipline neared its term of expiry, Goffman's work appeared, from within the cracks and joins of the solid masonry, issuing a voice that was indeed one of opposition, of small-scale resistance against engulfment, but which was no more capable than the functionalists of describing what might contradict the main structure, i.e. rise up as an alternative to it. Goffman seemed radical only by contrast with the conformist consensus which reigned in American sociology over the fifties. More charitably, his work may perhaps be taken as a herald or harbinger of the larger questionings which became common among social scientists as the Vietnam War and the black rebellion surfaced and then escalated. But the limitations of his small voice of protest should have been more obvious to those of us who enthused about the 'secondary adjustments' (i.e. surreptitious resistances) of the hospital inmates in *Asylums*, or about the 'role-distance' (i.e. the affirmation of personhood beyond mere status) displayed by the humane surgeon in *Encounters*.[17]

David Matza has offered a fascinating discussion of the relationship between the older traditions of American pathology and the 'Chicago school' of close, localised observations of low life that began with the classic slum studies of the 1920s, and found a recent continuation in the 'neo-Chicagoan' writers on deviance like Becker, Lemert and Goffman himself.[18] The functionalists had emphasised 'the functions – not dysfunctions – of deviant forms' and so had eliminated from the sociological canon any concept of social pathology in the analysis of such deviant enterprises as political racketeering or union corruption. Chicagoans and neo-Chicagoans also repudiated the distant moral critique of the deviant that is usually implicit in the category of 'pathology' and instead developed an empathising closeness towards their subject-matter which avoided the starry-eyed excesses of romanticism through marshalling the emotional resources of *pathos* and *irony*.[19] The older Chicagoan insistence on the pathetic features of the outcast's life – its loneliness, sadness, anonymity and misery – can obviously be found in abundance within Goffman's descriptions of mentally or physically handicapped victims; and, as with the other more recent Chicagoans, Goffman makes great use of the ironic strain, with its display of the mockery of circumstance and its impulsion towards the uncovering of hidden meanings behind everyday appearances. Thus, mental hospitals are really run for the benefit of the staff rather than of the patients; the general public thinks it is being kind to the handicapped but it is constantly putting them in an impossible position by asking them to provide a 'phantom normalcy'; the many ways in which we try to be nice while disappointing or denying somebody are to be seen as examples of 'cooling-out' technique, on lines roughly similar to the careful farewells constructed by gangs of tricksters to stop their victims from rushing to the police in anger once the fraud has been discovered. The interesting feature about all of Goffman's ironic discoveries as well as about most of his exercises in pathos is that the discovery reveals nothing that could alter the situation.[20] The secret behind social appearances – which usually amounts to a description of yet one more technique of saving either our own or someone else's 'face' – is a permanent structural feature of human interaction. Life after all consists of presenting and preserving face, in one or another setting, and since absolutely everybody is engaged in it, there can be no suggestion that we would take sides.

The older vision of the pathological in social problem-areas may have been patronising, dismissive, Salvationist, snobbish or plain naive; but it *was* able to take sides, to name good and evil, to imply prescriptions for action. Irony and pathos are not, indeed, in all their possible variants, incompatible with an activist political approach to social problems – the use of both ironic and pathetic modes in Marx's *Capital* or Brecht's *Caucasian Chalk Circle* are instances sufficient to be named here. Matza's analysis of the Chicagoans' literary motifs has a special force in Goffman's case precisely because pathos and irony are here used as emotional counterweights to an explicitly static social theory. With Goffman, we can be so attuned to the haunting psychological resonances – of bitterness, of worldly sophistication, of shocked recognition that leap from his pages that we can go for a very long time indeed without realising his ideological message.

Indeed, Goffman's fixed universe of social possibilities has proved to be an extremely poor guide to subsequent developments in the institutional field to which he has devoted his closest scrutiny: the treatment of the mentally ill. There is nothing in the outline of 'the moral career of the mental patient' as depicted by him in his paper of 1957 which would have enabled us to predict what has actually happened to the vast majority of patients newly entering psychiatric treatment since that date: namely, their speedy discharge, with treatment continued outside the institution's walls. The 'mortification' of the patient's civilian self through 'degradation ceremonials' and other institutional pressures is apparently far less intense, and certainly far from irreversible, compared with the period when the custodial ideology of the mental institution was at its peak. The change in the pattern of mental hospital admissions in Britain is well-known – the overwhelming bulk of psychiatric admissions are nowadays voluntary and short-stay, remaining on the wards only for a few weeks before they are returned – often with excessive rapidity, according to many observers – to the outside world. For the USA too, the available evidence shows a similar trend (see Part Two, below). Doubtless we have not said farewell to Goffman's 'betrayal funnel' of hospitalisation, whereby relatives of prospective patients collude with psychiatrists and other doctors to discuss practical measures for the care of their difficult dear ones, out of the latter's hearing. In fact, it is most unlikely that the enregistration of mental patients, with all the painful stages in the transformation of their identity, proceeds in any manner which is fundamentally different from that described in *Asylums*. For example, patients still have embarrassing personal details recorded in their files and discussed openly in situations not of their choosing. They have to take their meals and their leisure hours with many other patients, according to a common timetable decreed by the hospital adminstration. They lose privacy, and with it the capacity to compartmentalise or seal off from public view any serious aspect of their personal lives. Those basic characteristics of psychiatric hospitals which inspire Goffman to view them as examples of the Total Institution – namely, their all-encompassing inquisitiveness over their inmates, and their standardised timetabling of living arrangements – are still essential features of their nature. Yet a Total Institution which exerts so brief a hold over its residents – which, indeed, is usually successful in re-socialising them for an outside environment rather than in engulfing them within itself – cannot be so totally total. We can only understand the short-stay mental wards of our own era – and the transient (or sometimes recurrent but still less than permanent) 'moral careers' of modern psychiatric inmates – by conceding that something is missing from Goffman's picture. What, in fact, for Goffman are final and ultimate paradigms of mental hospital existence – since they reflect ultimate paradigms of human existence in general – can be seen instead as problems in institutionalisation or in mental care which may either find their own solutions or else call for further solutions either of a local (and perhaps personal) or a central (and thus political) character.

Walter Gove, for example, has pointed out that, even apart from the therapy provided as part of the official medical programme, the removal of a patient from home into the hospital may initiate processes which, instead of harming the relationships between family and patient, actively restore warmth and trust to a household threatened with collapse.[21]

> Hospitalisation interrupted a situation which was experienced as untenable and, by doing so, it blocked actions which threatened irremediable damage to family life… During and following hospitalisation there was a transition period of construction where the family evolved a new 'working consensus'… In some cases the removal of the patient and the conflict situation promoted a revival of positive ties and feelings.

Possibly, as Gove suggests, the relative brevity of psychiatric hospitalisation nowadays may enable these 'restitutive' processes to supervene in a patient's family relationships before the more personally destructive factors in long-stay hospitalisation have time to make their maximum impact. At any rate, it should be clear that the image of the 'betrayal funnel' may be misleading if it is taken to imply that the traffic of cumulative jolts leading from home into hospital is necessarily one-way. There is a path also that goes back up the funnel, leading from the hell of betrayal to the return of trust.

The 'mortification' of the patient's civilian identity would also appear to be a function of several factors, some of them alterable by human decision. The stripping of a sick person's possessions and personal clothing, the lack of privacy and seclusion, the lack of information and power concerning the inmate's rights, the present sharp and exclusive boundary between the society of the hospital and the society that uses the hospital: such identity-destroying features of hospital life are, in principle at least, changeable through the adoption of different policies by administrators, governments or publics. It is not easy to envisage how these constructive changes in mass psychiatric treatment might come about, given the present structure of institutions and values in our society. A more personal, more humane, more individual therapy for the mentally ill would cost money: money for the replacement of huge, overcrowded and isolated buildings by numerous smaller centres sited near the patients' home communities; money for the hiring and training of staff, especially an intelligent and responsible non-medical staff, since many of the abuses denounced by Goffman and other writers in this field spring quite simply from the necessities of an assembly-line handling of patients placed in the care of tiny numbers of staff who are on the whole discouraged from trespassing into the doctor's role by getting involved in detailed casework. One author has carefully contrasted the successive stages of a person's entry into the culture of, for instance, a mental hospital and a good hotel.[22] The provision of information and the answering of questions are seen as the key factors preventing 'mortification' in the hotel situation; but I remain unconvinced that sheer politeness, without massive mental health investment, will alter very much. A further reduction of the damage inflicted on patients by mental hospital would evidently require a radical re-structuring of the very category of 'hospital' itself. Such a step would entail gigantic social expenditures.

It is conceivable, that is, that a future society may maintain no specialised hospitals of any kind for the housing and treatment of the mentally disturbed. After all, more primitive societies than ours manage their mentally ill without the benefit of total institutions, usually by keeping patients within the community, though sometimes by expelling them altogether as outcasts and beggars. More acceptably for our own psychiatric ethic, it might be possible to maintain the residential mental hospital as a service institution of last resort, occupied only for a limited period by those patients who could not be tolerated as lodgers in family homes or communal households. The provision of informal small-scale living facilities for psychiatric patients is going to be much more expensive than the building and maintenance of a medical barracks whose services are costed down to a barely minimal outlay. And if the present thousands of inmates in mental institutions are to be taken from their overcrowded wards and redistributed around the community in small, friendly groups, the staffing of these psychiatric communes, even with part-time helpers, will obviously require a very considerable increase in public funding, as the ratio of staff to patients will obviously be going up.

Goffman's general assumption in *Asylums* is that there is no alternative to the way in which we treat mental patients in the public wards. This comes out quite openly in one or two passages:

> Once we have discovered the 'good functional reasons' for the deprivations and horrors of the total institution, I feel we will give less praise and blame to particular superintendents, commandants, wardens and abbots, and tend more to understand the social problems and issues in total institutions by appealing to the underlying structural design common to them all.[23]

A 'functional explanation' is here presented as a means of avoiding the questions of *policy towards inmates*, and of the moral responsibility both of society and of its official agents who administer the closed institution. An absolute limit is set by Goffman to any possible change in psychiatric policy: a limit which coincides with what has already been reached in our particular epoch of fear and exclusion directed against the mental patient. Thus:

> Nor... do I mean to claim that I can suggest some better way of handling persons called mental patients... mental hospitals are found because there is a market for them. If all the mental hospitals in a given region were emptied and closed down today, tomorrow relatives, police and judges would raise a clamor for new ones; and these true clients of the mental hospital would demand an institution to satisfy their needs.[24]

A daunting perspective, surely. If you oppose the mental hospital, then you have to be ready to take on the judiciary and the police as well: Goffman may well be right in tracing the links of social control as far as this. But it is not necessary to draw conservative, static conclusions from the portrayal of a repressive reality. We can choose to include all that Goffman tells us within a more radical political theory. Why is the image of the Asylum, with its multi-windowed blocks and the tall chimney of its furnace, so dismally compelling? Not, as Goffman would have it, because it bespeaks an immutable social imperative, but because it symbolises an ancient, indefinitely renewed tradition of neglect whose liquidation, in the face of so many entrenched moral and material interests, will require a large and dedicated effort.

Erving Goffman, then, is not to be classed as a critical social theorist. His method consists in a precocious sensitivity toward those elements of social living which involves the face-to-face adjacency of persons. On all other aspects of the social process, that is to say, on any institution or happening that receives its meaning from outside this immediately shared space among individuals within shouting distance of one another, he is virtually silent. His constant tendency is therefore to dissolve society into its 'settings', practising – in common with his rivals in the 'ethnomethodology' school and with the natural historians of small-scale behaviour like Roger Barker,[25] a *methodological localism* which has some interesting affinities with the better-known doctrine of methodological individualism as expressed in many introductory treatments of sociology.[26] Methodological individualism recommends, roughly, that all statements about social collectives be understood to refer to the individuals who comprise these sets, and to nothing beyond these individual human beings. Thus, if we discuss 'the army', we are referring to nothing else than a determinate set of people in various ranks, officers and soldiers: and so 'the army' is only a convenient summing-up term for *a, b, c... n* individuals. This recommendation has the worthy objective of avoiding the possibility of any 'surplus meaning' attaching to collective concepts, so that we will avoid being hypnotised by such resounding collective abstractions as 'the Church on earth', 'the Reich', 'the Party' and so forth. But a simple objection to it is that we cannot even specify the individuals concerned except by reference to the collective category that gives them their identity: the concept of 'soldier' has no meaning whatever without the concept of an army. The project of methodological individualism is therefore doomed to permanent failure if it is intended to express more than the platitude that only people make history. Methodological localism carries within it the failure of much smaller ambitions: far from explicating the grand social structures in terms of their component sub-units, it does not even attempt to raise its eyes from the merely local in order to incorporate any bigger view of things.

Yet, as I have argued in analysing Goffman's theory of the symptom, the pursuit of the local and the narrowly interpersonal will not provide us with enough grit even to digest the logic of the small-scale setting or encounter. The categories we bring to bear in perceiving and judging the actions of a present other are not themselves drawn, in the first place, from our exposure to face-to-face situations; thus, the concept of 'illness', or that of 'symptoms', while applied and specified within particular encounters between relative and relative, or doctor and patient, does not derive its principal meaning or force from such contemporary goings-on, but from an entire history which includes the development of scientific rationality, the evolution of medical institutions, and the learning of complaints passed on by sufferer to listener over successive aeons. The interpersonal has, in short, a chronological or more exactly historical aspect which Goffman overlooks. Microsocial radicalism of the kind which influences much of Goffman's readership, if not Goffman himself, is often founded on this confusion between the interpersonal and the face-to-face, between the ensemble of human relations and the cult of 'relationships': a few immediate friends and/or lovers. 'Relationship begins at home' is the repeated refrain of these miniaturists of the feelings: and to these, as to Goffman, it is necessary to reply sternly: No, relationship ends at home, and not in any cynical sense. Home, or any other directly interpersonal setting, is the summing-up of myriad currents of thought, emotion and action which originate far beyond the videotape of the microsocial researcher or anecdotes of observed encounters. The face-to-face location is not 'Where The Action Is' (despite Goffman's insistence, in a chapter under this title,[27] that such is the case); rather its action keeps the score, registers the running total, of all the rest of human activity, including that taking place in other countries and other centuries. Limited to the visible setting, the microsocial portrait is bound to be a still picture, or an endlessly repeated short movie whose ends are joined by its manufacturer; and the static and the cyclical visions of relationship are familiar in political theory as the basic philosophic framework for all forms of conservatism.

In the introductory preface to one of his more important books, *Frame Analysis*, Goffman offers a disclaimer which is intended perhaps to be a general reply to the critics of his earlier works:

> I make no claim whatsoever to be talking about the core matters of sociology – social organization and social structure… I am not addressing the structure of social life but the structure of experience individuals have at any moment of their social lives. I personally hold society to be first in every way and any individual's current involvements to be second; this report deals only with matters that are second.
>
> And Goffman hopes to anticipate the charge that 'to focus on the nature of personal experiencing… is itself a standpoint with marked political implications… conservative ones', by admitting disarmingly that:
>
> The analysis developed does not catch at the difference between the advantaged and disadvantaged classes and can be said to direct attention away from such matters. I think that is true. I can only suggest that he who would combat false consciousness and awaken people to their true interests has much to do, because the sleep is very deep. And I do not intend here to provide a lullaby but merely to sneak in and watch the way the people snore.[28]

The entire argument of my own discussion of Goffman may have suggested by now that it is illegitimate to offer a microsociological discussion of 'experience' which takes the macrostructure of social organisation for granted; and that in attempting so sharp a separation between the personal and the political, Goffman has joined the slumberers, and is thus in no position at all to watch other people snoring.

3. R.D. Laing: The Radical Trip

The anti-psychiatry movement required a whole train of concurrent, convergent influences before it could gather force. Some of these factors lay in the changing age structure of Western societies, as the prolongation and intensification of active life span, extending back into the teen-years as well as onward into maturity, encouraged unprecedented strains at the boundaries of dependency, both in youth and old age. The expansion of welfare facilities as part of the price of working-class consensus in all the capitalist democracies had encouraged a flow of expectations, mingled with rising disappointments, in matters affecting the public health – and, within this complex of recently assembled social rights, the standing of psychiatric provision was due for some serious challenge and scrutiny. Mental illness became an urgent source of welfare politics, but at the same time touched on deeper, more intimate political structures: the relations of authority between doctor and patient, between administration and clientele, between parent and child, between woman and man became open to fresh and simultaneous collisions in the post-war boom years, even as the authority relations between employer and worker became continually and centrally challenged in the politics of the factory. The sixties, in most countries of the West, constituted the high-water mark in the assertiveness of the various discontented classes.

But before the swing into counter-revolution which we have experienced since, consciousness was raised, and confidence was still relatively intact. The confidence arose from the strong trading position of a labour force and an electorate able to extract substantial benefits either from employers or from politicians. Consciousness changed partly through diffuse spontaneous changes in ideas refracted from altered circumstance, and partly through the propagation of militant alternatives to the status quo. Militancy in argument, in mood, in manners was the work of groups and leaders who offered, in various models and images, the outline of a logic that could vanquish the hallowed syllogisms of everyday banality. The movement for a critical psychiatry had (and still has) its leaders, its world-historic individuals who gathered the questionings and forged them into questions, who became prophets and sages. And amid the succession of psychiatric prophets who compelled attention through the sixties and early seventies it was R.D. Laing who dominated the scene longest, as arch-seer and prophet-in-chief. 'After Freud and Jung, Now Comes R.D. Laing. Pop-shrink, rebel, yogi, philosopher-king? Latest reincarnation of Aesculapius, maybe?' trilled the headline over *Esquire's* interview with him in January 1972. On his college lecture tour of America later that year, one university billed him as 'The Controversial Philosopher of Madness', and at another his arrival was greeted with bumper-stickers proclaiming 'I'm Mad About R.D. Laing'. 'Two chicks who dig Coltrane, The Dead and R.D. Laing' advertised for compatible guests to meet them at a party, in a back-page column of the New York *Village Voice* in the previous year: and Laing's assumed connection with the lifestyle of popular music had been earlier instanced in the assertion by a book reviewer (*Library Journal*, 1 June 1969) that he 'is reputed to have treated the Beatles'.

More serious and sustained attention was accorded to Laing by an unusual range of publics and specialists. The paperback editions of his main writings have been reprinted in most years since their first appearance, and the invocation of his name and work by philosophers, creative writers, and co-workers in the field of abnormal psychology was unabated even during periods when the mass media were angling their spotlights towards other celebrities. The reputation and rumour which has surrounded Laing has both eased and impeded his accessibility to intellectual audiences. The hundreds of thousands of young readers who bought and absorbed the scraps of psychedelic autobiography in *The Politics of Experience* found, for the first time in their lives, an apparently medical authority who, unlike most doctors and scientists, was not afraid of philosophising, or of quoting or writing poetry, or of expressing powerful and deep emotions that could variously either excite or shock his listeners. Others, from a more established vantage-point, felt outraged: one group of pro-medical polemicists even queried his right to speak as an accredited member of his profession:

> How much more serious he would seem if he gave up his medical identity... If Laing wishes to be a guru or a philosopher, there is no doubt a place for him, but young people who are suffering from schizophrenia may prefer to entrust themselves to a doctor who will treat their illness as best as he can.[1]

The resistance to Laing's ideas was not simply a matter of professional pique; the very idiom in which he couched his early contributions, a blend of psychoanalytic and existentialist concepts interspersed with close reportage on the inner experience of deranged patients, presented obstacles for those not fully attuned to these rather particular sensibilities. Professor Roger Brown, an experimental social psychologist from the Harvard laboratory, has remarked of *The Divided Self that* 'In the course of several years I read it three times – that is, all the pages passed my eyes, but nothing happened that I would call "understanding"'. The fact that Brown's fourth reading was much more successful, leading him to his choice of Laing's work to round off an introductory undergraduate psychology textbook, and to the conclusion that 'there is a sense in which Laing better than anyone else enables us to "understand" schizophrenia',[2] is a tribute to the power of Laing's ideas to work their way past what were clearly the entrenched methodological defences of a sceptical scientist. This experience of illumination, whether into mental illness or into a more general human situation, was common among those who followed Laing's writings. Equally frequent, though, was a blockage of comprehension like Brown's earlier response, or an irritated rejection either of Laing's own positions or of the manner in which they were being construed and used by his following.

A survey of R.D. Laing's intellectual history has to labour under certain special handicaps which I have tried to overcome without the hope of securing complete success. In the first place, Laing has performed some of his work in collaboration with others. One phase of his most important activity was conducted side by side with two other existential psychiatrists, David Cooper and Aaron Esterson, whose views cannot be assumed to be identical with his or to have remained in tune with the later alignment of his work after he ceased collaboration with them.[3] Esterson has maintained the interest in family networks which he developed in the book he wrote with Laing[4] and has gone on to produce more detailed sample descriptions of some of the very same families that were the subject of this old joint work.[5] In different ways, Cooper and Esterson have appeared in Laing's biography as the bearers of theoretical concerns which blended for a while with his – radical existentialism in Cooper's case, neo-Freudian family therapy in Esterson's – until the paths of the three began to branch separately. Although both Cooper and Esterson have intensified their 'Laingianism', the one as critic and the other as researcher of family life, Laing himself has moved on independently from them. Our analysis in this and the next chapter will deal with Laing rather than with his co-workers, disciples or camp-followers.

The second difficulty arises from Laing's habit of offering all at once several lines of enquiry which, pushed to any sort of conclusion, would yield obvious inconsistencies. The texts of his works are like the old Egyptian palimpsests, manuscripts with the first draft rubbed away and, while still partly visible, written over by another scribe – in this case Laing himself in a different ideological phase. We shall quote variant glosses from the canon of Laing's works in order to illustrate the way in which he sharpens (or tones down) an ambiguous rendering, much as a poet will re-shape the meaning of a key line through altering one or two of its words. In one particularly expansive phase of his development, roughly from 1964 to 1970, his writings and public activity consorted with a number of vanguard trends in society and politics – marxism, the counter-culture, psychedelic experimentation, romantic-expressionist literature, the critique of the mental institution, the critique of the family, transcendental meditation, Sartrean existentialism, Freudian psychoanalysis – which are normally, for quite good reasons, taken to be to a certain extent divergent or even dissonant. Laing's utterances held these disparate trends in intellectual suspense, counterbalanced in a kind of equilibrium that was bound to collapse once he advanced one particular element or argument to preclude certain others. During his lengthy balancing act he was continually misunderstood by those who saw him as more committed to one item – to marxism, let us say, or to meditation – than he was. The outline of Laing's career that we shall give is in the form of an account of developmental stages, a progression in which one stance is negated and transcended by a successor position. But Laing has at certain points refused to concede that any such progression took place, denying, for instance, that he had ever been a marxist, or that his involvement in mystical practice has 'represented any major switch of direction or change of any fundamental position... It was simply that what I did with my own time has become a little more publicly noticed than it used to be.'[6]

We may see in Laing's assertion of continuity in his intellectual development more than a convenient forgetfulness for awkward and outgrown phases. His strength, as well as his weakness, has come precisely from the wide span of his identities and from his capacity to entertain opposites as a prelude to marrying them off to each other.

Ronald David Laing (accurately pronounced '*Layng*', with *a* as in 'angel') was born in October 1927 and raised as the sole child of a family living at the edge of the Gorbals on the south side of Glasgow, in poor, cramped housing.[7] The family, lower-middle-class and strictly Lowlands-Presbyterian in religious outlook, was characterised by the mixture of moral repressiveness and occasional violence between male relatives which is normal among working-class puritans. Laing records that he was never let out to play with other children until he was sent to school, and that a programme of continued mystification and misinformation about sexual matters was conducted by his parents and school authorities until, near the age of 16, he himself was able to find and read a book on venereal disease with an account of the basic 'facts of life'. The solitariness of young Laing's conditioning was fortunately broken by the presence of the great books of religion and rationalism: Darwin, Thomas Huxley, the Bible, Mill, Haeckel and Voltaire. At 14, he says, 'I knew I was really only interested in psychology, philosophy and theology'; he became the initiate of 'a sort of Neoplatonic Christianity'.

Even during adolescence the moral idealism of this Christian outlook competed oddly with a gratuitous egocentricity. In 1972 his acolyte, Peter Mezan, heard Laing admit, while 'sitting on the floor of Suite 608 (of New York's Algonquin Hotel) in a terry-cloth bathrobe', to having been 'very much motivated by the whole fame complex, especially in my teens'. Thus, he decided he would produce his first book by the time he was 30, and stuck to that with the date of publication of *The Divided Self*. He resolved early on that the kind of fame he craved was 'the fame of a wise man', and to this end 'I decided at the age of 13, for instance, that I would make a point of forgetting anything that was painful.'[8] We do not know what sort of intellectual dialogue touched him during his education, with a 'Classical' emphasis on ancient languages, at a state-supported boys' grammar school; but Laing was 18 before he met with astonishment, for the first time in his life, people of his own age 'who had never even opened a Bible'.

Domination by religious questions was shortly succeeded by an exposure to the anguished secular humanism of French post-war literature. In January 1948 he came across a translation, in the magazine *Horizon*, of extracts from Antonin Artaud's vigorous attack on psychiatry and psychiatrists, 'Van Gogh, le suicidé de la société'. This early anti-psychiatric polemic, the product of Artaud's resentment as a confined lunatic in an appalling French asylum and of his strong identification with Van Gogh as a fellow-artist and fellow-victim, came to Laing as 'a revelation' which played a decisive part in his development.[9] Sartre is another noteworthy influence in the same period: it was through *Being and Nothingness* that Laing was introduced to Husserl, Hegel and the European phenomenological tradition that would inform his own psychiatric enquiries.[10]

However, this preliminary involvement in the humanities had to compete with the lengthy rigours of a medical training organised around the empirical natural sciences. The contradiction sensed by Laing between a humane theory based on 'the whole person' as subject and a scientific practice dealing in inert part-objects is a common theme in his work, and partly explains his repeated insistence on the necessary autonomy of a separate 'science of persons' distinct from the medical sciences. His writings are scattered with grisly stories of the pathology he encountered in patients and – more usually – in doctors during his years as a medical student, and he has come to believe that 'at its very best, medical training was bedeviled, and still is, by its own insane theory and insane practice'. The textbook descriptions of schizophrenia struck Laing, when he first read them in these days, as 'a very good description of much of medicine itself, including psychiatry. The heartlessness, the divorce, the split between head and heart. The fragmentation, indeed disintegration behind all that, and its disavowal and projection.'[11]

In 1951 Laing took his medical degree, and chose to specialise in psychiatry, like nearly all of his student friends, as a refuge from 'the medico-surgical lunacy all around'. After six months on duty as a junior doctor in a neurosurgical unit, he was conscripted, working immediately as a practising psychiatrist in the British Army's Central Hospital. It was here that he began to develop his renowned capacity to enter into prolonged and meaningful relation with individuals regarded as hopelessly 'mad' by the rest of the world – one of his first such encounters being with a young patient of 18 with delusions of being Julius Caesar and Hamlet, kept in the padded cells of the military hospital where Laing used to go and talk at length with him, sharing his fantasies of robbing the gold from the vaults of the Bank of England.[12]

From this posting, he returned to civilian life as a psychiatrist in the National Health Service, working in the 'female refractory ward' of Glasgow's Royal Mental Hospital. Here he made special efforts to get to know the most neglected and apparently hopeless patients, resuming the padded cell visits in which he could sit and listen to what others had dismissed as ravings, and eventually enticing both patients and staff into the construction of an experimental day-room in which a dozen of the most withdrawn 'chronic schizophrenic' women on the ward could go for occupation and recreation. Laing's approach was still to a large extent formed within a conventional natural-scientific framework: he accepted the current view of his milieu that schizophrenia was the name of a disorder in individuals, possibly genetic or biochemical in origin and manifested as the result of some innate intolerance towards stress. He selected the patients for this study through drawing up detailed 'sociograms' of the ward's relationships, counting the number of times each inmate addressed or paid attention to another. Even a short exposure to the bright humane regimen of the day-room produced encouraging results. The women opened up socially, losing at a stroke the 'withdrawnness' that had been inscribed indelibly in their case-notes for year upon year. Laing, together with members of a research team working in the same ward with a rather more formal psychoanalytic perspective than his, hastened to have the immediate results published in a medical journal.[13] However, it turned out that the progress of the patients was fairly short in duration. All 12 were discharged from the hospital within 18 months; but within another year they were all back inside again.[14]

Such an outcome would nowadays be considered unsurprising by many psychiatrists, since most of the discharged patients would be returned to a family environment in which the other members were much too involved with the patient for anybody's good. The period of innovation in British social psychiatry that had generated the work of Laing and his colleagues in Glasgow was at this very time on its way into a series of researches that would demonstrate, in terms independent from Laing's own orientation, the pathogenic character of the family nexus into which many schizophrenic ex-patients were being discharged.[15] However, at this stage, Laing did not respond with a direct challenge to the reigning orthodoxies on 'the schizophrenia question'. Instead, he worked over some case-material from his Glasgow experience, adding recollection to theoretical reading in a draft that would become the basis for two books, *The Divided Self* and *The Self and Others*. In 1957 he moved to a post at the Tavistock Clinic in London. Here he would discover a particularly close affinity to the psychoanalytic ideas with which he had long been fascinated even when in the toils of physiological medicine. His training analysis was undertaken with a Freudian psychoanalyst attached to the Tavistock, Dr Charles Rycroft; and he was soon to be influenced by the analytically informed services of marriage and family counselling that are undertaken at the same centre. Soon after the move to London he completed his manuscript of *The Divided Self*, offering its preliminary text to several Tavistock colleagues for their comments. It was published in 1960 by Tavistock Publications. By the time it entered a paperback edition, five years later, the New Left had arrived on the British scene, and Laing had progressed into political radicalism and the status of celebrity. In the moment of its first appearance, however, the impact of *The Divided Self* was far from sensational.

Looking at the work now, we can see how hard it was for many of its readers to take bearings on the many intellectual origins that had helped to compose it. Laing's use of existentialist material was most unusual for a writer born and nurtured within the Britain of that time.

It is striking that he was able to extract fertile insights into psychotic and allied states of mind not only from clinicians of the European phenomenological school (Binswanger, Minkowski, Boss), but from theologians (Tillich, Bultmann), philosophers (Sartre, Heidegger, even Hegel) and writers (Beckett, Lionel Trilling) who dealt in non-pathological, indeed fundamental, situations of human existence. These concepts, in partial conjunction with those of Freudian psychoanalysis, were applied to the knotted thought processes and behaviour of an obscure group of severely disturbed mental patients, who had been hitherto regarded as inaccessible to rational comprehension. One of the most difficult of philosophies was brought to bear on one of the most baffling of mental conditions, in a manner which, somewhat surprisingly, helped to clarify both. Existential philosophy, with its reputation of introverted cloudiness and speculative indiscipline, was here set working in a concrete, practical and socially urgent context – the understanding of the mentally ill. Conversely, a major form of psychosis was elucidated as a mental system possessing lawful shape and sequence, comprehensible in existential terms as the outcome of rational strategies adopted by the patient in the face of an ambiguous and threatening personal environment. The clinical descriptions in *The Divided Self* are set in a vivid, clear style, often with an unobtrusive poetic skill, as with the portrayal of the patient Peter's imaginary smell ('the sooty, gritty, musty smell of a railway waiting-room') or the images of desolation (like 'the ghost of the weed garden' or 'the black sun') which haunt the remnants of personality inside the young hebephrenic Julie.

As we begin *The Divided Self*, Laing informs us that he personally as a psychiatrist finds great difficulty in detecting the 'signs and symptoms' of illness in psychotic patients, since their behaviour actually appears to him as meaningful and appropriate rather than as odd or irrelevant. He then provides us with a stunning demonstration of what it means to understand patients as human beings rather than to classify them as instances of a disease. He gives a long quotation from the nineteenth-century psychiatrist, Emil Kraepelin, who reported a spate of excited talk produced, in front of an audience of students, by a young catatonic patient in response to the doctor's questions. Laing is able to show very convincingly that, through the adoption of only a slightly more sophisticated vantage-point on the patient's behaviour (i.e by assuming that he is capable of discreetly ridiculing his interrogator), almost all of the young man's utterances, which have struck Kraepelin as the inconsequential ramblings of an organic disease process, can be seen as comprehensible responses to the immediate situation he is in.

What is particularly noteworthy about Laing's use of this example is the fact that Kraepelin's interpretation (or rather, non-interpretation) of his patient's behaviour has been on record for decades in several countries as a classical case-note of psychiatry without anybody, apart from Laing in 1960, trying to re-value it.

The final chapter of *The Divided Self*, a 30-page discussion of a single schizophrenic patient named Julie, introduces what will be a characteristic theme of Laing's theorising: an extended analysis of the patient's family background. Julie's relatives have developed a sequence of definitions about her which runs, throughout her lifetime, roughly as follows: as an infant, Julie was a 'good' girl; later, particularly in adolescence, she became a 'bad' girl, negative and rejecting towards her parents; finally, in her present condition, her behaviour has overstepped even the bounds of 'badness' and she is 'mad', mentally ill, a patient. This sequence forms, in a number of ways, a prototype of the analysis of schizophrenia that will be developed by Laing in future works, where the Good–Bad–Mad progression will be seen as the usual pattern for the 'election' of an individual into the role of madness by other members of his or her insidiously demanding family.

However, this first book of Laing's can be distinguished from his later work on at least three counts. There is not a hint of mysticism in it, not the faintest implication that there is any further world of being beyond that described by natural and social science (phenomenology being included in the latter). There are no intimations of an innermost substance or grounding of all things and appearances, lying perhaps in some core of inner personal reality beyond the probings of the clinician. Laing has in fact been at deliberate pains, in his borrowings from the more opaque existentialist writers, to de-mystify their categories. The floating, abstract concepts of Being and Not-Being, the whiff of dread before death and the hints of the supernatural, characteristic of Kierkegaard and Heidegger, are replaced by transparent, empirical usages. 'Ontological insecurity', which is said to lie at the heart of serious mental illness, simply means a profound personal uncertainty about the boundaries between the self and the world, which can be contrasted with the differentiation of ego-boundaries that takes place in normal child development. 'Being-in-the-world' means social interaction between persons, and Kierkegaard's 'Sickness Unto Death' is not the loneliness of the soul before God but the despair of the psychotic. Laing is, in short, naturalising the mystical elements of continental existentialist thought.

The second cardinal feature of *The Divided Self* follows from this. Since there is no super-reality beyond the here and now of actual people, psychotic patients are not seen as the mystics or prophets of this supersensory world. They are not, as in the later Laing, pioneers in the exciting endeavour of exploring 'inner space'. The only inner space that is ever even hinted at in the text amounts simply to the set of private coordinates which map out the fantasies of the psychotic. Material and interpersonal reality is the only one we have got: consequently it forms the only standard against which the schizophrenic's experience can be tested. By this criterion, the schizophrenic has failed, has fallen short of normal, healthy sensory and emotional achievement: we are left in no doubt, in fact, that she or he is in a thoroughly bad way. Laing's reluctance to use the term 'disease' (because of the implication that a 'disease' may have discrete and impersonal 'symptoms') does not imply any refusal to admit the disturbance, disorder and profound alienation of the psychotic state.

Thirdly, this disturbed state is an attribute, at least in large part, of the individual as the patient. The condition called 'schizophrenia' by doctors is, in Laing's terms, still very much like a syndrome, i.e. a set of characteristics attributable to an individual, cohering typically and meaningfully with one another and demarcating this person from other conditions which are given different names (such as 'hysteria' or 'normal development'). These defining, co-existing characteristics are not impersonal or subpersonal attributes of individuals, isolated bits of behaviour like a high temperature or a twitching leg. They are, on the contrary, deeply personal in quality, occurring at the highest level of integration of the individuals' behaviour, and related to their whole fundamental orientation towards the world they perceive and move in. All the same, 'schizophrenia' is still a pattern of responses manifested by individual persons: it has not vanished, as it does in the Laing of five years hence, into the criss-cross of distorted and distorting signals that typifies Laing's description of the patient's family in which no individual is 'ill' or 'schizophrenic' at all. Even the patient Julie of the last chapter of *The Divided Self* (with all its detail of the family cross-press at work upon the patient) is presented unmistakably as a disoriented individual operating with a complex repertoire of psychotic mental gambits. Her 'existence', and the modes in which she construes it, form the basic material of the narrative. By contrast, the schizophrenic women of *Sanity, Madness and the Family* (1964) have no existence separable from that of their relatives: it is not they, but their families as a whole (though it is not always clear whether the women themselves are included) who bear the basic attributes of the syndrome.

Laing has himself recognised this important shift in his thinking, and has even apologised for his earlier concentration on the individual patient. In the preface to the 1965 Pelican edition of *The Divided Self*, he wrote that while the book did entail an understanding of the social context of the patient, 'especially the power situation within the family, today I feel that, *even in focusing upon and attempting to delineate a certain type of schizoid existence*, I was already partially falling into the trap I was seeking to avoid' (italics added). If 'schizophrenia' is not a name which refers to any kind of a personal condition, then any attempt to describe it, even in very sensitive terms, must be a 'trap'. However, Laing has not gone on to explain how far he still regards as valid the mode of analysis practised in *The Divided Self*; it is doubtful how much of the early Laing could be reconciled with the radical scrutiny of the later books.

Laing leapt ahead of the theoretical framework of his first work very soon after it was published. In 1960 Jean-Paul Sartre issued the 750-page Volume One of *Critique de la Raison Dialectique*. The *Critique* marked a sharp turn in Sartre's philosophy in that it purported to offer a new foundation for a general science of man, an 'anthropology' in the broadest sense which was intended to expose the basic nature of all thinking about society (including both sociological and historical thought), to outline the structural prerequisites for the formation of all social groups, and to state the laws governing the succession of one form of social organisation by another. At this time, from 1958 to 1962, Laing was settling into a research programme at the Tavistock Institute dealing with interaction inside families (both with and without a schizophrenic member). His research now tended to emphasise the interdependence between a subject's outlook on other people and their perception of her or him, especially within a closed social group: the main ideas of the *Critique*, with their emphasis on the formation and bonding of groups, lent themselves to assimilation by this theoretical perspective. Laing's next book *The Self and Others* (1961, revised as *Self and Others*, 1969) was a collection of essays partly reaching into his new preoccupation with family communication patterns, partly developing his earlier analysis of the world-view of the psychotic patient. It owes no debt to Sartre's *Critique*, but in the following year Laing published an article ('Series and Nexus in the Family')[16] which, for its analysis of family interaction, drew on Sartre's newest ideas as well as on the early findings of the Tavistock project.

Laing's work was now becoming closely associated with that of Cooper and Esterson. Cooper had come to London following his medical training in Capetown and was working as a doctor in British public mental hospitals, in one of which he was to supervise a research programme of treatment based on Laing's theory of schizophrenia.

In the early sixties he cooperated with Laing on a more literary enterprise, the production of a short book summarising for English readers the gist of Sartre's recent philosophical writing. The fruits of this intense labour of exegesis appeared in 1964 as *Reason and Violence: A Decade of Sartre's Philosophy*. It is a straightforward condensation of Sartre's *Critique* to one-tenth of its original length, so compressed as to be virtually incomprehensible to anyone seeking an introduction to Sartre's thought, and resembling a précis for private study rather than a popularisation for any intellectual audience. (Cooper's chapter in the book on Sartre's *Saint Genet* forms a clear contrast to the rest of the text in its liveliness and clarity.) At any rate, the intellectual collaboration of Laing and Cooper was well under way by the early sixties, and was soon to result in more creative forms of common writing and therapeutic practice.

Esterson has been a shadowier figure, less associated with public occasions (such as the 'Dialectics of Liberation' conference) than the other two. He had graduated in the same year as Laing from the Glasgow medical school, and then became a British general practitioner, a doctor on an Israeli kibbutz and a hospital psychiatrist back in Britain. In 1958 there was published the report of a research collaboration between Laing and Esterson on the effects of 'collusive pairing' among members of a psychotherapeutic group.[17] Through the author's existentially interpretative glosses, the group comes through as an uneasy, abrasive gathering of seven small-time con-men, but the report does offer a foretaste of the later Laing-Esterson work on human ploy and counterploy in small social settings. Esterson joined Laing as a research associate in the Tavistock family project, publishing its main report with him in 1964.

On Laing's thinking in the Tavistock Clinic programme, influences now converged from two widely separated quarters: Paris and Palo Alto, California. Terror and engulfment had defined the schizophrenic's personal desolation in *The Divided Self*; engulfment and terror, exercised overtly or insidiously by the familiars of the mental victim, were now specified as crucial agents of human derangement both in Sartre's essays in psychoanalysis and in the contributions of the Palo Alto school of schizophrenia research headed by Gregory Bateson. (Research groups in the United States led by Theodore Lidz and Lyman Wynne had come to a similar viewpoint on the origins of schizophrenia, but Bateson's approach must be credited with some priority in time as well as a more general influence.)[18] Sartre had produced case studies illustrating his new sensitivity to pathological social pressures for some years before the *Critique*: both the Genet of *Saint Genet* and the main character of the play *Altona*, the war criminal Franz Von Gerlach, are shown as experimenting with mental strategies of self-definition in response to the ignominious labelling which society has affixed on them. Suffocating in a web of competitive, exploiting relationships, Genet and Franz both express and evade their human responsibilities by performing intense mental work (involving a criminal and homosexual career in the former case and a sort of voluntary psychosis in the latter) on the demeaning and degrading social categories ('thief' or 'murderer') which they know to constitute the terms of their appearance in the eyes of others. The omnipotent unconditioned ego of the old Sartre is now an 'alter ego': Self and Others (to crib from Laing's terminology) now mutually and ferociously impinge on the most critical areas of personal choice. The parallelism between the vision of human bestiality given in Franz's death speech at the end of *Altona* and the history of the normal social bond outlined in the *Critique* has often been pointed out: in both, humanity is a cruel, malignant species lying in wait to thwart and destroy humanity itself. And the *Critique's* version of human evolution is basically a detailing of this social cannibalism, which is an ineluctable historical imperative in a world of scarcity, accompanying all social transitions and transformations so long as individuals are replaceable by one another in the struggle for scarce resources.

Laing's *New Left Review* article of 1962, 'Series and Nexus in the Family' makes use of two of Sartre's basic group categories, applying them in the context of family behaviour. The *Critique* visualises an initial, minimal stage of group formation in which the members share a common goal but do not depend on each other for its practical achievement. They may, however, fabricate a crude sort of group identity through their awareness of one another's behaviour, or by being able to name a single target as the subject of their separate hostilities. A bus queue, a bunch of anti-Semites and the world's system of stock exchanges are examples of this type of group, which Sartre terms a *series*. A deeper and more solid form of social unity is attained in the *bonded group*, whose members each take a decision or 'pledge' before the others to join together in linked activity for the achievement of the common group goal: revolutionary cells, football teams and lynch mobs are examples of bonded groups. The basis for this fusion is always *terror*, registered within each individual as the fear of what the other group members will do to the member who secedes or betrays.

Laing describes two family patterns which correspond to Sartre's identification of human groups. There is one domestic situation which is essentially a 'series'; the members of such a family lack any personal concern for one another though they may make a great display of concern for the likely effects of scandal, thereby showing that the basis for their group's existence lies in an anticipation of 'what the neighbours will say' rather than in any shared relationships within the home. Laing also describes a family constellation, termed a 'nexus,' which like Sartre's bonded group is held together by fear, anxiety, enforced guilt, moral blackmail and other variants of terror. The nexal family is like a criminal society where mutual protection is only the obverse of mutual intimidation. Another Sartrean distinction which Laing now emphasised in his analysis of families is the difference between 'praxis' and 'process' in the explanation of human action. *Process* refers to events that appear to have originated from no particular person or persons: they just happen or proceed, with no identifiable human decision or wish at the back of them.[19] (Most people perhaps regard every-day politics in this light, as something that just happens to happen, like the weather.) In contrast, *praxis* is action that can be traced to definite decisions undertaken out of definite motives by definite people; social analysis should undertake to show praxis at work where apparently only process exists. That is, social events can be rendered *intelligible* (a term of some importance in the later Sartre and Laing) by showing that they are the outcome of decisions taken in a social field by motivated actors; and Laing is issuing notice of his purpose to seek intelligibility and praxis in quite gross and grotesque forms of human pathology.

Laing had already written, in *The Divided Self*, about the necessity for understanding in the interpretation and treatment of psychotic behaviour. Even before his baptism in Sartre's *Critique*, he was emphasising the potential intelligibility of much that was apparently crazy. But the type of understanding that Laing sought after 1960 was distinct in its concern for the anchoring of explanation in the social setting of the patient. The psychotic 'symptoms' of the schizophrenics in *The Divided Self* can be rendered intelligible (in a broad, non-Sartrean sense) by viewing them as expressions of a fragmented or split Self. They do not have to be converted into forms of 'praxis,' i.e. of human communication within a set of people, in order to be understood. In his first book, Laing translates psychotic behaviour into the terms of action, which may include inner or mental action; subsequently he insists on a translation into the terms of *re*action, or of action in the flux of others' actions on the subject.

But the neo-Sartrean framework was only a general specification of the type of understanding which Laing had already begun to accept and seek in the clinical field. The American research groups who were working on the family backgrounds of their schizophrenic patients were also situating the 'process' of psychotic illness within the 'praxis' of communication from parents to their children (even though they did not use the terminology of Sartre in describing their work). In his second book *The Self and Others* Laing drew heavily on the work of these researchers; their concepts become interwoven with those of Sartre in later writings by Laing and his collaborators. Here we will provide only a short composite account of the hypotheses and findings of the American teams.

The pathology of family communication has become one of the great research enterprises of American science. Hundreds of families have trooped into the laboratories of academic institutes and hospitals, there to have their entire verbal output tape-recorded over many sessions, their gestures and eye movements filmed and their biographies unearthed in depth by interdisciplinary panels of doctors, psychologists, sociologists and technicians. The families inhabit this select theatre for a period of hours or more, enacting a kind of real-life TV serial based on their usual domestic interchange, and then depart. They leave behind them a mass of sound-tracks, videotapes, behaviour, checklists, completed test-sheets and other revelatory material, a huge deposit of past praxis which is then worked over for months by the bureau of investigators, and in due course delivered to the interested public as a journal article. The cumulative bibliography of the Schizophrenic Family forms a veritable saga of modern home-life, running in repeated instalments through some half-dozen scholarly channels over about 25 past years, and with no end yet in sight. The origin of the series is usually traced to Bateson's 1956 paper[20] outlining what has become known as the 'double bind' theory of the origins of schizophrenia. The expression 'double bind' refers to a specific pattern of disturbed communications, detectable within pathological families, in which one member is subjected to a pair of conflicting injunctions or 'binds', both of them highly unsettling or traumatic; a third injunction, implicit in the situation, may prevent the threatened party from leaving the field and so avoiding the conflict. The unfortunate recipient of these messages is lost whatever s/he does, and if the ordeal is repeated tends to opt out of social interaction and to lose confidence in the accuracy of her/his perceptions of other people.

The 'double bind' mechanism, is, however, only one of many modes of violence and fraud which have been seen to operate in disturbed families. A double-bind household constitutes, in the very cast-list of its *dramatis personae*, a group whose principal characters, both separately and together, would bode ill for domestic peace, even independently of the discovery of any specific types of intimidation in their language and behaviour. Mr Doublebind is reported to be a shifty, spineless, passive father, impoverished and rigid in his mental processes and bewildered by tasks involving quite elementary social graces. In the enactment of the family drama, he is constantly upstaged by his spouse, a domineering dragon of a woman who sets unrealisable demands on the life-style of her children and is then insecurely reproachful to them when they fail to live up to her immature stereotypes. The suffocating, spiky embrace of Mrs Doublebind, her tiresome niggling obsession with conventional manners, her intellectual and emotional dishonesty and her incessant moral blackmail are all repeatedly documented in the literature. The Doublebind children are a dependent, weedy brood, mentally unstimulating and mutually disloyal. If they are ever more than bit players in the tribal charade, it is through their role in ganging up, in coalition with their unspeakable parents, against the unlucky fall-guy or -girl of the house: Charles (or Clarissa) Doublebind. It comes as no surprise to note that Charles/Clarissa, a naive and dithering but basically rather sweet personality, has been driven into a spiralling psychosis through this unholy conspiracy of pressures from his/her nearest and purportedly dearest. The Doublebind menage is a blood-besmirched arena for internecine assaults and insults, a telephone network of crossed lines, scrambled messages and hung-up receivers. The research agents who have eavesdropped on Doublebind conversations and painstakingly decoded their obscure content have let us know just what has been going on in this grim parlour. The Doublebind family is duly incriminated as a *pathogenic communications system* or *nexus of mystification*. They are convicted in the fact of their disagreement one with another, for such discordances of outlook are to be taken as attempts to *disconfirm*, *disqualify* and *invalidate* the autonomous personal experience of the other, especially of the victim Charles/Clarissa. Let them not, on the other hand, try to escape the charge by agreeing with one another: the common assent of the Doublebinds is a *collusion*, and any mannerisms of warmth or co-operativeness should be seen as expressions of *pseudo-mutuality*, a false front of domestic solidarity tricked up for the outside world by this collection of competitive, mutually suspicious individuals. Any counter-move by Charles/Clarissa against this onslaught of mystification is met with a successful counter-counter-move which places him/her in an *untenable position*. (No younger Doublebind has ever been found to be in possession of a tenable position: on this the witnesses are unanimous.)

The climax of this vicious campaign against an offspring is reached when the Doublebind family decides to 'elect' Charles/Clarissa as an insane mental patient, thereby expelling him/her from their totalitarian kingdom. The chorus of false attribution and impossible injunction, orchestrated by the monstrous Mrs Doublebind (who at this stage exercises the wily stratagems of a Goneril or Regan against the combined Lear-Cordelia figure of her child) rises to a crescendo of rejection; at this point orthodox psychiatry affixes the label of 'schizophrenic' upon the family scapegoat, in a degradation ceremonial of hospital admission which inaugurates a lifetime's career as a mental patient.

In the last sentence of this dramatised account of the theory, the incrimination of psychiatric medicine comes from Laing and his London colleagues; the American researchers have in the main refrained from any radical indictment of psychiatry's own collusions. For the American teams tend to regard 'schizophrenia' still as the name of a behavioural and cognitive disorder attributable to individual patients (though caused by their family circumstances); the notion of 'treating' such a disorder by appropriate medical or psychotherapeutic means is not usually queried in their analysis. Laing, on the other hand, is sceptical about the very existence of a schizophrenic malfunction from which the patient can be said to be suffering: 'schizophrenia' means, if anything, the communications disorder of the whole family, so that the language of 'diagnosis' and 'treatment' of sombody called 'a schizophrenic' would simply mask the web of familial connexions which is the real truth of the matter.

The framework outlined above, admittedly in the bold strokes of caricature, but not, I believe, with any essential infidelity to those authors' meaning, takes us from the Laing of *The Divided Self* to the stage his work had reached by 1963–64. *The Self and Others* (1961), *Sanity, Madness and the Family* (1964) and the *New Left Review* article of 1962 are the products of this stage, which still refrains from any celebration of a supersanity achieved by the psychotic in his voyage into inner space. (The first indications of what has been termed Laing's 'psychedelic model' of schizophrenia appear during 1964.) The book *Interpersonal Perception: A Theory and a Method of Research*, written by Laing with two Tavistock team-mates, H. Phillipson and A. Russell Lee, also belongs in the phase under present review (despite its date of actual publication in 1966) since its focus is on the perception of family members by one another.[21]

In *The Divided Self*, the boundaries of Laing's existential analysis have been drawn around the patient: its typical chapter headings run Ontological insecurity', 'The embodied and unembodied self', 'The inner self in the schizoid condition', 'Self-consciousness' and 'The self and false self in the schizophrenic'. The space of the patient's self is not of course uninfluenced by other people, but its topography is mapped as that of a relatively closed system. By contrast, *The Self and Others* is nearly always inside relationships involving at least two persons; its second part deals with those stratagems of small-group action which may 'drive the other person crazy', while its first section is a *tour de force* which tries to establish the social, interpersonal content of such apparently private modes of experience as masturbation and psychotic depression. The change in Laing's standpoint for the analysis of schizophrenic behaviour becomes quite dramatic. *The Divided Self* had achieved its comprehension of madness by entering the apparently fractured logic of the patient's world-view and supplying the missing terms. When the hebephrenic Julie speaks, in her disjointed way, about 'a told bell', 'the occidental sun' and 'Mrs Taylor', these utterances are rendered meaningful by construing them as puns: Julie is a 'told belle' (a girl told what to do and be); 'accidental son' (because her mother had half-wanted a baby boy); and 'tailor-made by her parents'. But in the 1964 book by Laing and Esterson, interpreting the family patterns around 11 schizophrenic women as variations on the theme of Clarissa Doublebind, none of the patients is ever reported at any point as uttering 'schizophrenese'. There are no word-salads or schizoid puns to be interpreted. At any rate none are transcribed in the text out of nearly 200 hours of recorded interviews with these patients. The symptoms have become totally dissolved in the flux of social praxis. One patient, Lucie, displays what might be thought to be a rather hesitant speech style, with an abundance of rambling qualifications to her remarks, but most of us have come across a fair number of interviewees with the same style and no psychotic diagnosis. The parents of these young women are scarcely less confused and 'thought-disordered', in the quoted transcripts, than their disgraced and labelled offspring. The insane patients of *The Divided Self*, with their dislocated body-images, splintered self-systems and depersonalised fantasies, sound as though they need some kind of specialised and continuous attention; Laing does not object to the provision of this attention under medical auspices. But with the 11 women of the 1964 series, one is at a loss to understand why they were ever sent into hospital at all, unless on the assumption that the medical authorities are in collusion with their rejecting families. For we are given no reason to suppose that anything is actually the matter with Maya, Lucie, Claire, Sarah, Ruby, June, Ruth, Jean, Mary, Hazel or Agnes.

The disappearance of the symptom can be indicated from Laing's changing attitude towards schizophrenic speech. In *The Divided Self* he admits, in effect, that he is unable to understand, or translate for others' benefit, everything that a schizophrenic patient has to say:

> A good deal of schizophrenia is simply nonsense, redherring speech, prolonged filibustering designed to throw dangerous people off the

> scent, to create boredom and futility in others. (Penguin edition, p. 164)

Compare this with the conclusion to the preface of the 1970 edition of *Sanity, Madness and the Family*:

> Surely, if we are wrong, it would be easy to show it by studying a few families and revealing that schizophrenics really are talking nonsense after all. (Penguin edition, p. 14)

The pawky sarcasm here comes from a new confidence. Incoherence and confusion will vanish into comprehensibility once the family context is supplied. It is no longer 'simply nonsense', to be explained as the outcome of a deliberate effort to talk nonsense.

At several points during Laing's argument in this period, one could encounter a constant and serious ambiguity over the applicability of his ideas to 'normal' families. It was not even clear whether, within his terms, 'normal' families could be said to exist at all. Part of the uncertainty arose from the way in which Laing took over some of Sartre's descriptions of the social bond in non-pathological groups, and used them to explain developments within what must have been rather severely disturbed family settings. It will be recalled that Sartre accounts for the more intense kinds of group affiliation by positing the internalisation of violence or 'terror' among the membership. Laing's construct of the 'nexal family' outlines a similar process of bonding through terror, but he widens the category of terror so as to include within it virtually any form of concern felt by one member of a family over the effect that another member's actions may have personally on her or him.

> The highest ethic of the nexus, then, is reciprocal concern. Each person is concerned about what the other thinks, feels, does.
>
> My security rests on his or her need for me. My need is for the other's need for me. His or her need is that I need him or her. My need is not simply 'need' to satisfy biological drives. It is my need to be needed by the other. My love is a thirst, not to satisfy my love, but a thirst to be loved. My solitude is not for another, but for another to want me… And in the same way, my emptiness is that the other does not require me to fulfill him or her. And, similarly, the other wants to be wanted by me, longs to be longed for by me. Two alienated loves, two self-perpetuating solitudes, an inextricable and timeless misunderstanding – tragic and comic – the soil of endless recrimination.

> In such families it is assumed that to be affected by the others' actions or feelings is 'natural'.
>
> ... If Peter is prepared to make sacrifices for Paul, so Paul should be prepared to make sacrifices for Peter, or else he is selfish, ungrateful, callous, ruthless, etc. 'Sacrifice' under these circumstances consists in Peter impoverishing himself to do something for Paul. It is the tactic of enforced debt.[22]

The blindness of these passages is unbelievable. This is Laing's description of the life-style of families living in a sort of 'family ghetto', involved in a 'reciprocal terrorism' as 'gangsters' caught in a mutual-protection racket. In a knowing tone not free from a certain lofty satire, Laing is attacking any human relationships which have built into them some anticipation of exchange, or some sense of a limit that will be violated if the exchange is unreciprocated. Such assumptions of a continuing reciprocity, along with anticipations of a possible limit to the relationship in the event of a non-return of affection or action, are of course very common outside family ghettoes and even outside families.[23] The agony of unrequited sexual passion; the feeling of 'unwantedness' in infirm parents dependent on their children; the unease aroused by oblivious guests who overstay their welcome; the unpopularity of the non-union worker who accepts a wage increase won through the activity of organised mates; our disillusionment in fair-weather friends who are on hand for social pleasantries but absent in times of distress – all these, on Laing's analysis in this period, are targets just as eligible for criticism as the nexal family. To 'invest in' another being's anticipated response is seen as literally capitalistic and hence disreputable: the 'debt' of a relationship has to be 'enforced', a deliberate tactic:

But can expectations of reciprocity be dismissed so easily? Are women liberationists simply wrong to rebel against the endless impoverishment of culture and personality which has been women's traditional lot? May not parents ever decide that they have had enough insufferable presumption from their children, or children from their parents? Would not, in short, a little more 'terrorism' in the cause of reciprocal concern be a highly desirable outcome in many homes? And is not recrimination ('comic' or 'tragic' as the case may be) some times a more progressive state of affairs between two partners than the submissiveness of one partner? For it seems inconceivable that new demands for equality in personal relationships could ever be founded without some expectation of the very reciprocity which is so frowned on here by Laing.

The mystery of the 'normal' family becomes more perplexing when we look at the home lives of the schizophrenic women reported in the

Laing-Esterson book. The original perspective of *Sanity, Madness and the Family*, on its first publication in 1964, appeared to be straightforwardly comparative: it was subtitled *Volume I: Families of Schizophrenics*, a formula with the clear implication that a Volume Two would follow dealing with families untenanted by a schizophrenic member.

Laing did in fact report that the Tavistock programme was making comparisons with the patterns of communication in non-schizophrenic, 'normal' families.[24] Both elementary scientific method and common curiosity would dictate the choice of a comparative framework for this research; in the absence of a control group drawn from non-schizophrenic households, how could any behaviour of the patients' families be said to explain the origins of schizophrenia? Yet the descriptions of the families in the 1964 study contain remarkably little that might be specifically schizogenic. These are rigid, demanding parents, setting unrealistic, overweening standards which block their children's autonomy; they define the approved behavior-patterns for their daughters in ways which stifle the women's self-images; and their expectations for the family's future are often contradictory and incoherent. But all this is true nowadays of many households that display feuding between generations, suppression of young personalities – and a complete absence of schizophrenic children. Laing's and Esterson's account of the Abbotts and the Lawsons is striking not because it presents unfamiliar material but because we have seen it or heard about it all before. And the theoretical framework outlined in the introduction is again non-specific to schizophrenia: 'we are interested in what might be called the family *nexus*... The relationships of persons in a nexus are characterised by enduring and reciprocal influence on each other's experience and behaviour.' The concept of 'nexus' is now used to include not simply the disturbed family but any family at all (or, for that matter, any close and enduring face-to-face group). Laing seems to have resolved the ambiguity of his earlier description of 'the nexal family' by taking a decision that all families must be nexal.

In the later re-issue of *Sanity, Madness and the Family* (Penguin, 1970) the effort to sustain a comparative explanation without resorting to a comparative research method appears to have been abandoned. For the work is no longer presented as the first instalment of a series that will deal in turn with schizophrenic and non-schizophrenic families. The subheading *Volume I* has been dropped, and it is made clear in the new preface that no comparative data from other kinds of families are ever going to be presented: 'Would a control group help us to answer our questions? After much reflection we came to the conclusion that a control group would contribute nothing to an answer to *our* question.'

Laing and Esterson posed the 'question' that was the topic of the investigation as follows: 'Are the experience and behaviour that psychiatrists take as symptoms and signs of schizophrenia more socially intelligible than has come to be supposed?' They claim that they are not out to test the hypothesis that certain family interaction patterns cause schizophrenia (a project that would indeed, they admit, have required a control group) but simply concerned to show that the patients' experience and behaviour 'are liable to make more sense' when viewed in the family context than outside it. Yet, even if we were to take at its face value the authors' disclaimer of any interest in a causal investigation, it by no means follows that comparative evidence 'would contribute nothing' to illuminating the problem of social intelligibility in schizophrenic behaviour. Supposing it were found, on examining normal families, that these displayed interaction patterns of mystification that were precisely similar to those found in households with a schizophrenic member: would not the vision of schizophrenic behaviour as an intelligible reaction to such mystification become rather more uncertainly founded? Or supposing that we were to analyse the family processes surrounding patients with an acknowledged organic diagnosis of mental disorder (epilepsy, say, or Down's disease) and found that the reactions of the patient 'made more sense' within the domestic context than when taken in isolation from it. We might conclude that there was some general syndrome of interaction within handicapped families, affecting schizophrenic and other diagnoses in roughly parallel ways, where the initial disability and the parents' reaction to it, the child's reaction to the parents' reaction and the child's physiological deficit were deeply intermingled and confused. This would tend to tell against a view of schizophrenia that regarded it as a reactive condition pure and simple, requiring no organic predisposition in the patient. If the demand for 'intelligibility' in the description of human action means more than a preoccupation with telling stories – *any* stories – about the person cast as subject, we must be careful to check the stories that we tell about that person with the stories that might be told just as easily about quite different sorts of people. Laing cannot evade the requirements of comparative method by an appeal to 'intelligibility'.

This lapse is all the stranger because Laing's other published study from the Tavistock Programme (*Interpersonal Perception*, 1966, jointly with H. Phillipson and A. Russell Lee) pays explicit tribute to conventional scientific canons in its use of empirical control material and tests for the statistical significance of comparisons. The Interpersonal Perception Method (or IPM), devised by these three authors on the basis of a hypothesis by Laing on the supposedly greater interpersonal insight displayed by schizophrenic patients vis-à-vis their relatives, is validated in this study by comparing the test scores of couples from disturbed marriages with those produced by relatively trouble-free couples. The assumptions of the book are by and large those of orthodox marital counselling: we do not have here a radical-nihilist critique of the lie at the heart of human relationships, but a liberal-reformist statement that some relationships are discernibly better than others. The better ones, within the terms of the IPM, are those where the parties achieve a close matching in their perceptions (a) of the way in which they are perceived by one another (b) of the fact that their partners perceive them correctly as perceiving something or somebody. Disturbed couples, on the other hand, exhibit constant mismatchings, or disjunctions between what each thinks the other perceives or feels. The postulates of the study could hardly be in greater contrast with the rest of Laing's work. 'Reciprocal concern' (in the case of the untroubled couples) here hardly implies terror, but rather an achieved harmony. The possibility of a mutually benevolent 'nexus' is conceded, and the anticipation of violence as the cause of social bonding is totally absent from the analysis.

Interpersonal Perception does not, however, represent a break or interlude in the development of Laing's thought. Despite its rather kindly inconsistency, its uncharacteristic hint of mellowness in the understanding of intimate relationships, it does follow through his earlier emphasis on the spiral of interlocking perspectives in the transaction between persons. We have suggested that, as Laing's theory progresses, this vision of interlocking others tends to take precedence over any attention of those characteristics of an individual which are not defined in terms of his immediate peers' perception. The 'vanishing of the symptom' is only part of the disappearance of the subject, the displacement of 'the self' from an internally structured space to a group-directed field. The couples who get tested on the IPM are asked about their judgement of their partners purely in relation to those aspects of behaviour which are manifested within the couple itself: other characteristics of the person remain unchallenged. The husband and the wife will rate themselves and each other on such statements as 'He finds fault with me'; 'I take her seriously'; 'He is wrapped up in himself'; and so on. It is out of bounds for them to consider whether one or the other of the pair is a depressive, a spendthrift, hysterical, career-minded or even sexless. In the world of the IPM, marital disharmony depends not on whether Mr Smith is a drunken good-for-nothing but on whether Mrs Smith thinks that he thinks that she is bitter towards him and on whether he actually does think that she is bitter. In the marital case-history provided as an illustration by the authors, the focus on, so to speak, the outer leaves of the onion is remarkable. 'Mrs Jones' is reported to be very unhappy with her husband, largely through her (unfounded) suspicion that he has slept with another woman. The IPM questionnaire sheets completed by the Jones couple establish (a) that she does not love him; (b) that he is conscious of the fact that she does not love him. But these (on the face of it, plausible) indicators of marital rupture need not be taken as definitive, since they are drawn only from the first windings of the perceptual spiral. They matter less than the fact that Mr and Mrs Jones are in considerable agreement at the higher, more indirect levels of attribution: thus, she correctly perceives him as perceiving her as feeling disappointed in him, and so on. The Jones's perspectives on one another may be at odds, but their meta- and meta-metaperspectives concur: they may be out of love, but *at least they know it.* And on the strength of these disillusioned, bitterly refracted awarenesses, the authors conclude that the unloved Mr Jones and the unloving Mrs Jones have a hopeful marital prognosis, with 'a good capacity to work with and contain their conflicts'. It needed an awful lot of statistics to produce that avuncular twinkle.

Up to the mid-sixties, Laing's conceptual journey had been from Self to Others: it was soon to concentrate once again on the charting of an individual rather than a social space. From 1964 onward he was associated with an interpretation of schizophrenic experience which was not entirely original (Gregory Bateson had a few years earlier hinted at a similar perspective),[25] but that has since become identified as Laing's personal vantage point on the field; schizophrenia was henceforth to be seen not as a psychiatric disability but as one stage in a natural psychic healing process, containing the possibility of entry into a realm of 'hyper-sanity'[26] as well as the destructive potential of an existential death. This view was developed in a number of articles and speeches and then in *The Politics of Experience.* Psychiatric medicine offered, at best, a mechanistic bungling which would frustrate the lawful progression of this potentially natural process; at worst, it drove its patients insane with its murderous chemistry, surgery and regimentation. Instead of the 'degradation ceremonials' performed on patients by doctors and nursing staff (a degradation inherent in the very act of diagnosis and examination no less than in the impersonal processing of mental hospital admission), what was needed was a sympathetic 'initiation ceremonial, through which the person will be guided with full social sanction and encouragement into inner space and time, by people who have been there and back again.' Schizophrenic experience was, at any rate in some patients, no more than the first step in a two-way voyage which led back again into 'a new ego' and 'an existential rebirth'.[27] Laing's therapeutic community (Kingsley Hall) was organised between 1965 and 1970 in an attempt to provide just such a sympathetic setting for the completion of the schizophrenic's cyclical voyage; hospitals, with their formalisation of roles and their traditions of interference, could not be expected to furnish the conditions for successful 'initiation'.

The novelty of these views, measured against not only orthodox psychiatric theory but also against Laing's own previous writings, should be apparent. Their introduction was both sudden and confident: fully fledged statements of the position appear in lectures and articles presented by Laing in the course of 1964 and 1965, often before a non-medical public. The Institute of Contemporary Arts, the *Psychedelic Review*, the radical journals *Peace News*, *Views* and *New Left Review*, the London weekly *New Society*, and an inconsequent jamboree dignified under the name of 'First International Congress of Social Psychiatry' (which met in chaotic conditions in a large London school) were the first recipients of the new message. Laing also presented his case to the writers and artists who were working with him in the 'sigma' project: Kingsley Hall, and to some extent David Cooper's schizophrenia research ward at the Shenley Hospital outside North London, were in this period part of the scene frequented by this wing of the cultural left.[28] Laing's presentations before medical audiences were to continue in the vein of his pre-1964 theorising: he did not usually try to tell doctors and psychoanalysts that their schizophrenic patients were super-sane voyagers into aeonic time, but rather developed (often with impressive skill and clarity) his classifications of misleading family talk and his notations of the psychotic's layered fantasies.

Laing's sharp turn towards the celebration of the schizophrenic condition was accompanied by two developments in his thought whose conjunction appears as something of a paradox: his language becomes at once both *more socially committed* and *more mystical*. The schizophrenic's experience is seen as an indictment of the conventional world's standards of what is sane or insane; and his incarceration and punishment in the mental hospital necessitates a critical appraisal of 'the larger context of the civic order of society – that is, of the political order, of the ways persons exercise control and power over one another'.[29] In his 1965 preface to the Pelican edition of *The Divided Self*, Laing insisted that his critique should be taken as a condemnation not simply of the micro-world of the family but also of the larger social order, the civilisation of 'one-dimensional men' which 'represses not only "the instincts", not only sexuality, but any form of transcendence'. 'The statesmen of the world who boast and threaten that they have Doomsday weapons are far more dangerous, and far more estranged from "reality" than many of the people on whom the label "psychotic" is affixed.'[30] Two years later, in his contribution to the 'Dialectics of Liberation' conference in London[31] (which he sponsored with three other psychiatrists) he again juxtaposed the small-scale assaults of modern psychiatry and the huge lunacies and systematic violence perpetrated by the world system of imperialism.

However, in this period, from 1964 until seven or eight years later, Laing enjoyed a degree of appreciation among the marxist left which was perhaps excessive in relation to his own rather guarded commitment to political radicalism. The British playwright David Mercer, who collaborated with Laing over much of this period (and wrote the scripts of a TV play, *In Two Minds*, and a film, *Family Life*, exhibiting the causation of a psychotic illness in a young woman through 'double-bind' pressures from her parents) has recounted how

> There was one particular instance when he [Laing] gave what was in effect a private lecture to a group of friends, which lasted about four hours, in which he, first of all, declared himself as a marxist and said that he wanted to try to relate the question of Marx and marxism to his ideas in psychiatry; and there's no doubt that for Laing the two are very closely interwoven.[32]

The impression of a marxist commitment in Laing was reinforced by the appearance of his name among the signatories welcoming the May Day Manifesto, a campaigning pamphlet coauthored for the socialist-humanist New Left in Britain by Stuart Hall, Edward Thompson and Raymond Williams[33] in 1967. This was a militant and developed anti-capitalist statement; it was in the same year that Laing wrote the short introduction to his collection *The Politics of Experience and the Bird of Paradise*, with its somewhat elliptical denunciation of the capitalist system[34] and its acknowledgement of the importance of Marx's work (along with that of Kierkegaard, Nietzsche and assorted other thinkers) in the critique of modern alienation. By 1970 a commentator on the British New Left could assert that 'Ronald Laing must be accounted one of the main contributors to the theoretical and rhetorical armoury of the contemporary left'.[35] Outside Britain the link between Laing and the far left seemed a strong one in the later sixties. A laudatory reference to '*el trabajo psiquiatrico de R.D. Laing, D.G. Cooper y sus asociados*' appeared in a literary magazine produced in Havana at a time when the Castro regime was still interested in appeasing the intellectuals;[36] and, arriving in the wake of the 1968 'May events', the French translations of

Laing's and Cooper's work came at exactly the right moment to detonate an explosion of interest in 'l'antipsychiatrie' among an enlarged and confident left public.

The other and contrary move, towards an apparent celebration of mysticism and the inward-looking delights of the psychedelic 'trip', took place in the same period of left-wing politicisation in Laing. Jeff Nuttall, the chronicler of project 'sigma', has described how, in a room of the large country house where the first conference of the group took place in 1964, 'Laing enacted a catatonic ceremonial, summarily describing its magical function'.

> 'It's a question,' he said, 'of coming down from the surface of things, down to the core of all things, to the central sphere of being in which all things are emanations.'[37]
>
> Laing started to talk about this coming down to a place of being where there was no differentiation between separate entities, to a place of being where there was a total unity in the universe... And in doing that he related it to catatonic behaviour by suddenly standing up and walking quietly to the middle of the room, saying 'One might almost only have to do this to maintain one's relationship to existence.' And he turned right towards the window and he looked at the ceiling; and then he returned to his place.[38]

In Laing's published work from the 1964–67 period a number of pronouncements can be found with a distinctly otherworldly flavour.

> Orientation means to know where the orient is. For inner space, to know the east, the origin or source of our experience.
>
> There is everything to suggest that man experienced God... It seems likely that far more people in our time neither experience the Presence of God, nor the Presence of his absence, but the absence of his Presence. With the greatest precautions, we may trust in a source that is much deeper than our egos – if we can trust ourselves to have found it, or rather, to have been found by it. It is obvious that it is hidden, but what it is and where it is, is not obvious.[39]

Occasionally we even find an explicit analogy drawn between the role of the psychoanalyst and that of the religious celebrant:

> I believe that if we can begin to understand sanity and madness in existential social terms, we, as priests and physicians, will

> be enabled to see more clearly the extent to which we confront common problems…
>
> Among physicians and priests there should be some who are guides, who can educt the person from this world and induct him to the other.[40]

Laing, in short, regarded the psychotic's experience of an alien reality as something akin to a mystical apprehension: it is not 'the effulgence of a pathological process' but the faithful reflection of another actuality which is concealed from us by the blinkers of our mundane civilisation. The lunatic can be 'irradiated with light from other worlds', and partakes of 'those experiences of the divine which are the Living Fount of all religion'.[41]

What is the nature of the apprehension achieved by the mystical lunatic? It appears that the psychotic condition may enable one to overcome a deep rift in the human personality, characteristic of 'normal' people in our type of society. Modern civilisation has created a fissure between the 'inner' and the 'outer' layers of existence, between 'me-here' and 'you-there', between 'mind' and 'body'. These divisions of personality are not inevitable or natural, but the outcome of 'an historically conditioned split'; we can conceive of a point in human existence before this lapse from fusion occurred, an 'original Alpha and Omega of experience and reality' to whose one-ness the mystic and the schizophrenic both manage to return.[42] It is not the psychotic who is 'alienated' or has the 'split personality', in Laing's terms, but the so-called 'normal' person: alienation and splitting are indeed the basic conditions of our repressive normality and its apparatus of anti-human institutions.

Schizophrenic patients, then, are engaged in a lonely voyage back towards the primeval point of one-ness: it appears that they are in some sense re-tracing the steps taken by the whole course of human evolution, and that once they have regressed far enough they will be able (just how or why is not at all clear) to advance back again into the world of common twentieth-century normals. Laing's description of the destination of the backward voyage is picturesque if imprecise: 'in and back and through and beyond into the experience of all mankind, of the primal man, of Adam and perhaps even further into the being of animals, vegetables and minerals'; 'to temporal standstill… to aeonic time… back into the womb of all things (pre-birth)'. The psychotic return is recommended to all who are able: 'we have a long, long way to go back to contact the reality we have all long lost contact with'; and, 'This process is one, I believe, that all of us need, in one form or another. This process would be at the very heart of a truly sane society'.[43]

This perspective on psychosis is, of course, unique in psychiatry. There are moments when Laing appears to approach the thought of Carl Jung in his emphasis on religious archetypes, necessary to the integrity of the personality and deeply embedded in the collective memory of the human race: as when he speaks of 'the emergence of the "inner" archetypal mediators of divine power, and through this death a rebirth, and the eventual reestablishment of a new kind of ego-functioning, the ego now being the servant of the divine, no longer its betrayer'.[44] But neither Freud nor Jung nor any neo-Freudian or neo-Jungian, nor for that matter any other existential analyst has taken the stance that psychosis is a higher form of sanity. Schizophrenia is breakdown, sheer affliction, for virtually all psychiatric schools; only for Laing does it mean also breakthrough and blessing. Both of Laing's movements, towards social criticism as well as towards a mystique of psychosis, are intelligible only as the systematic development of some elements in his earlier perspective on madness. *The Divided Self* had taken the first step of viewing schizophrenic experience in goal-directed terms. Laing went on to extend the area of meaning in the schizophrenic's world-view, which was to be seen now not simply as shot through fitfully with intention but as a valid vantage point in its entirety. Psychotic reality is in essence a competitor, a rival, a challenge to the reality defined by the normal and the sane. The sane and the normal eliminate their rival by declaring it to be madness, a deviation to be visited with legal and other penalties. Peaceful co-existence between the normal and the psychotic ideologies is impossible, and it follows that any person who accepts the psychotic vision as authentic must at once declare war on the world-view of the normal consensus; at the very least she or he must declare a critical suspension of judgement on the received social values which decree the limits of sanity and insanity. At times Laing seems to be saying that one cognitive system is as good as another, that your 'delusion' is my 'reality' and nothing can adjudicate between us. At other times it looks as if the patient is right in perceiving as he or she does, and the rest of the world is blind or wilfully ignorant. In Laing's celebration of the schizophrenic we sometimes find hints of the traditional literary figure of the Holy Fool, the crazed seer, the Cassandra or Poor Tom whose disjointed prophecies condemn a society ripe for judgement. This is of course only a limited and rhetorical radicalism: it is saying 'How dare a crazy world label me as crazy?' But then, if his movement towards critical social analysis was primarily a consequence of his identification with patients, one would not expect it to develop the intellectual energy of a more committed politics.

The sympathy with mysticism followed naturally from Laing's position of solidarity with the schizophrenic. We may see the growth of his ideas as a sequence of challenges to the whole catalogue of schizoid 'symptoms' which is customarily presented in psychiatric textbooks. Each manifestation of behaviour that in orthodox medicine is offered as a 'sign' of clinical pathology is taken by Laing to be a comprehensible act which, when aligned against its social context, appears as eminently reasonable and sane. Does the schizophrenic utter a 'word-salad'? Well, it isn't quite as mixed-up and incoherent as that: here, here and here it makes rather good sense, with one or two poetic turns of phrase that are pretty striking. Besides, the schizophrenic does start talking stark nonsense every now and then, quite deliberately, just in order to throw the likes of you and me off the scent. Does this patient present 'inappropriate affect', grimacing when he should keep his face still and reacting coldly in situations demanding a show of emotion? Only according to that mother of his, an unreliable and partisan witness; and besides, who wouldn't grimace at that old tyrant? If that patient hears voices inside her head, it is because she lacks the personal confidence that would enable her to claim ownership of her own thought-processes; if she retreats into the waxy automaton passivity of the catatonic state, we can understand her withdrawal from a responsibility and an agency she feels to be impossible.

So far, so good: all the symptoms have been validated as meaningful and even worthy forms of behaviour. But what are we to make of that peculiar syndrome of the dissolution of personality itself, the 'loss of ego-boundaries' characteristic of so many severely deteriorated schizophrenics who literally do not know where they themselves leave off, and a reality exterior to themselves begins? Up to his psychedelic phase, Laing accepted the typical medical and psychoanalytic description of these states of being; his existential accounts of 'depersonalisation' and 'boundary-loss' augment rather than contradict the orthodox texts of clinical psychiatry. But if the schizophrenic experience was to become completely validated, to enter the realm of health and normalcy rather than of sickness and handicap, ego-loss and de-realisation had to become positive virtues, or at least viable alternatives to our common sense, interpersonally bonded realism. Laing called this identity-anchored, space-and-time-bound mode of experience, common to most members of society, *egoic experience*. The ego is 'an instrument for living in this world', and as such is scarcely an unmixed blessing. Characteristic of the modern age is an overemphasis on egoic adaptation to exterior realities, a drive to control 'the outer world' at the cost of forgetting 'the inner light' of imagination and fantasy. Laing appears to concur with traditional mystic philosophy in regarding the egoic mode as 'a preliminary illusion, a veil, a film of *maya*… a state of sleep, of death, of socially accepted madness, a womb state to which one has to die, from which one has to be born'.[45]

The alternative to downgrading the 'egoic' (which appears to be a synonym for humanity's perception of and activity in the world of nature and society) would have been to admit that the loss of the boundary between 'inner' and 'outer', 'ego' and 'world', was a terrible misfortune; and this Laing could not do if he was to pursue his project of out-and-out solidarity with psychotic experience.

Thus, Laing's phase of apparent mysticism must be seen as part of his rationale for non-intervention in a schizophrenic's delusions; it sprang from his insistence that all human experience is potentially valid and potentially intelligible, that none of it should be shunted off into a garbage heap for incineration by sanitary technicians. The analogy between the psychotic and the psychedelic states, between the schizophrenic's withdrawal and the mystic's other-worldliness, was an inevitable move in his campaign to upgrade the status of the apparently abnormal and insane. It was a crucial move, because if we refuse to follow Laing this far we are left with the position that the schizophrenic is a disabled victim – of precisely what set of circumstances need not be considered here – whose basic perceptions and reactions can only to a limited degree be understood in the terms of 'intelligibility'. Laing could maintain this total suspension of judgement on 'egoic' rationality only at the cost of losing his own professional and personal identity. His position at the end of the sixties therefore confronted him with the choice of joining some of his patients and followers in a mystical or psychotic 'boundary-loss', or else of moving on, away and back, from anti-psychiatry to psychiatry.

4. R.D. Laing: The Return to Psychiatry

These mid-sixties transitions in Laing's thought, with their double load of social radicalism and personal mysticism, are still widely regarded as permanent elements in his contribution to psychiatry.[1] Nonetheless, he was to go to great pains to repudiate any taint either of socialism or of transcendentalism in the work he did during the seventies. The claim for any kind of privilege in psychotic perception was now scarcely made, except insofar as the experience of such patients was taken, among sundry other items of fantasy material, as showing the central importance of foetal implantation and of birth itself as precipitants of identity and later trauma. In the earlier Laing, both the movement towards the political left and the flirtation with psychosis as a heightened and heightening experience were logical progressions from his identification with the schizophrenic patients as society's ultimate underdog. He took measured steps from an empathising psychiatry into an apparent marxism and a mysticism of solidarity – and then re-traced his route back again into a psychiatric posture. The journey from psychiatrist to marxist was in part a matter of some temporary emotional alliances, between himself and David Cooper, between the Laingian working group as a whole and the *New Left Review* circle; but it probably developed in the main through his interest in devising a language to encompass power relationships. 'Questions and answers', wrote Laing in the sixties, 'have so far been focussed on the family as a sub-system. Socially, this work must now move to further understanding… to the meaning of all this within the larger context of the civic order of society.'[2]

These larger questions never extended in Laing much beyond a certain wonderment at the existence of destructive or violent sociopolitical structures in nations or in the world system. Laing deplored the hydrogen bomb and the Vietnam war at a time when hundreds of thousands of the vaguely liberal-minded took much the same attitudes. When the Campaign for Nuclear Disarmament receded and the Americans made their peace with Hanoi, he behaved no differently from the rest of his intellectual generation in forsaking the world of dissident politics. His sole political role now is that of an occasional moraliser, as on Watergate:

> We are liars. Believe us. The president, the vice-president, the secretary of state, the chief of staff, all represent vast complexes of deception and self-deception, apparently.[3]

Or on the politics of psychiatry in Russia:

> When a book like this [on dissidents in the USSR] is on sale in Russia in Russian – that'll be the day! In the meantime I hope that President Carter does not cut down on R. and D.[4]

References to Marx in the sparse publications and more frequent interviews which Laing produced in the seventies are very rare. He now denies ever having been a marxist in the political sense.[5] In an interview some years ago on an American tour he could recall Lenin and Trotsky, along with other marxist authors, as having been formative influences in his reading;[6] in a later American dialogue his view of the founders of Bolshevism is much more jaundiced:

> Lenin carried Machiavelli's *The Prince* around in his pocket and went to sleep with it under his pillow – I think he died with it under his pillow. His closest associates were ferocious creatures like Trotsky. There's no question about the ferocity of the game.[7]

Laing's retreat from socialism is tragic for his left-wing admirers. But it is particularly shocking for those who took it as fact that there were genuine radical implications in his work of the mid-sixties. In retrospect, the radicalism was less an implication than an obscure insinuation. Somewhere in a forthcoming volume, we were led to believe, or at least in an ongoing draft, or at the very least in the barest hint of a conception, Laing was going to deliver a theory encompassing and criticising within its single span every type and kind of interference by one human being with another. The napalming of peasants would be shown as related to the suffocating love of parents; the manipulation of psychotic delusion through phenothiazines would be linked with the suppression of political dissent through bludgeon or gallows. But the evidence is thin that Laing was ever seriously on the way to delivering so comprehensive and extraordinary a synthesis. In his speech to the 'Dialectics of Liberation' conference of 1967 he indeed linked the interpersonal insults of families and mental hospitals with the larger atrocities of the United States military in Indo-China. But the concepts that leap the gap from micro-terror to state-sponsored violence are of a peculiarly general order. It is the propensity of people to discover enemies in external groups, or rather to *invent* external groups as a focus for their enmity, to which Laing (in this speech as well as at other points of his more radical period) refers for the explanation for advanced capitalism's military forays into the Third

World. The categorisation of 'Us' and 'Them', which he here terms 'collective paranoid projection systems that operate on large scales'[8] and is elsewhere analysed as 'a sort of social mirage' created by a particular group to reinforce its own identity,[9] marks the limit of Laing's knowledge of social institutions larger and wider than the family or face-to-face group. In the speech to the 'Dialectics of Liberation' conference, Laing expressly foregoes any attempt to comprehend the international social order as a whole,[10] or even any of its major sub-systems. The 'almost total social scepticism' about macro-systems which Laing confessed even at the peak of his political radicalism should have warned his socialist followers.

One of Laing's most sympathetic commentators, Martin Howarth-Williams, has convincingly described the inherent limitations of Laing's social theorising, guided as it was above all (in his radical phase) by concepts drawn from Sartre's portrayal of bonding among small groups rather than by marxist insights into the formation of whole socio-economic systems.[11] The incrimination of 'Us and Them' as the prime source of political alienation and conflict finds its climax in the concluding pages of the 1969 lectures on *The Politics of the Family.* Here it seems to be no longer any specially Sartrean process of group bonding but socialisation itself, the inculcation of positive and negative value-judgements in small children, that causes such phenomena as 'racism; semitism; anti-semitism; anti-antisemitism. Blacks and Whites. Black Anti-Whites, White Anti-Blacks. White trash and Niggers.'

> As long as we cannot up-level our thinking beyond Us and Them, the goodies and the baddies, it will go on and on. The only possible end will be when the goodies have killed all the baddies, and all the baddies all the goodies, which does not seem so difficult or unlikely since to Us, we are the goodies and They are the baddies, while to Them, we are the baddies and they are the goodies.[12]

The Olympian relativism of this position, reducing all social antagonisms to 'this knot that we seem unable to untie... tied *very very* tight – round the throat, as it were, of the whole human species' was open to obvious objection. As Vernon Reynolds commented,

> Are good and bad to be so simply conceived of? Are fascist political philosophies and all the good-bad rules that stem from them ethically on a par with the good-bad rules that stem from political philosophies based on the spirit of democracy? They are not. Some 'goods' are better than others; some 'goods' are worse than some 'bads.'[13]

Unfortunately Laing's cryptic ventures into social analysis cannot be pursued further. Since emerging from his phase of radical politicking he has made no further general pronouncements on the nature of society. He has repudiated the printed version of his talk to the 'Dialectics of Liberation' conference, stating that it 'was used without his permission'.[14] And he has resolved the problem of the 'goodies and baddies' section in *The Politics of the Family* by excising it from the paperback edition first published by Penguin in 1976.

In his relation to mysticism as well as to psychedelic experience, Laing once again offered hints of a more profound reorientation than he actually came to make. The autobiographical fragment, 'The Bird of Paradise', invited his readers to believe that he himself had made the journey to that 'beginning of beginnings that is nothing at all... that Alpha and Omega' which precedes the tawdry dualisms of ordinary existence.[15] Timothy Leary himself, the sixties' principal guru of transcendental chemistry, reported one session of apparently psychedelic bliss around 1964 with Laing, when Laing became 'stoned high in a Sufi ballet' and 'gone, spun out of time'.[16] Laing's version of this interesting meeting has not been vouchsafed to us. But Baba Ram Dass (formerly, as Dr Richard Alpert, Leary's colleague and co-celebrant of LSD in Harvard's Psychology Department) relates a long acid-session in London involving Leary, Laing and himself: Laing 'was so far out. I mean, the minute we took LSD he took off his clothes and started to do yoga. This was three or four years ago.'[17]

Much of his reading public assumed that Laing was, like Leary, a high priest of LSD (although, as Howarth-Williams points out after a careful review of Laing's published material, including interviews, any references at all to 'acid' are very hard to find).[18] Laing was subsequently at pains to normalise any impression of psychedelic deviancy which the ecstatic 'Bird of Paradise' passage might have conveyed. He told one American interviewer in 1970 that the chapter was not the record of an LSD trip but 'merely a description of some of the things that make up my inner life'[19] and he explains the famous final sentence of the chapter ('if I could turn you on, if I could drive you out of your wretched mind, if I could tell you I would let you know') by referring to its connexion with some lines from a poem by W.H. Auden which long pre-dated any possible reference to LSD.[20] By October 1972 he was telling the *Times* interviewer that 'he was never an apostle of the drug experience like Timothy Leary and had in fact been a restraining influence on the drug culture in London'. It seemed that Laing would not be caught again by anyone, tripping with his clothes off.

In regard to mysticism, too, our guru is to be found discreetly covering any possible embarrassment with the very 'veil of *maya*' or worldly appearances which he had previously toyed with discarding as an unnecessary wrapper for the innermost essence of knowledge. His BBC broadcast of March 1970 on the theme 'Is there a future for religious belief?' gave only an ambiguous answer to a question which might have tested the degree of his commitment to an immaterial reality: 'until, or if, from a religious point of view, there is a new dispensation giving rise to new forms of revelation, those of us who cannot help ourselves are compelled to continue the impossibly absurd project of keeping these alive.'[21] To his American follower, Peter Mezan, just before his departure for South Asia in 1971, he proffered several hints confirming the purpose of his intended Vedic and Buddhist meditations in the East. He was especially keen on acquiring the capacity to divorce the self from any of its social attributes, and to achieve a 'release from mindfulness. And beyond release is *nirvana*, which as I understood it is some kind of perpetual bliss, beyond life and death'. Between Mezan and Laing on these occasions there was much bandying of the Brahma Sutra, the Diamond Sutra of Mahayana Buddhism, and even the *Mystic Theology* of Dionysius the Areopagite, not to mention the Zen *koan* and the works of Gurdjieff; but the extent of Laing's own endorsement of the religious content of these texts is left strangely unresolved in Mezan's report of these interviews.[22]

Once he was in Sri Lanka, Laing undertook a six-week course of intense meditation in the Theravada-Buddhist training monastry at Kandubodda, where one observer reported him to have been 'doing better, much better, than long-time meditation experts, Sinhalese Buddhist as well as foreign'.[23] Laing also spent a month in India half-way up a Himalaya mountain in the company of a swami, experiencing hunger, cold and further meditation. Once back in England, Laing made considerable efforts to present his involvement with Eastern mystical practice as an urbane, Westernised episode. He told the *Sunday Times* correspondent that his visit had been 'the most relaxing holiday I ever had'.[24] A later interview with the Paris *L'Express* reproduces the 'holiday' interpretation of his Theravadist and Brahminical sojournings:

> The East, I repeat, was the best place for me to get away from it all… I found it very restful to be in a place where I could escape from my own social system into a system where I didn't have to shoulder any responsibility, where my involvement was minimal.[25]

Equally Peter Mezan, the fan to whom Laing had offered his intimations of *Nirvana* just before going East, was told back in New York that the Four Foundations of Mindfulness, his chosen path of meditation out at

Kandubodda, had 'nothing especially mystical about it, it required no particular beliefs, was without ritual, was consistent with his notion of what psychoanalysis was really about, and it did, in fact, calm his mind considerably, at least for a time.'[26]

Laing's campaign of normalisation has been conducted on all fronts – madness, the medical model and the critique of the family as well as mysticism, drug-tripping and socialism – where he had stood in the vanguard of the sixties' counter-culture. While his old comrade David Cooper developed the critique of domestic relationships (first outlined in the collaborative work he undertook with Laing and Esterson) into a full-scale onslaught entitled *The Death of the Family* (published in 1972), his late mentor went all out to prove that the family was, on the contrary, alive and well and living near Belsize Park, London. Of his former radical supporters he complained in 1972 that

> it suited them to use me in the attack on families. I'm not against families. I have a very nice one here. And although I have tried to show how families have gone wrong, I think they are one of the best relics of a crumbling system we have to hang on to.[27]

And when the paperback edition of *The Politics of the Family* was issued four years later, any reader who turned to it for fresh confirmation of those horrors of maternal and patriarchal tyranny which, after all, have kept countless psychiatrists, novelists and playwrights in business for some while would find it prefaced by a new free-verse exercise by Laing, of a quite contrary tendency. The verses begin:

> A family.
> a place of peace and quiet
> a place to laugh and cry and dance and sing
> a place to eat one's bread in gladness

One looks in vain here for even an ironical qualification of Laing's eulogy of domesticity, the '*cosy nests/where no eyes are pecked out... with a nice mummy and daddy*'. The Laing who now dissents from any implication that 'madness is superior to true sanity. I'm sorry if I put that idea into people. I would never recommend madness to anybody,'[28] is a safer, cooler character than the Laing of extremities and ecstasies who saw the Bird of Paradise, the Lotus and the 'cosmic froth and bubbles of perpetual movement of Creation Redemption Resurrection Judgement Last and First and Ultimate Beginning and End.'[29] The habitué of Sartre,

Marx and the New Left has reached the point where he feels impelled to declare for the record that 'he especially resents the implication that he is a guiding light of the extreme left, that his psychological insights somehow support revolution.'[30] It is a laundered and sanitised Laing who now faces an audience which has itself become conservative by comparison with the Vietnam demonstrators, the flower children and the assorted radicals of his readership in the sixties. Ronald Laing was a timely writer for that epoch; and since then, it appears, he has been moving with the times.

The task of evaluating Laing's work has been made both easier and more difficult by his increasingly moderate posture.

With the seventies, his creative development reached a distinct and lengthy pause. His published corpus was enlarged only by some slighter volumes of whimsy on personal relationships (*Knots*, 1970, *Do You Love Me?*, 1977 and *Conversations with Children*, 1978), by the diffuse autobiographical fragments in *The Facts of Life* (1976), and by a large number of interviews and lectures which, along with some collaborative work in film, or musical recording, served to popularise and authorise the more conventional reading of his past work which Laing now wishes to gain credence. As a further essay in the construction of a 'science of persons', Laing employed some of these occasions to advocate the LeBoyer method of infant delivery (which avoids any precipitate severing of the umbilical cord) and to canvass, elliptically, his own theory that the earliest traumas afflicting the integrity of the person can be sited, not merely in these early moments of inadequate midwifery, but in the very implantation of the fertilised ovum in the womb of an unwilling mother. A serious discontinuity between this latest approach[31] and the whole of Laing's previous intellectual career is striking; it affords no connection with any general social theory, it is removed from any concern with the linguistic symbolism of violence and exploitation, and neither the Freudian nor the Sartrean premises which informed most of Laing's previous work have the slightest relevance to it. Insofar as Laing still retains any radical values in this present approach, it is the radicalism of one more 'alternative technology' – a technology of obstetrics rather than of energy supply or goods manufacture or of food production – divorced from the history, the sociology, the economics and the politics that have made some of the authors of counter-technology into compelling prophets for our century. Laing will be remembered for more important reasons than his late interest in ante-natal and post-natal complications of this idiosyncratic sort. Stripped of their political and transcendental pretension, the sequence of ideas which he developed around psychiatry from

The Divided Self to *The Politics of the Family* forms a connected complex of arguments which can be appraised in their own right irrespective of Laing's fleeting attempts to widen their scope into marxism, mysticism or the physiology of the uterus.

The critic of Laing is now, indeed, faced with the task of defending those elements of his work which their author now wishes to repudiate or at least downgrade. So long as Laing chose to take his empathy with schizophrenic patients to the lengths of a mystique of insanity or of a radical-sounding relativism which implied that one cognitive standpoint was as good as another, he fell into the polemically convenient category of the Romantic Idealist, the heir to a long line of anti-rational and subjectivist thinkers who have formed the target for radical obloquy from the *German Ideology* and *Holy Family* of Marx and Engels through to Lenin's hack-job *Materialism and Empirio-criticism*. When the far left as a whole was caught up in the cult of Laing, a critic could expose the threat posed by his work for the scientific-rationalist tradition of the Enlightenment – a tradition ambiguous it is true, but worthy of defence against cultism and unreason.[32]

Paradoxically, however, in the period when Laing has moved towards the criteria of everyday commonsense in his approach to drugs, the family and mental illness, it becomes necessary to present a somewhat sharpened and radicalised version of his case with which to combat some of the reigning biochemical orthodoxies in the world of psychiatric medicine.[33] A writer as nervous of any taint of the left as Laing is now cannot do other than pull his punches in any major ideological confrontation. But the battle against clinical positivism remains as urgent as ever, even if he now tends to evade it.[34] Laing's capacity to entertain and dramatise alternative models of psychic deviancy remains a valuable resource, the weapon of the sceptic against categories which tend to congeal in the hands of classifiers with vast social, chemical and even surgical powers over those classified.[35] But once he departs from scepticism – and of course he does so very frequently – he becomes open to some very damaging evaluations of his own positive philosophy and practice.

Some of the criticisms offered by commentators on Laing during his earlier over-extended and over-exposed phases retain their force now that he has opted for a narrower, more conservative identity.[36] It will be recalled that, at one point in the early sixties, with the production of *Self and Others* and *Interpersonal Perception*, Laing became fascinated with a multiple-refraction perspective on individual selfhood. Human collectives were seen essentially as social fantasy systems manufactured by a virtually infinite regress of projections from Self to Other.[37] The fictional parody of a Laingian doctor's utterance by Clancy Sigal, who consorted with Laing's group during its most radical period, is an only slightly exaggerated rendering of the refraction perspective:

> If the person being mirrored by the other person sees nobody but the mirroring person he fails to reflect his Oneness into the Other's Otherness which mirrors to the unmirrored person only the mirror-Person's self-mirror. And so it goes, spiralling down the staircase of untold generations.[38]

But the vision of the Self's disappearance into a meta-world of diffracting Others, an over-socialised conception of personhood, always co-existed in Laing with a pre-social vision of the Self. What was portrayed in the earlier writings as a schizoid construction, with an authentic 'inner' self resisting engulfment by a socially implicated false 'outer' self, became Laing's basic contribution to the definition of the human subject. The 'different perspectives, educations, backgrounds, organisations, group-loyalties, affiliations, ideologies, socio-economic class interests, temperaments' that are characteristic of different persons are not part of the very fabric of their humanity but 'so many *things*, so many social figments that come between us.' It is conceivable that 'we could strip away all the exigencies and contingencies, and reveal to each other our naked presence' and 'take away… all the clothes, the disguises, the crutches, the grease paint, also the common projects, the games that provide the pretexts for the occasions that masquerade as meetings.'[39] Only such a role-less encounter would be authentic – though somewhat ineffable.

Russell Jacoby's strictures on the post-Freudian humanists of America are relevant also for Laing:

> To them the concept and fact of roles are a violation of humanity. The role is a facade, consciously assumed so as to hide the real self… society is conceived as an external factor, an outside force acting on the individual but not decisively casting the individual from within and without… The neat division between roles and real selves reduces society to a masquerade party.[40]

In Laing, the role-masquerade is a robbery perpetrated by society on 'our own personal world of experience' – which pre-dates the social. 'We have all been processed on Procrustean beds' – Procrustes, it may be remembered, being the character in Greek myth who took people of a definite natural shape and size and then either stretched or truncated their limbs in order they might fit the mattress he provided. Or: 'We are all fallen Sons of Prophecy, who have learned to die in the Spirit and be reborn in the flesh.'[41] The episode of the Fall is variously dated in Laing's account: as the point of critical role-acquisition it shifts in his work from adolescence to early training, from birth to after-birth. The most logical point at which to mark the lapse into socialisation has always been the birth experience: even in his more immaterialist phase, he described the necessary voyages of the schizophrenic shaman as 'from being outside (post-birth) back into the wombs of all things (pre-birth)' and back again 'from a cosmic foetalization to an existential re-birth'.[42] In latter years the journey of recovery back to the old lapse is presented differently, in that the crucial foetalisation, the womb entry (and exit) have become less cosmic and much more literal. But much of Laing's progress has consisted in his elaboration of womb fantasies, and in his increasingly serious attitude toward the results of his fantasising. It is as though he had come across Rousseau's dictum that 'Man is born free, and is everywhere in chains' at some early stage in his intellectual formation, and made it into a permanent slogan for a lifetime's work. As with Rousseau, innocence pre-dates the Fall into social slavery. But, unlike Rousseau, Laing does not correlate the loss of Paradise with the institution of private property. It is self-division itself, some primal act of psychic differentiation, which expels us from the intra-uterine Eden: 'once the fissure into self and ego, inner and outer, good and bad occurs, all else is an infernal dance of false dualities.'[43]

It is important to note that, in developing his imagery of pristine birth and social violation, Laing used a language that appeared to overlap with the more sociological and political critiques of socialisation offered within the modern left. For example, at one stage he inveighed passionately against the mutilation of the individual's experience through the conformist pressures of the family. But his criticism of the family's agency has only a coincidental relationship with the attack on the family that is produced, for example, by feminism or by the psychologically sophisticated varieties of marxism. You will search Laing's writings in vain for any critique of the family as the repository of patriarchy;[44] or as the gatekeeper opening doors leading out to different positions in the larger social division of labour; or as the temple of private acquisitiveness and consumer sovereignty. It is the family as the agent of socialisation, interposing its drab screen of categories between the infant and his or her birthright of ecstasy, to which Laing objects (or did object, in his more radical days). Laing never based his description of micro-social violences in any historically specific account of (say) the bourgeois family or the nuclear family. At the stage when Laing started to consider that there might be several distinct sorts of family in history, so that 'we needn't identify the family with any particular exploitative form that families have tended to take',[45] he was also moving the blame for the suppression of the child's transcendence away from the parents and on to the midwife and doctor. When, for a mixture of psychological and logical reasons, he could not continue with the schema of a pre-social Self raped by an ahistorical violator, he did not abandon the schema: he simply found another instrument of violation, framed this time in medico-biological terms even further removed from a social and historical appraisal.

The marxists who applauded Laing's apparent convergence with their doctrines during the sixties ('R.D. Laing is *one of us*,' the editor of the *New Left Review* remarked to me when Laing was just coming into public attention) must now wonder just what continuity exists between yesterday's anti-capitalist prophet and today's denouncer of Umbilical Shock. The truth is surely that Laing took from Marx and from the New Left only what he needed for his own purposes of argument. From Marx he selected a number of concepts and phrases that accorded with his vision of a primal Self spoiled by social mismanagement: the notions of *ideology*, *alienation*, and *mystification* are introduced by Laing into a family context, along with a general sensitivity to the existence of relations of oppression behind the smokescreen of consensus or complacency. But the main contention of Marx that 'social being' determines 'social consciousness' was never accepted by Laing: if anything, 'social being', the presence of structures of social organisation which can be at odds with the consciousness of the individuals comprising these structures, is dismissed by Laing and his followers as the outcome of a plurality of 'praxes' or individual-subjective projects.[46] The largest social unit that Laing is able to handle is that of the extra-familial personal network of a family, a potential face-to-face assembly which the good therapist will strive to reconvene;[47] further contexts to these lower level networks can be suggested until we reach what is termed 'the context of all social contexts, the total social world system' – but on these reaches of society Laing has always professed a virtually complete agnosticism.

Laing was, in short, part of the Cult of Immediacy in the latter 1960s.[48] That is, he was among those for whom small-scale structures and relationships were more real than the larger complexes of society because the former were more direct, more 'personal'. At one moment in his left-wing period he did advocate the prosecution of 'revolutionary change' through 'sudden, structural, radical qualitative changes in the intermediate system levels' such as 'a factory, a hospital, a school, a university', etc.[49] To this extent he shared the concern of the New Left of that time with micro-social transformation as 'the little motor that sets the big motor running': the guerrilla *foco*, the Red Base of college or factory occupation, the questioning of the immediate institutional context as a prelude to the seizure of more central structures. But for the most part, Laing has concentrated on small social arenas as containers of relationship in their own right. It is the family living-room where the double-binds are bonded, or else the therapeutic commune as the place of 'sanctuary, asylum, where life-in-relation can flower',[50] which has been his long-term channel of interest. The promise that the investigation of schizophrenic symptomatology would culminate in a scrutiny of 'the civic order of society – that is, of the *political* order'[51] did not refer to an impending discussion of class, bureaucracy, the state, the economy, or even sexism. The 'civic' and 'political' order meant more families, more hospitals, more networks of the immediately repressive agencies that check fantasy, exploration, experience. The 'non-immediate social configuration' (Jacoby's useful term) which is the ground for all face-to-face relations of authority, whether of boss and worker, or of parent and child, was never theorised in Laing. The allusion to Marx and marxism was only one element in a roll-call of sundry thinkers who had, in very varied ways, stated the view that 'humanity is estranged from its authentic possibilities'.[52]

The insertion of some terminology drawn from marxism – an intellectual system with a massive stake in the analysis of the total social order – into an approach whose sole interest is in the dynamics of face-to-face groups does not suffice to constitute a synthesis. Laing is not a synthesiser so much as a collector and populariser of ideas from intellectually diverse quarters. It has often been pointed out, for example, that his coupling of psychoanalytic language (for which the unconscious is a clearly indispensable concept) with the project of a Sartrean intelligibility is methodologically suspect (since no Sartrean account of human motives can leave room for unconscious processes). Patch upon patchwork is Laing's record as a thinker: Sartre upon Freud, and then a scrap of Marx. Continuity lies not in his particular propositions, but in his repeated demand for 'life-in-relation' and for a place of sanctuary for the harassed soul.

It is to Laing's career in this provision of asylum and sanctuary that we must now turn. Apart from Laing's early experiment in the chronic schizophrenic ward in Scotland in 1955, the first therapeutic setting of a specifically Laingian kind appears to be 'Villa 21', a unit in the National Health Service mental hospital at Shenley, Hertfordshire, set up in 1962 by David Cooper. Forty-two patients under the age of 35 were treated on this ward (whose work terminated when the research project associated with it was wound up). Although the ward staff undertook considerable efforts to divest themselves of routinised institutional role-playing, Cooper felt that the hospital setting (and in particular the anxieties of senior staff outside the unit) generated coercive pressures upon the nurses which prevented the development of a patient: staff solidarity.[53] A more independent unit, free of institutional pressures of this kind, was clearly the next step. In 1965 the Philadelphia Association, a charitable trust chaired by Laing, and involving Cooper, Esterson and several other associates, obtained a five-year lease on Kingsley Hall, a former community centre in the East End of London. The Association acquired premises for other therapeutic group households both during and after the tenure of Kingsley Hall. By 1974 there were seven such communities in London, ranging in size from seven to 11 rooms. The Philadelphia Association took over an estate at Seaton, in Somerset, in late 1977 in order to found a farming and craft community with 'a balance of disturbed and undisturbed people'.[54] There have been other reports of centres for the exploration of psychotic experience on lines deriving from Laing's work: the Arbours Association, established as a dissident unit (after Kingsley Hall had closed) by some of his co-workers there who split with him, and some similar or parallel projects begun in the United States.[55] Differences in method or orientation make some of these collateral ventures hard to compare with Laing's work; but on Villa 21 and on some Philadelphia Association projects enough news is available to reach the beginnings of an evaluation.

One distinguishing feature of the Laingian group setting for schizophrenics or their befrienders follows naturally from the theory discussed earlier: all the partners of the community are encouraged to forego their usual social roles, and in particular those roles that fall along the hospital divide of 'staff' and 'patients'. A brochure put out by the Philadelphia Association stated:

> At Kingsley Hall everyone's actions could be challenged by anyone. With no staff and no patients – with the ultimate breakdown of the binary role system of the institution – no resident has been given by any other resident any tranquillisers or sedatives. Experience and behaviour which could not be tolerated in most family or psychiatric institutions made heavy but finally tolerable demands on the community.[56]

Similarly, progress was measured in Cooper's Villa 21 by the degree to which – in an admittedly incomplete way – the professional behaviour usually attaching to the position of psychiatrist or mental nurse was eliminated. It is true that some tranquillising drugs were administered, but a quarter of the patients received no tranquillisers at all. While the project began with a fairly structured regime, encompassing community meetings, small group meetings, 'family meetings consisting of a patient, his nuclear family and a therapist', organised work programme and occupational therapy, these structures were progressively abandoned in favour of a staff withdrawal from all tasks involving the supervision and 'treatment' of the patients. Dirt, disorganisation and unpredictable absences by certain patients inevitably followed; the staff re-imposed some controls while Cooper was away on holiday, but even this assertion of authority by rank-and-file staff can be seen as a 'de-centring' from the hegemony of the psychiatrist that is more usual in the mental institution.[57]

However, a de-centring is not the same as a de-structuring: and here there is some confusion in the work of Laing and the Laingians. For while staff and patients may have dropped their conventional roles in both Villa 21 and the Philadelphia Association communities, it by no means follows that they abandoned all roles and all structures. Laing and Cooper, after all, both argued that their community settings should be used to allow the open display of psychotic experience that is normally suppressed or repressed in the hospital; and the attentive acceptance of such episodes by the other members of the community clearly constitutes highly skilled and sophisticated role-performance. The 'family and milieu therapy' offered in Villa 21 (to quote the term used by Cooper, Esterson and Laing in reporting on the project) can only refer to a pretty definite set of arrangements. And Laing has admitted, in a conversation with the Italian psychiatrist Giovanni Jervis, that Kingsley Hall was unable to eliminate the problem of psychiatric violence, citing one incident in which a refractory member of the community was put inside a sack which was carefully tied up and left at the bottom of the stairs.[58]

Not everybody at Kingsley Hall found that there was 'no external structure, or authority, or formality to fall back on to decide if you ought to do anything';[59] others were clearly struck by the medical infrastructure of relationships in the communes.[60] 'It was cold, and it was an institution,' remarks a dissatisfied expatient of Villa 21, who also recalls of one of the Philadelphia Association's households:

> One or two people there were seen as being more responsible and capable. And there was a doctor, Dr Crawford, who was not supposed to be in control, but who was on call, and he *was* called. And we all knew him as Dr Crawford. He was a doctor so I called him 'Doctor'.[61]

Laing's recent insistence on his own medical role, where he has 'publicly stated, explicitly and repeatedly, that he is not an "anti-psychiatrist" but a physician and psychiatrist',[62] accords oddly with the earlier portrayal of a non-medical framework for the asylums he helped to institute. But there is nothing necessarily non-medical or anti-medical about Laing's methods in the handling of schizophrenia. True, he and his co-workers minimise the use of the drug treatments that almost all other practitioners employ; but to abstain from medication is potentially as valid a choice for a doctor as to administer a medicine.[63] Even the most extreme propositions of Laing on the course of psychosis have, in the demystified form in which they are at least sometimes offered, nothing intrinsically anti-medical about them; the model of a condition that will terminate itself if left to run its natural limits, and will only be worsened if the physician meddles with it, is an ancient but reputable concept in medicine, even if the tendency in our modern, technologically based therapies is to stress intervention almost as the rule of the healer's art. An explicit convergence between the treatments offered by mainstream psychiatry and some newer developments in Laing's own approach may be seen in the Philadelphia Association's plan for a farming and craft community to house its 'disturbed and undisturbed people'. Occupation in handicrafts and agriculture has, after all, been recommended by eminent psychiatrists as an indispensable therapy for mental patients from the age of Pinel to our own day.[64] It was always implausible to suppose that the inhabitants of a Laingian commune would do nothing with their time there except engage in psychic voyaging and the unravelling of double-binds.

In electing to stand on the terrain of medicine, Laing is asking to be assessed by the standards of natural-scientific enquiry. Like any other psychiatrist, he must expect his work to be judged by empirical studies on the subsequent fate of the persons he treats. From this standpoint, there are two major problems in evaluating Laing's practice. In the first place, there is a continuing uncertainty as to what this practice is. Some years ago, it was clear that he advocated the encouragement of a regression in which the patient is permitted 'to collapse back into an undifferentiated, unintegrated state',[65] presaging a reintegration into social living through a lawful sequence of stages. Mary Barnes, the most publicised example of this regressive method, was one of the first members of the Kingsley Hall commune, joining it in mid-1965 as the long awaited 'place where I could "go down" and grow up again'.[66]

It is remarkable that both Laing and his co-therapists who report on Kingsley Hall have concentrated on this single completed case of therapeutic regression. Information about other cases is scarce. In 1972 Laing told an American enquirer that 'I've known of only two or three such experiences that people have actually had through to completion. Otherwise, I've seen it in bits and pieces, here and there.'[67] A year later, answering an enquiry from a distraught husband as to what it was that got people out of psychotic episodes (the wife concerned having long overstayed Laing's own forecast in a destructive insanity that would end in her painful death through self-inflicted burns), he replied: 'I feel that I know that less than I did 20 years ago as a young doctor.'[68] The centrality for Laing of the method of emergence from psychosis laid down in his writings of the latter sixties must now be in some doubt; the years of practice have led not to a cumulation of evidence and theory but to a growing inconclusiveness. Secondly, the follow-up material provided for public scrutiny by Laingian centres is far from encouraging. When the 'Villa 21' experiment was being wound up, a report was published by Laing, Cooper and Esterson which claimed a relapse rate of only 17 per cent for patients discharged from the unit and followed up after one year.[69] The *British Medical Journal*, which published this report, devoted an editorial to it in the same issue, commenting that the particular index of relapse chosen in the study – namely, re-admission of the patient into mental hospital – is an administrative measure which may reflect the policies of psychiatrists rather than the patients' own state of mental health. G.M. Carstairs also pointed out, in a letter to the same journal, that an earlier study in Edinburgh on a sample of schizophrenic patients discharged from hospital had revealed a very similar one-year relapse rate (taking re-admission to hospital as the criterion again) to that shown in the 'Villa 21' report, and without the benefit of the 'systematic clarification and undoing' of 'schizogenic' family communication patterns offered by the Laingians.[70] Carstairs suggested that both the patients from 'Villa 21' and those from the Edinburgh sample were benefiting in a non-specific manner from an increased amount of personal attention rather than through any specific therapy, Laingian or other. The general tendency in British hospital policy towards schizophrenic illnesses since the time of that debate would suggest an even greater caution in the use of the re-admission rate as an index of health. If a patient is discharged from a mental hospital and subsequently is not readmitted, we should not conclude without further evidence that his or her mental condition has improved. The hospital may have believed that 'community care' facilities existed which were in fact absent; the patient may be barely surviving outside the hospital, or indeed may not have survived at all;[71] there may have been a cutback in hospital places even for serious emergencies; or the adminstrators of the institutions may be discouraging new entries as part of their ideology of de-hospitalisation.

The standard of reportage from the subsequent communities organised by Laingians is even more patchy. The Philadelphia Association's brochures have provided statistics for the persons entering and leaving the various households from year to year, with further details of their sex, age, length of stay and presence or absence of a previous psychiatric diagnosis or period of hospitalisation. For example, the 1974 brochure states:

> From June 1965 to September 1974, 316 people, 197 men and 119 women, have stayed in our households; of the 316, 142, 80 men and 62 women, have been psychiatric in-patients; of the 316, 288, 182 men and 62 women, have left.
>
> The usual length of stay has been between three months and one year; of the 288 who left, 29, all of whom had been psychiatric in-patients, 9 men and 20 women, have been back in hospital once, or more, since leaving, as far as we know.[72]

We can tell from these facts that the majority of the household's residents have no previous record of being in a mental hospital; but we cannot distinguish how many of the 288 leavers had been mental patients, nor whether mental patients tended to stay for longer in the households than the period of up to a year which is cited as the usual stay for all residents, nor whether residents with a 'schizophrenic' diagnosis tended to stay for longer, or to experience more re-hospitalisation, than others. Indeed, although the Association's articles specify that one of the primary purposes is 'to relieve mental illness of all descriptions, in particular schizophrenia',[73] there is no means of telling from the brochures whether its households are principally concerned with an alternative therapy for schizophrenia or with living arrangements for a more mixed group of normal, neurotic or diffusely disturbed people. The statistic which reports that a mere 29 of the residents have entered hospital again is encouraging at first sight, but we do not know how far Laing and his coworkers have succeeded in discovering any further information about the fate of their discharged residents. Institutions normally lose touch with the people who pass through and out of them, unless they enjoy special funding and staffing for follow-up work. Depending on whether the 29 re-hospitalised former patients represent 10 per cent or 50 per cent of those on whom the Association actually has some reliable later details, we would be to different degrees impressed or discouraged. Finally, we have no picture at all of the extent to which the Association's ex-residents, particularly those who entered its facilities as active schizophrenics, have been holding down jobs, hallucinating, landing up in prison or dying in obscure basements. The capacity to stay out of a mental hospital is no more than one indicator of sanity or survival.

Even with this extra information, it would still be hard to draw effective comparisons between Laing's methods and those of orthodox psychiatry. The medicine of the National Health Service is available, for what it is worth, to all comers; but it can be assumed that the Philadelphia Association's patients are drawn from a more educated stratum than that constituted by the general run of people with a severe mental illness. Laing's clientele is formed in part through a process of ideological self-selection which requires a prior exposure to his writings, if not from the patient personally then from some close contact who is wise to Laing and his ideas. Since the Association's practice is financed on a fee-for-service basis,[74] the middle-class character of its constituency will be further reinforced.

A much more serious uncertainty in judging the work of Laing and his associates lies in the very description of the schizophrenic career which they have offered to the public. The course of the illness and its recovery is presented as a two-stage process beginning with disintegration and culminating, after the climax of the first, regressive phase, in a restitutive journey towards an authentic self and a non-repressive relatedness towards others. The process may have its own agonies of detour and false dawning: but, once completed, the recovery of the essential person marks his or her entry into a 'kingdom of freedom' quite as distinct in individual history as the advent of the communist society is held to be in the marxist vision of emancipation in social history.[75] For anyone with a knowledge of severe mental illness and the fate of its victims, the only possible conclusion can be that Laing is talking about a 'schizophrenia' quite different from the range of the disorders encountered under that label by other practitioners. The course of schizophrenia as described by Laing for those patients who have been treated by his methods resembles only one type of schizophrenic career: the case of the acute psychotic episode, the long burst of delirium which clears up after its first appearance without any further sequel in the patient's life. A minority of schizophrenic cases has always presented this uncluttered outcome, even before the advent of modern phenothiazine drugs; and just as conventional psychiatrists, ignoring the possibility of a spontaneous remission, may ascribe their patient's recovery to the blessings of the pharmaceuticals industry,[76] so Laing may be boosting his own claims of success with the aid of a number of patients who in any case would have worked out their own salvation. But the majority of patients with a schizophrenic diagnosis do not display this once-and-for-all remission of symptoms. They continue, at varying intervals, to become disabled in their personal and work relationships and highly eligible for the mental-patient role. For the counsellor or befriender of the schizophrenic with a recurring state of illness, Laing's work appears as either misleading or irrelevant. 'Whoever he has been seeing, they are not our patients,' remarked Peggy Pyke-Lees, who as the general secretary of the National Schizophrenia Fellowship has for many years been in close touch with groups of relatives and patients from all over Britain.

It is true that, for Laing, the permanency of the schizophrenic career is a social artefact, the result of those repressive institutions that block the development of the acute phase from its native solution in the psychotic 'voyage', and instead launch the unfortunate patient into a lifetime's career of sedation and confinement.[77] But it is implausible to suppose that the great bulk of people who have to manage their own periodic outbreaks of schizophrenic illness only have to do so because they have not had the privilege of experiencing a spell of existential rebirth in one of the Philadelphia Associations's households.[78] The continuation of a psychotic illness cannot, in general, nowadays be ascribed to the repressive effects of the psychiatric hospitalisation or the 'chemical straitjacket' of neuroleptic drugs; for large numbers of relapsing schizophrenics have spent only a brief time in hospital, if they have had in-patient experience at all; and discontinuance of prescribed medication is extremely common (by up to one-third of patients, according to good evidence).[79]

Since Laing's early work in the Scottish Health Service, which accorded closely (as we have seen in the previous chapter) with the research concerns of mainstream social psychiatry, he has not published on the problems of management in chronic schizophrenic disorders. Owing to his single-minded focus on the phenomenology of certain aberrant but transient subjective states, he has contributed nothing on, for example, the type of work a disabled schizophrenic could be encouraged to undertake, nor on the strategies a relative or other co-resident of such a patient should try to adopt in order to minimise distress and relapse. Absent from Laing's work, and that of his co-workers, is any consideration of the 'extrinsic' handicaps – i.e. those which would operate even if the person were not ill – such as those arising from lengthy unemployment or lack of money. Nobody would guess from Laingian writing that a well-meaning therapeutic intervention can precipitate disaster in a vulnerable patient, even though this important fact has been publicised in the literature for some years. There seems to be a near-total oblivion in Laing, Cooper, Esterson and Berke to the amount of social pressure – not necessarily at a helpful level of intensity – involved in the organisation of a psychotic voyage with its train of attendants. The entry into and exit from the inner world of psychotic experience is said, in the classic Laingian case, to be 'as natural as death and giving birth or being born'.[80] But whatever is 'natural' in the ordeal of a psychotic episode is likely to be overlaid by many determinations of suggestion and expectation once it is undergone in the context of a Laingian commune. A reading of Mary Barnes's narrative of Kingsley Hall, or of Clancy Sigal's fictional but informed account of 'Meditation Manor' in *Zone of the Interior*, reinforces one's impression that the 'nature' of the Laingian psychosis is, in part, that of an elaborately staged artefact. We are left wondering whether it is always beneficial for patients to be inducted into a social network marked by such evident therapeutic zeal. The merit of the Philadelphia Association and its collateral bodies may, when some of the dust has settled, be seen as that of devising – in common with many projects both outside and within the publicly funded services – arrangements for housing psychiatric patients rather than for healing them. Meanwhile, those who involve themselves in work with schizophrenia sufferers will find Laing's romantic conception of a pristine, pre-social equilibrium formed in psychosis less useful than the dictum of John Wing: 'It should be clear that there is no such thing as a "natural history" in a disorder as reactive as schizophrenia.'[81]

5. Michel Foucault: The Anti-History of Psychiatry

For one venerable and still influential school of writing, the history of psychiatric treatment can be seen as a progressive unravelling of those anti-scientific errors which have stood in the way of a modern medical appreciation of the psychic calamities. Act One of the diagnostic psychodrama commences with the Dawn of Enlightenment, that point in Greek antiquity when Hippocrates attacked the view that epilepsy was a 'sacred' affliction and insisted that it was a naturally caused disease. Following Asclepiades' discovery of the Rest Cure (conducted so that the patients' internal atoms could be got to settle), the Alexandrian physician Soranus emphasised the doctor–patient relationship and Aretaeus drew attention to manic-depressive psychosis and the specifically senile states. The curtain then falls on the Dark Ages of Psychiatry, when magical explanations and witch-burning replace any clear understanding of the natural origins of psychosis. In the lengthy interlude, the distinguished Arab clinicians, Avicenna, Averroes and Rhazes, revive the organic traditions of Galen, and Johann Weyer in 1563 produces the first clinical descriptions of auditory hallucinations and persecutory ideas, as well as inventing the vaginal speculum and denouncing the witch-hunters' handbook *Malleus Maleficarum* with the demand that witches should be sent for medical treatment instead of being killed. His book is placed on the Index, and eclectic alliances between demonology and medicine continue to hold the stage until in the seventeenth century a new overture announces the Age of Reason. Despite a sudden entrance by King James I whose *Daemonologie* of 1597 is a superb plea for anti-psychiatry (in the form of witch-burning), Descartes, Hobbes and their fellow-rationalists produce a machine-like image of the human mind which triumphs over all supernatural explanations: in the epoch of mechanistic medicine, a misleading but necessary framework for the advent of the modern physiology of depression, all psychopathology is ascribed to commotions of the animal spirits, the nerve fibres or other tributaries of the central nervous system. The neuro-anatomical dissections of Thomas Willis (*Pathologiae Cerebri*, 1667) unseat the uterus as the causative organ of hysteria and, as the humours of antiquity are at last banished from the working of the body, the brain itself becomes progressively localised as the regulator of thought and emotion.

Meanwhile, in an obscure but significant subplot, a classification of disease, mental as well as physical, is being hatched, from the seventeenth to the eighteenth century, that will set the terms for the more scientific nosologies of the modern era. The celebrated seventeenth-century physician Thomas Sydenham recommends the subdivision of illnesses into determinate species according to the accurate procedure devised by botanists for the plant kingdom, and Linnaeus' own table of the *Genera Morborum* of 1733 – which includes 11 mental illnesses in the scheme of 325 distinct maladies – is only one episode in the march of the diagnostic schemata. The fruits of this prodigious labour of classification – the trances, passions, vapours, hypochrondriacal or hysterical distempers, vesaniae, syncopes, paraphrosynes and apoplexias, all marshalled under various degrees and orders – soon disappear from the psychiatrist's catalogue.[1] What remains for our subsequent history is only William Cullen's great category of neurosis, announced in 1769 and referring then to any disorder whatsoever of the mind, brain or nervous structure: that, and more importantly the very project of a standard psychiatric classification. This survives to the present in the constant revision of diagnostic manuals and inventories, as 'neurasthenia' slips in and out of the list of psychoneuroses available in the United Kingdom and 'homosexuality' ceases to be a personality disturbance for the Americans.

Meanwhile, within the eighteenth century, the scenes of current psychopathological interest have revolved from the clinical philosopher's interrogation of lunacy to the more sensational topical questions aroused by the treatment of the deranged, both in private and in public practice. King George the Third delivers his 'My lords, ladies and peacocks' oration to the opening of Parliament and is whisked off to be bled, blistered, strait-jacketed, knocked about, dosed with bark and saline, confined to Windsor Castle, and publicly debated in pamphlet and Parliamentary Committee – an airing which, while of doubtful benefit to His Majesty, assists in the establishment of psychiatry as a recognised medical profession. The mental illnesses and psychiatric confinements of Christopher Smart and William Cowper, and later of the Marquis de Sade and John Clare, effect a powerful charge of sympathy from the literary public to the plight of asylum inmates. The condition of the latter is suddenly improved, and a new therapeutic era of Moral Management ushered in, through a train of humane impulses converging from the Enlightenment and Revolution in France and from religious and secular liberalism in

Britain. In 1792 William Tuke joins forces with other Quakers to gather funds and support for the opening of the York Retreat, the mental hospital without bars or restraints that would become the exemplary asylum. In 1793 Philippe Pinel strikes the chains from the insane patients entrusted to his superintendence at the Bicêtre; in the words of a recent commentary, 'Pinel abolished brutal repression and replaced it by a humanitarian medical approach which in mid-nineteenth century culminated in the great English non-restraint movement and which made possible psychiatry as we know it today'.[2] A similar message was announced in the editorial Prospectus for the opening issue of *The Asylum Journal*, published by authority of the Association of Medical Officers of Asylums and Hospitals for the Insane in November 1853:

> From the time when Pinel obtained the permission of Couthon to try the humane experiment of releasing from fetters some of the insane citizens chained to the dungeon walls of the Bicêtre, to the date when Conolly announced that, in the vast Asylum over which he presided, mechanical restraint in the treatment of the insane had been entirely abandoned, and superseded by moral influence, a new school of special medicine has been gradually forming... Pinel vindicated the rights of science against the usurpations of superstition and brutality; and rescued the victims of cerebromental disease from the exorcist and the gaoler...
>
> The physician is now the responsible guardian of the lunatic, and must ever remain so, unless by some calamitous reverse the progress of the world in civilisation should be arrested and turned back in the direction of practical barbarism.

The nineteenth-century reforms in hospital management had a profound effect on the terms of diagnosis, by bringing thousands of fresh cases, ambulant and untrammelled by exterior fetters, within the gaze of the 'new school of special medicine'. Phrenology and mesmerism, false guides to the theories their discoverers claim, still disclose a route to the structures of the brain and the deeper unconscious. The way is now open for Kraepelin and Freud, the originators of modern concepts of psychosis and neurosis respectively, to chart the contemporary era of psychiatric medicine: the naming of dementia praecox follows from the isolation of dementia paralytica and persists, in the new shape of the schizophrenias, to the present day. Kraepelin also groups together the affective psychoses, carves out the psychogenic neuroses (an area soon to form the interface between psychoanalysis and medicine), promotes psychopathic personality from an afterthought to a species of disturbance, and reinforces an organic tradition of treatment whose continuation, in various chemical, electrical and surgical forms, we see in most clinics and hospitals today. After many long diversions and retrogressions, the torch of psychiatry is passed forth along the straight track of the modern diagnostic and curative science, earning the plaudits of the historian. One historical commentator has ventured a distant retrospect to the ancients of the discipline:

> It is interesting at this point to look back at the civilisation of ancient Greece and Rome, and see how long it took for the ideas of the great classical thinkers to be brought to fruition.
>
> Aesculapius developed a form of sleep-therapy... Hippocrates considered the brain the centre of mental activity... Plato's concept of the soul's struggle parallels Freud's descriptions... Aristotle's awareness of the potential for change and his image of a self-actualised person accords with Erich Fromm's description... Aretaeus antedates modern concepts of mental disease as an extension of normal personality traits...
>
> It has taken 2000 years for psychiatry and social consciousness to build up the courage to pick up the flag of awareness where the ancient great minds left it.[3]

The basic perspective of this variety of psychiatric history is, roughly speaking, liberal, evolutionist and sympathetic to modern diagnostic categories as the criterion of reality against which earlier discoveries are to be tested and found wanting. An alternative variant is to be found in the historiography of Richard Hunter and Ida MacAlpine for whom psychiatry as a distinct discipline from neurology is a sheer aberration, and history's punctuation marks are to be found in the clinical signs of extrapyramidal disorder or other neurological lesion, revealed in eighteenth-century verse or seventeenth-century portraitures: thus an illustration of a madman on the title-page of Burton's *Anatomy of Melancholy* is said to reveal 'abnormal arm and hand postures... associated with choreoathetosis'.[4]

Both varieties of institutional psychohistory treat the social past as a slope tending towards the medical present, which becomes the apex of all previous endeavours: an incomplete and provisional peak, to be sure, but one whose incompleteness does not mar the grand conception of the long ascent itself. This liberal, evolutionist history of psychiatry is distinguished by a special emphasis on the barbarism of past ages;

not only the cruel treatment of the insane at the hands of their keepers but also the persecution of the witches during the medieval period occupies a prominent place in the account.

In fact, the history of witchcraft and witch-hunting has only a very small overlap with the history of the mentally disturbed. Persecutory attitudes towards women, as well as to the old, the heretical and physically awkward, are much more incriminated in the medieval fever of the witch-hunt than is any specific hostility towards the insane, or any ignorance of the possibility of naturally caused disorder among the accused.[5] The mentally ill were involved in the witch-trials not primarily as defendants (those adjudged to be deluded were often removed from the court's jurisdiction) but as evidence of the witchcraft practised by others, since explanation of psychopathology was commonly cast in the terms of spirit possession.[6] Even James I, in his treatise of 1597 *Daemonologie*, did not deny the existence of 'Melancholie… folie and Manie' but claimed that witches behaved 'directly contrary to the symptoms of Melancholie'.[7] Yet the story that 'during the Witch Hunt of the Middle Ages the mentally disordered were engulfed in the flames of the Inquisition which swept Europe'[8] is repeated from text to text[9] as part of the self-congratulatory account of the march of progress from the *ancien régime* of lunacy to the Enlightenment brought by the therapeutic *philosophes*, and from thence to the modern Psychiatric Republic. Szasz,[10] indeed, has traced the witch-as-mental-patient theory from Esquirol and Pinel down to modern psychiatric historians like Zilboorg, Alexander, Selesnick, and Albert Deutsch, and has convincingly refuted it. As he observes, horror stories from the past serve to make the present condition of the mentally ill somewhat more palatable. If we have so little to boast about in the overcrowded back wards, with the lockers that are all the patient's privacy placed only a few feet from one another, we can at least hark back and congratulate ourselves that blood-letting, fetters and the stake have gone out of fashion.

Against the complacencies of the uncritical medical chronicle of psychiatry, a number of rival accounts, explicitly composed as formal history or implicit within the formulation of a theory, have made an appearance in recent years. Not every critique of psychiatric diagnosis involves historical analysis. Thus, while Thomas Szasz contends that the history of psychiatry 'is largely the account of changing fashions in the theory and practice of psychiatric violence, cast in the self-approbating idioms of medical diagnosis and treatment',[11] he locates the causality of this violence in the age-long urge of man to seek a victim by making the

Other into an outcast. The mental patient just happens to be the latest representation of 'the perennial scapegoat principle', replacing the Jew, the witch and the black slave in a long line of persecution. When Szasz states that the modern 'mental health movement' is the Inquisition in a new disguise, he contests the orthodox psychiatric history not by an alternative history of events but by an historical transposition of motives from one epoch to another, making social institutions into the mere bearers of a timeless impulsion which is 'basic to man's social nature'.[12] Similarly, in another passage, the evils of diagnosis in psychiatry are ascribed to the logic of classification, which is appropriate for the natural sciences but when applied to human beings can only be designed for the constraint and control of their behaviour.[13] No events actually occurring in the world are of consequence for this stricture on diagnosis, which is invalidated in virtue of its logical character as a classificatory action.

With an equally unhistorical bent, Laing's critique of diagnosis rests, not on an incrimination of any determinate part of the medical project, but on a conviction that all human categorisation, all subdivision of the '*prima materia* of the given' in experience is a splitting 'from the stuff of our original selves': the violent enterprises of psychiatry, with its electroshock and surgery, are used 'only if the *normal social* lobotomy does not work' (italics in the original),[14] and the 'knot' that is tied 'round the throat, as it were, of the whole human species' was placed there not by psychiatry but by an age-long habit of attributing good and bad qualities to one's fellows.[15]

But so lofty and ahistorical a vantage point on psychiatry is far less common in the literature than the attempt to construct a counter-history of psychiatry, where the present diagnostic era is contrasted either with past alternatives or with other possible approaches. Foremost among these is the prodigious work of Michel Foucault: a vast and dense enterprise begun with a provocative history of insanity in 1961,[16] broadened into a reconstruction of general medical practice in 1963,[17] revised further in a methodological text six years later,[18] and more recently extended from the exclusion of the mentally sick to the exclusion and incarceration of the criminal classes, in a resounding book on the origins of prisons.[19]

It may, in fact, be argued that there is little or no connection between Foucault's more recent output and the usual project of history writing as an attempt to reach 'the truth of the past'. He is now a self-proclaimed dealer in fictions, seemingly unconcerned with accuracy and evidence. As a moraliser and critic for our own time, he analyses the 'discourses' of the past solely in order to uncover our present-day strategies of power and manipulation. Such, at any rate, is the persuasive reading of

Foucault offered recently by Allan Megill, who is at pains, however, to single out *Madness and Civilization* as the one, of all Foucault's works, which stands closest to a genuine historical endeavour.[20]

Other interpreters of Foucault still see his later work as a very high level sort of historiography, focusing on 'the general signification of the history of particular forms of rationality and scientificity'.[21] But we must confine our attention to his admittedly historical version of the uses of insanity and its institutions, summarising and quoting from the somewhat shortened English edition.[22] In it, no interest is shown in the medicine and psychiatry of antiquity or the Arab Enlightenment: we begin with the Middle Ages, at a point where the scourge of leprosy is beginning to regress, leaving behind it a host of vacant lazarhouses in all the countries of Europe. Over the succeeding epochs, the psychic and material structures of shame and horror formerly applied by society to the leper will be awoken and exercised afresh on the poor, the criminal and the 'deranged minds'. The leprosaria themselves, 'from the fourteenth century… would wait, soliciting with strange incantations a new incarnation of disease, another grimace of terror, renewed rites of purification and exclusion' (p. 3).

The beginnings of the new ban on insanity occur before the Age of Reason itself. We see it in the late Middle Ages and the Renaissance, where the mad are packed away on 'ships of fools' and made into an object-lesson for the public by ironists like Cervantes and tragedians like Shakespeare. Folly is no longer of permanent human significance, something that is true for all, like sin or vice; still less is it a symbol of cosmic disorder, the 'witches' sabbath of nature' that is portrayed by Bosch and other painters of monstrosity as an analogue of God-sent doom. The mad of Renaissance literature are already tamed by a secular, moralising focus on their individual misfortunes: and before long madness will lose even this qualified licence to stand and rave in public. In what Foucault terms 'the classical age' of bureaucratic rationality in the seventeenth century (the French title of his work is *L'Histoire de la folie à l'âge classique*), there takes place *le grand renfermement des pauvres*, the 'Great Confinement' in which, in the main countries of Europe, not only the poor but the wandering insane are swept from the streets and hedgerows and locked away in special institutions: the *Hôpital Gènèral* in Paris and 32 provincial cities, the Zuchthaus or house of correction typical of Germany, the workhouses and bridewells of England. The insane are caught up in a general proscription of idleness and beggary (though, inside the houses of confinement, they are still rendered into a spectacle for the visiting public to come and peep at). They are caged but not treated, or even diagnosed. The rigid, sectarian rules of the institution express for Foucault the triumph of Reason over its vanquished, controlled opposite: 'here, order no longer freely confronted disorder, reason no longer tried to make its own way among all that might evade or seek to destroy it.'

> Here reason reigned in the pure state, in a triumph arranged for it in advance over a frenzied unreason. Madness was thus torn from that imaginary freedom which still allowed it to flourish on the Renaissance horizon. Not so long ago, it had floundered about in broad daylight: in *King Lear*, in *Don Quixote*. But in less than half a century, it had been sequestered and, in the fortress of confinement, bound to Reason, to the rules of morality and their monotonous nights. (p. 64)

The origins of psychiatric diagnosis are traced by Foucault in other manifestations of seventeenth-century and eighteenth-century 'classical thought'. Within the institutions of confinement, incarceration rather than therapy is the rule; but outside them, in the medicine of private practice, a mechanistic, manipulative therapeutics brings to bear upon deranged patients a whole range of violent, exterior methods which seem to form the forerunner to modern electro-shock treatment and psychosurgery. The demented are dosed with iron filings, purged through the injection of scabies and the ingestion of vinegar, dipped into cold or hot baths, and (more leniently) subjected to the undulations of sea travel. Because the madman's 'subjectivity' is seen, in the classical age, as containing nothing but unmixed error, a non-psychological treatment is inflicted on him.

But, terrible as are the depredations wrought upon the bodies and minds of patients by classical rationalism, it is not until the very late eighteenth and the early nineteenth century, during the very epoch favoured in psychiatric history as the seedbed of progressive trends in therapy, that the worst and most thorough expulsion of the mental deviant occurs. Pinel and the Tukes, in different but parallel ways, replace the fetters and bars of the old madhouses by the closed, sealed order of an asylum system founded on a 'gigantic moral imprisonment' (p. 278), that of the medical superintendence of insanity. In the York Retreat and Pinel's Bicêtre, which were to become the exemplars for the most advanced mental institutions of their time, the patients are subjected to a continual scrutiny and judgement from their keepers and doctors; in this latest age of reason, madness is allowed no voice of its own, except in the marginal instance of the mad artist or philosopher, the Van Gogh or Artaud or Nietzsche; for the mass of the insane, medical science in the asylum relies not on specific diagnoses or therapy but on the authority of the doctor's personage, an authority expressing the power structure of the society outside. The institution is

> a microcosm in which were symbolised the massive structure of bourgeois society and its values: Family-Child relations, centred on the theme of paternal authority; Transgression-Punishment relations, centred on the theme of immediate justice; Madness-Disorder relations, centred on the theme of social and moral order. It is from these that the physician derived his power to cure. (p. 274)

Foucault argues that the Pinel-Tuke medical model of confinement for the insane persists to the present day. A number of authors have taken *Madness and Civilization* as a text of decisive importance for the understanding of psychiatric history down to modern times. The theory that mental institutions evolved as a psychological replacement for the long-vanished leper hospitals has been repeated rather uncritically,[23] even though in Europe the old asylum buildings had earlier been monasteries, almshouses or military buildings rather than leprosaria; and in America a whole gamut of total institutions – penitentaries, workhouses, orphanages and reformatories, as well as insane asylums – were constructed during the Jacksonian period as part of a general ideology of correction through confinement that owed nothing to the ancient lazar-house.[24] And, while the seventeenth and eighteenth centuries do evidently form a turning-point in the extension of bureaucratic and bourgeois rationality over the insane and other deviants, it is illegitimate to conclude, as some marxist readers of Foucault have done, that 'mental illness is a "new" feature of the beginning of capitalism'[25] or that 'houses of confinement for the insane first appeared on a significant scale during the late seventeenth century in response to the need to eliminate the main source of political and social unrest in the period.'[26] The mentally afflicted, viewed as 'ill' within a medical framework, had been confined in custody or therapy for centuries before the 'Great Confinement' in Europe. The well-off insane, from antiquity down to modern years, were cooped up in their relatives' homes, often receiving specialised (if ill-considered) medical attention. Well before the seventeenth century, various hospitals had accommodation to care for the insane, and historians are beginning to unearth detailed records kept by some of these.[27] The nation-wide chain of special charitable hospitals for the mentally ill in Spain – a society hardly likely to be touched by the spirit of an enveloping rationalism – dates from the pre-bourgeois fifteenth century, even before the unification accomplished by Ferdinand and Isabella.[28] For Spain, too, the invocation of population pressures to explain the herding of the indigent into asylums will hardly work, since the number of Spaniards dropped by a third, as a result of epidemics, between 1365 and 1497.[29] Medieval or late medieval psychiatric history is now much superior to Foucault's hazardous hints about such practices as 'the ship of fools' which never actually existed.[30] From a large variety of medieval literary, legal and scientific sources, we now have evidence of the highly medical – indeed, crudely physiological – view of mental illnesses that was current in pre-rationalist Europe.[31] Both in the domestic management of the insane and in the charitable hospitals, as well as in the private madhouses, which are documented for England as far back as the early seventeenth century,[32] a medical tradition based in large part on an exterior, mechanical intervention upon a passive patient has been passed on from one century to another.

For the fate of the demented sufferer has been, in certain typical modes of care, unchanging over successive epochs and modes of production. He or she was placed under the domination of other, superior persons, within the confines of an obscure cubicle whose interior scarcely interested the general public; here he or she was always the prey to faddist remedies, inflicted sometimes harmlessly and sometimes brutally upon a prostrate but living body and on a mind whose consent was rather rarely elicited. Others, the chronically disordered of their day, were left variously to rove or to rot, in the public space of Skid Row or in the back wards of silent institutions. Foucault's (and Rosen's) suggestion that there ever was a historical period in which Reason engaged in an equal dialogue with Unreason is a useful counterpoint to our modern ways of dismissing the insane; but is unlikely to sample any further behaviour from the past than that of an intelligentsia, which has always preferred to toy with 'madness' as a literary or artistic spectacle rather than to rearrange society's dealings with the common insane, who live outside the safe distance of a poem, a tract or a painting.

Thus, in his time, King George III was bled repeatedly by his keepers, as was the mental patient in the seventeenth, sixteenth and previous centuries back to the time of Galen. 'When the whole body abound with melancholike bloud, it is best to begin the cure with letting of bloud, and you must cut the lyver vein of the arme', writes the physician and surgeon Philip Barrough in 1583,[33] and adds 'of the frenisie' that 'if he be riche let servauntes hold him, if poore, bind him, for inordinate moving deminisheth strength'. Bleeding was a psychiatric panacea for all the major forms of mental illness (phrenitis, melancholia and mania) right through the Dark Ages and the early Middle Ages;[34] this most organic of therapies received a further final impetus in the butcheries perpetrated by the founder of American psychiatry, Benjamin Rush (whose practice amounted to 'the almost complete exsanguination' of his patients),[35] and in the less complete but still flagrant cuppings and leechings that went on well into the 1830s.[36]

The washing of the shaven head with vinegar is similarly described by Foucault as a sovereign remedy typical of 'classical' rationalism's rituals of purification on the insane; yet the pre-rationalist use of vinegary purgations on the scalp can be exemplified from the psychiatric sections of the thirteenth-century scientific encyclopaedia *De Proprietatibus Rerum*, circulated from manuscripts by the friar Bartholomaeus Anglicus, translated into English in 1495, and reaching a wide audience through repeated editions across Europe in the next century of printing. In the words of a sixteenth-century English edition of Bartholomaeus, 'the medycyne is... that in the begynnynge the pacyentes heed to be shaven; and washed in lukewarm vynegre, and that he be well kepte or bounde in a darke place'.[37] Purgatives and other evacuants of the digestive system are recommended for the mentally ill over all the aeons of psychiatric medicine from the Byzantine to the bourgeois – Jackson (1972) quotes the early medieval reliance on Oribasius, the Byzantine Galenist purger; Skultans (1975) is good on Victorian vomitants and laxatives; and Hunter and MacAlpine (1963) ease us along the intervening therapeutic epochs with 27 references to evacuant methods. In all this long psychiatric exploration of the gut, both the diagnostic system for the classification of the illnesses and the accepted causal framework for their explanation was, of course, changing several times over.

The form of shock treatment which is achieved by ducking the patient in cold water was another treatment founded in antiquity, which enjoyed a special revival in the seventeenth and eighteenth centuries,[38] well before its introduction as a punitive measure in the mental hospital of Pinel's tradition. As it forms an important topic in Foucault's case, we shall return to the matter later. Even the 'rotatory machine' of the early nineteenth century, on which the melancholic was centrifuged into oblivion by a purely mechanical effect, was given a very similar rationale in the early form (the whirling chair) devised by Arab medicine for posterity: Avicenna (in the eleventh century) had recommended its use in melancholia 'to direct the blood into the proper parts'.[39] It is a pity that Foucault insists (pp. 182–83) that the rotatory method in psychiatry expresses a philosophy distinctive to the years following the arrival of the Age of Reason.

What is particularly striking about the long history of psychiatric medicine is its capacity to produce quite different rationalisations for a relatively constant practice. Foucault's infatuation with the terms of each stage in therapeutic logic – an indulgent reconstruction, which sometimes goes well past the evidence of available texts – does not form a patient's-eye-view of psychiatry so much as a doctor's account of what, in any particular epoch, he thought he was doing.

From the ancients to the moderns, the constancy and continuity of mechanistic medical practice is evident. What innovations there are have come in technique or in the hardware of technology rather than in basic method; from the douche of cold water we move to the plunge of electro-shock, from trepanning to psychosurgery, from the chemical correction of humoral imbalances to the inhibition or stimulation of nervous action. Even the immeasurable leap from the consolations of philosophy or religion to the insights of psychotherapy takes place within the long trajectory of mechanical medicine, so long as it remains in a mere juxtaposition with treatments designed to influence physiology directly. Foucault's critique of the psychiatric cure of classical rationalism as 'a series of partial destructions, in which psychological attack and physical intervention are juxtaposed, complement each other, but never interpenetrate' (p. 178) can be extended forward to the eclectic pills-and-sympathy dualism of contemporary mainstream therapy. But it applies with equal force to the psychiatric epoch of antiquity which Foucault never examines as an adequate baseline for his comparisons. In the version of medico-social dualism practised, for instance, by Soranus of Alexandria, verbal interaction (in the form of cheerful chat and the admonitions of philosophers) takes its place next to such mechanical modalities as bleeding (yet again), fasting, mild rotation (in a hammock or sedan), careful diet and suitable anointing.[40]

The continuities of the mechanical tradition form neither an unfolding tale of progress (as in the liberal-evolutionist history) nor the irruption of a bureaucratic rationalism into a preceding Golden Age of permissiveness towards insanity (as one is tempted to conclude from Foucault). As measures directed towards suffering patients, they can be performed well or badly, in scientific as well as humanitarian terms. But the record of their insertion into successive historical epochs does not match the rise and fall of class relationships in different modes of production or contrasting political systems. The medical attitude has its own autonomy, deriving from the craft of the physician and surgeon: its Age of Reason occurred, to be sure, in the hey-day of bourgeois rationality, but it also flourished earlier in the societies of Mediterranean antiquity that founded the craft in the West, as well as in the imperial civilisation of China with its distinct and lengthy lineage of medical and scientific rationalism. Within the appalling alternatives offered by vulgar marxism, medicine – including psychiatric medicine – constitutes neither base nor superstructure. It is a separate instance of the domination of mental over manual labour, undertaken as part of the conditions of any society's reproduction.

As a social art, it is subordinate to class ideologies and institutions of whatever epoch. As applied science, it moves within the theory–practice web of experimental method whose long-term role is to improve the implements of production. We can speak of the emancipation (never, doubtless, complete) of psychiatry *from* ideology: to regard psychiatry only *as* ideology is to detach it from its relation to the history of science, or else to fall into a larger relativist trap of science-as-ideology, which means denying all the conquests of experimental reasoning.

Foucault's critique of psychiatric history is a welcome alternative to the complacencies of the evolutionist account, and an antidote to that tempting empiricism which documents the birth of medical facts as the virgin offspring of pure sense, without parentage in the evolving structures of reason. Even in *The Birth of the Clinic*, his later, rather skimpy account of the ideological roots of medical research in the eighteenth and nineteenth centuries, Foucault asks a number of searching questions about two sorts of methodological inadequacy: the ludicrous mis-observations of these empiricist pioneers in their approach towards the ascertaining of physiological facts; and the flaws in any history of medical discovery which views the record primarily as one of good, bad or indifferent data collection. Rosen[41] and more recently Hay[42] have produced serious exposures of the limitations of an empiricist or Lockean method in the evolution of medical and psychiatric ideas. An awareness of the medico-philosophical rationales (or rationalisms), that precede and structure observation in any epoch, is clearly necessary. But, in *Madness and Civilization*, Foucault incriminates, not so much one method of reasoning against another, but Reason as against Unreason (or madness). This identification of Reason as the true author of psychiatric discovery, the principal jailer of deviants and foremost instigator of capitalist values becomes, paradoxically, enclosed within the very rationalism he denounces. In his account, the remedies and institutional measures against insanity seem to take their origin from the logic of certain medical or scientific ideas, which are too often seen divorced from concurrent social pressures. As another eminent historian of the asylum has put it:

> The explanation here is so caught up with ideas that their base in events is practically forgotten. Reason acts as an independent

> force, seeking victory for its own purposes. Foucault, to be sure, states that the asylum is an expression of bourgeois morality... But such a declaration does not in itself link ideas and the society in a convincing way. Ultimately in *Madness and Civilization* the goals of the asylum are purely intellectual; the combat is between perceptions and visions, not classes. Foucault's institutions bear only a slight relation to the society that built and supported them.[43]

These strictures are perhaps a little sweeping: the account in *Madness and Civilization* of the seventeenth-century 'Great Confinement' is indeed grounded in the contemporary economic conjuncture of wage reduction and multiplying vagrancy, as well as in the secularisation of attitudes to poverty and – more dubiously – in the age-long 'social sensibility' of banishment that had hounded the lepers (pp. 45–49).[44] But Foucault's overwhelming concern with the logic of 'classical' (i.e. seventeenth-century) diagnosis overlooks some of the older, subterranean traditions of psychiatry, which always functioned as a minority option for some of the mentally ill during the darkest ages of exclusion for the great bulk of the insane. The relation of psychiatry to social and economic imperatives is visible less in the internal logic of diagnosis than in the differing classes and roles of patients that become available to psychiatric inspection over successive epochs of the organisation of medical care. The psychiatry of public assistance is kept going over centuries in the charitable institutions of Christendom; the psychiatry of 'management' and medical domination (for example, through the doctor's 'catching the eye of the madman') will be established in private madhouses and the domestic regimen of wealthy patients shortly before it is extended to the public asylum of the Tuke-Pinel era, as is obvious from several of the eighteenth-century excerpts in Hunter and MacAlpine's anthology.[45] We must try to remember that the evolution of the medical model of intervention against insanity and the development of the total psychiatric institution have somewhat separate histories. When the asylum for the specialised catchment of the insane is founded, it is in response to a broader sanitary movement that includes paupers and criminals within the orbit of state-guided correction; and, as well as investing the physician-superintendent as the custodian of bourgeois values, it will receive madness from the secular arm of capitalism's correctional institutions, medicalising its definition in accordance with ancient maxims and remedies which becomes available, for the first time, on a mass scale.

The first 'Great Confinement', that of European absolutism, removed or reduced the charitable role of medieval Christendom and swept the indigent insane out of the mainstream of medical practice. (English Tudor rule, as Wallerstein[46] reminds us, was less successful and less centralised in its projects of pauper control.) The second 'Great Confinement', that produced by the medically based asylum over the course of the nineteenth century, follows a path more ambiguous than that narrated by Foucault. By the latter part of the century, the transition to the custodial barracks for insanity was complete, and medical authority had lost anything but the semblance of therapeutic interest for the vast mass of long-stay inmates contained within the buildings which still form the tangible infrastructure for society's disposal of its chronic failures. But the coming of the late nineteenth-century asylum amounted to a negation of the Pinelian institutional ideals as well as its bureaucratised continuance. The part accorded to industrial occupation in the management of the patient's daily life – evident in all the documents of the Tuke-Pinel renaissance[47] – restored to the mentally sick a sheltered position within a national community founded on industry, as some kind of recompense for their loss of status in the now-eroded village society. The motifs of fear and surveillance that are visible in the writings of the founders of Moral Management are still subordinate to other, more therapeutic goals; and in the case of the most eminent British physician associated with this trend, John Conolly, are discounted in favour of principles of treatment that have scarcely been improved in all the succeeding epochs of vanguard practice: the involvement of friends of the patient in treatment; the proper training of hospital attendants; the foundation of a domiciliary service in which the majority of the mentally ill would receive solely out-patient care from a visiting doctor or nurse.[48]

But from Conolly's heritage, as from other, less enlightened Moral Managers, far more was bequeathed in the way of precept than in practice. Through the vast ingathering of the pauper lunatics that took place in mid-century, in both Britain and the United States, the small model hospital was turned into a teeming asylum-barracks without medical content. In 1831, for example, Hanwell Asylum for Middlesex County was opened as a small institution of 300 beds; Conolly joined it in 1839 as Superintendent, and there pioneered his principles of non-restraint. By 1846 it had expanded to over 900 places; the local justices wanted to double even this, but Conolly warned that 'individualised patient care' was already wearing thin and would become impossible. To house the overspill of the insane from London's workhouses or private asylums, the county constructed a further thousand-bed institution at Colney Hatch; by 1897, its patient-complement was 2585.[49] In America, identical custodial pressures from local State authorities in the 1840s and 1850s were compounded by the dumping of foreign-born (especially Irish) patients, victims of the stresses of migration and urbanisation. Pioneer Tukean institutions like the Bloomingdale Asylum of New York were now filled with overcrowded chronic wards, becoming indistinguishable from the public asylums with their heavy load of jail-hardened deviants.[50]

Doctrines of moral management and the momentum of therapeutic zeal inevitably gave way to theories of the incurability of mental derangement, the hereditary predisposition to insanity, and the special psychiatric vulnerability of social groups held in disfavour by different medical authors: Irish and blacks in the United States, the lower classes generally in Britain.[51] In psychiatry, as in politics generally, the nineteenth century sees a betrayal of the individualist ideals of the bourgeois revolution by a statism deriving from the requirements of a later stage of capital growth. Foucault misses this movement, having been captured by the concept of a timeless bourgeois rationality which seeks the control of rebellious Unreason quite outside the complex of social contradictions characteristic of different periods.

We have reason to take Foucault's own self-criticisms very seriously; there is evidence that he has forsworn some of the larger, trans-historical ambitions of *Madness and Civilization*. More recently, he has remarked that in this book 'one was still close to admitting an anonymous and general subject of history', and he has satirically repudiated the quest, explicitly undertaken in *Madness and Civilisation*, 'to reconstitute what madness might be, in the form in which it first presented itself to some primitive, fundamental, deaf, scarcely articulated experience'.[52] However, despite its many provocative and dazzling insights, the ethos canvassed in this particular early work of Foucault's has accorded all too well with the glorification of mania and the dismissal of scientific logic that were fashionable during the mass cult of 'anti-psychiatry' in the latter 1960s. More recently, the scholarly achievement of Foucault's later scrutiny of institutional medicine, *The Birth of the Clinic*, has been rendered into an important weapon of Ivan Illich's polemical armoury, attacking the scale of modern medical provision.[53] In the latter case, Foucault can be validly dissociated from his following; he has written expressly that the book 'has not been written in favour of one kind of medicine as against another kind of medicine, or against medicine and in favour of an absence of medicine'.[54] *The Birth of the Clinic* does not moralise on the historical attitudes it discloses, in sharp contrast to the tenour of its anti-psychiatric predecessor, where every development in the therapy of the mentally ill is denounced as a fresh addition to Reason's despotism.

An elaborate case is mounted by Foucault, for, example, against Pinel's use and advocacy of cold water shock treatment for the insane. It is admitted that cold immersion was an ancient nostrum, dating from antiquity and the Middle Ages; water has been credited with properties of inward purification which long antedates the Age of Reason. All the same, in Pinel's time the application of water 'could no longer be anything but mechanical'. It is the sudden shower of cold water on the head, or the plunge into the surprise bath, that becomes 'the favoured technique' in preference to the milder ablutions or the mere drinking of water practised in earlier regimens. Esquirol's description of the rough methods in vogue at Charenton hospital is retailed: 'the sufferer came down the corridors to the ground floor, and arrived in a square vaulted room in which a pool had been constructed; he was pushed over backwards and into the water' (pp. 167, 172). Moreover, Pinel's punitive use of the cold douche marks 'the conversion of medicine into justice, of therapeutics into repression' since it is employed as a regular coercive measure against work-shy or refractory patients. The Pinelian asylum is a courtroom and guardhouse recognising the permament culpability of its inmates; 'moral treatment' is in this context a sly expression for punishment, and the cold water jet baptises the madman into a thorough subordination unknown in previous therapeutic eras (pp. 266–67).

But the ducking of the demented was not a modern invention: Foucault himself cites instances of its occurrence from the period before the Revolution as well as in van Helmont's seventeenth-century euphemism of 'hydro-therapy'. Although he attaches a special significance to its discovery or revival in the Age of Reason, we have here another element of continuity with medieval practice. The following is a description of a traditional English water treatment long in vogue over various parts of rural Cornwall:

> In our forefathers' days, when devotion as much exceeded knowledge, as knowledge now cometh short of devotion, there were many bowssening places for curing of madmen… The water running from St Nunn's well fell into a square and close walled plot, which might well be filled at what depth they listed. Upon this wall was the frantic person set to stand, his back towards the pool, and from thence with a sudden blow in the breast tumbled headlong into the pond, where a strong fellow, provided for the nonce, took him and tossed him up and down, alongst and athwart the water… but

if there appeared small amendment he was bowssened again and again, while there remained in him any hope of life for recovery.[55]

Here the similarity with Esquirol's administration of the 'surprise bath' at Charenton appears almost uncanny (down to the prescription that the sufferer stand with his back to the water). However, Pinel himself is far from being another inheritor of the long tradition of aquatic shock treatment. He is at pains in his *Treatise* to insist that the therapy of immersion is of extremely limited applicability: 'The real utility of bathing in maniacal disorders remains yet to be ascertained,' while the bath of surprise 'however successful in some instances might in others be extremely dangerous, and… can only be resorted to in cases almost hopeless and where other remedies are ineffectual.'[56] He lauds cold water shock not as a medical prescription, for there are 'numberless inconveniences attaching to this practice,'[57] but as a simple measure of coercion in the maintenance of order. Therapy and repression are seen as distinct, not confounded or substituted in the way that Foucault suggests. It is the greater good of the institutional community, not the personal benefit of the patient, that guides the physician's hand on the cold water tap.

We may indeed deplore Pinel's recommendation of a method so easily misunderstood as a mystifying therapy. But in *Madness and Civilization*, he is given as little credit for his less punitive endeavours. Like the English pioneers of moral treatment, Pinel was convinced of the value of 'interesting and laborious employment' in the management of the insane: 'I am very sure that few lunatics, even in their most furious state, ought to be without some active occupation.'[58] But industrial therapy for the mentally ill is mentioned by Foucault only as a capitalistic exaction, and even the sheltered, agrarian work programme of the Saragossa asylum hymned in the *Treatise on Insanity*[59] is rendered into a tyrannous celebration of a forced order 'in which nature is mediatized by morality' (pp. 196–97). It is hard to know what to make of the incessant demand in *Madness and Civilization* that Reason should proceed to establish some 'dialogue' with Unreason; for the terms of dialogue apparently exclude any ascription of responsibility, in the form of blame or punishment, from the sane to the insane, as well as any reintegration of psychiatric patients into an industrial, economic role. Dialogue has to be restored also without the mediation of psychotherapy, which is seen as the twentieth century's own extension of moral-medical authority over the victims of diagnosis. 'To the doctor, Freud transferred all the structures Pinel and Tuke had set up within confinement'; and 'focussed upon this single presence… all the powers that had been distributed in the collective existence of the asylum' (pp. 278, 277).[60] In passages like this Foucault is playing a game against psychiatry in which the opponent is allowed no chance of scoring points.

We do not insist on Fair Play for Psychiatry purely out of an abstract spirit of good 'gamesmanship'. The goal of a dialogue with unreason that has been sketched by Foucault is an admirable one. Unlike Foucault, however, we propose that it actually be implemented, through specific transformations in the structures – social, political, economic and therapeutic – of latter-day capitalism and (in the case of Russia and Eastern Europe) state capitalism. The restoration of society's dialogue with its unreasonable members cannot take place other than through a concrete and historical critique of social practice and through the parallel evolution of political programmes designed to maximise the acceptance of the mentally ill in work and social intercourse. The mobilisation of the mentally ill (at periods when they are well enough to act publicly) as well as of their friends, relatives and partners in treatment, forms an indispensable part of this dialogue, which cannot exclude medicine from the range of material that it must encounter and transcend. The character and course of mental illnesses is nowadays shaped irrevocably by medical intervention. One central task of a radical political programme for the mentally ill is to enable them to appraise and select the judgements of the medically qualified (for example, over chemical therapies or spells of hospitalisation) rather than to confirm their own passivity by obedience to the doctor's writ. The blanket dismissal of 'the medical model' by anti-psychiatric writers and practitioners renders impossible the intelligent discrimination of medicine by its consumers; the chronic or recurrent sufferer from a schizophrenic illness, for instance, has to learn to manage a disability that may be accentuated by the wrong drugs, relieved by correct medication, compounded by unwanted side-effects and variously enlarged or reduced by social relationships such as those with a nurse, a relative, an employer, the police or a social security official. There is no primal Arcady into which mental patients can slip, away from modern institutions of care and intervention. If they slip anywhere away from it all, it will be into the gutter or the graveyard.

Dialogue with unreason is possible, and necessary, on terms fairly similar to the dialogue of society with other handicaps and misfortunes. The 'lucid intervals' characteristic of most mental infirmities indeed distinguish them from the conditions of permanent communicative handicap, such as deafness, sclerosis or terminal coma. 'The key,' writes one chronic schizophrenic patient of his own career, 'lies in how I think of myself when I am well.'[61] The mythology of madness which is canvassed by many psychiatrists as well as by anti-psychiatrists has the unfortunate effect of reinforcing a blanket judgement whereby mad people, saintly or awkward, persecuted or treated, are seen as mad all the time. Foucault never presents an intelligible account of any particular psychological syndrome. We are invited to reflect on a number of distressing and unsatisfactory cultural stereotypes of insanity, and then to enter into a human relationship with these unfortunate figments of past or present diagnosis. It is true that the demolition of inaccurate stereotypes may be a preliminary to real dialogue, but we are left without much of a clue how to proceed after Pinel, Tuke and Freud have done their worst.

To reject Foucault's anti-psychiatric romanticism is not to endorse the liberal Public-Relations history of mental medicine. The virtues of the non-restraint and moral-management schools were largely negative, in undoing the havoc of age-long persecution wrought on the bodies and minds of the mentally infirm. By their proclamation of the unique benefits of seclusion away from the normal community in an enclosed and special environment – an emphasis stemming directly from the crude Associationist psychology of the Locke-Hartley school – the most influential founders of modern psychiatry lent a potent impetus to the long and baneful tradition which would, for decade after decade down to our own modernity, regard the removal of the mental patient from his own familiar surroundings into a hospital setting as the treatment of first resort. So long as their emphasis on medical surveillance and dominance was combined with an active and varied regimen for manageable numbers of patients, even their class-divided, paternalistic institutions produced therapeutic results of a high order.[62] But the early superintendents cannot be exempted from responsibility for the hideous extension of their hospitals in the wake of the pauper-dumping campaigns conducted by the Poor Law and Lunacy Commissioners in England and the philanthropic followers of Dorothea Dix in various State legislatures of America. The Moral Managers' philosophy of seclusion and even the imposing scale and design of their asylum architecture could be turned all too easily into the grounding of a depersonalised, repressive internment. To resist the dumping demands of the sanitary bureaucracy would have required positive and sustained political struggle outside the narrow channels of medical influence, challenging the broad assumption and policies of welfare provision in the Victorian and Jacksonian periods. David Rothman has commented on the acquiescence, in the American case, of asylum superintendents and administrators in the mid-century's retreat from psychiatric to custodial goals.[63]

The growth of this epoch of an anti-therapeutic nihilism, in synchrony with broader hereditarian and pessimistic ideologies of control for society's dangerous classes, reflected the physician's alliance with the bourgeois of that day. The contrary alliance, of clinical authority with radical politics and working-class discontent, would have possessed a singular potency. To pose the question of this alliance for the nineteenth century is doubtless an anachronism: we can only indicate the lessons of its absence for the present day.

It is around 25 years since I sat waiting in an ante-room within a gigantic British mental institution, where the adoptive mother who had reared me since my early infancy lay in a condition of passive dementia. When it was time for me to enter the ward, the nurse in charge drew from her pocket a bunch of keys, and unlocked the door to admit me into the large hall, filled with row upon row of beds, in one of which, scarcely recognisable, lay my parent. The keys tinkled in the silence of that corridor; and it is still easy for me to hear the sound of their metal. It is a sound that reverberates back over the centuries of locked doors and futile dormitories of the neglected. In physical, material terms, the locks have all but gone: but in these matters the human mind still finds it hard to unlock itself. Foucault's work will be measured to the extent that it can aid in the formation of an informed political practice, the key which can both open and destroy the locks, bars and fetters of psychiatric and social confinement.

6. Psychiatry and Politics in Thomas Szasz

For over two decades Thomas S. Szasz has been conducting a continuous, single-minded and stylish battle against mental-health ideologies and institutions, along a gamut of media from the scholarly to the popular, between the covers of 15 books and across the pages of some hundreds of articles and reviews. Goffman began his influence in counter-psychiatric theorising at the same starting point as Szasz, i.e. the later fifties, but is better known as a general sociologist of the small-scale encounter than as a theoretician of mental health issues. Laing came into public attention during the psychedelic sixties, arriving with a sensational impact that has faded given the ensuing changes in modern cultural styles and in Laing's own personal outlook. Foucault now reigns almost supreme in the modish avant-garde of Paris, London and New York, having achieved his eminence through the passing of the revolutionary or radical social aspirations that structured intellectual life in all three centres after 1968. In these successions of ideological fortune, Szasz's stance as a critic of psychiatry has been unwavering. He is at the same time the *doyen* of the movement of mental-health revisionism and the herald of the newer orthodoxies of right-wing thought on welfare in the post-collectivist epoch of Ronald Reagan and Margaret Thatcher. From a position of apparent marginality, situated on the fringe of the right-libertarian grouplets associated with American individualism, he has emerged as a thinker fully concordant with the mainstream of conservative thought on social policy; and, paradoxically, in his transition from fringe figure to conservative luminary, he has often received the approbation of the socialist or radical New Left, which has seriously misunderstood the implications of Szaszian anti-collectivism.

Yet any reader in the literature of mental health revisionism, will find Szasz's work uneven, occasional, lacking even in the structure of a schematic overstatement. Two books by Szasz may be taken as the pillars of his theoretical edifice: *The Myth of Mental Illness*, published back in 1961, and *The Manufacture of Madness*, which appeared in 1970. The former consists of a fundamental attack on the logic of the concept of mental illness, in terms remote from any purchase on the actual institutions of psychiatric treatment; the latter is a critique of the operating social and political functions of psychiatric ideology. Yet the two works fail to form a natural complement to one another. *The Myth of Mental Illness* is only seldom militant despite its polemical title. In the main, it fulfils the promise of its sub-title 'Foundations of a Theory of Personal Conduct', providing a reworking of psychoanalytical categories of normal and abnormal behaviour along the lines of a game-playing model of social interaction which is zestful and insightful, but neither particularly uncommon nor particularly iconoclastic by the standards of recent social-psychological theorising.[1] The text is enriched with a host of clinical and conceptual observations whose value stands independent of whether one accepts the author's main case: that 'mental illness' is an invalid and perilous idea. For instance, Szasz perceptively points out[2] that the orthodox-psychoanalytic ideal of 'genital primacy', as a desirable goal for adult functioning, omits to state whether the successful genitality of 'king and concubine, master and servant, soldier and prostitute, or husband and wife' is considered the model to be followed. Again, the observation that much personal misery arises not simply through loss of a person or persons but also and even more through 'the loss of game'[3] neatly integrates clinical empathy with the sociological discussion of 'anomie' (loss of norm) which is usually applied to whole groups of the displaced rather than to individual victims. Much of Szasz's text is concerned with elucidating the many cases in which people can be said to be following rules, or learning to follow rules, in either a socially acceptable or a socially deviant manner; it would be relatively easy for an adept of psychoanalytically-guided psychotherapy to accept Szasz's general theoretical discussion of game-playing and rule-following without thereby concluding that the argument had destroyed the utility of 'mental illness' as a structuring concept.

Since in this work Szasz is more concerned with the construction of a game-analysis of human action than with the destruction of the pretensions of medical psychiatry, many polemical ideas which will later be developed much more vigorously are to be found stated here in less bellicose fashion. The targets of his critique are large, portentous and heterogenous. Marxian 'historicism', health insurance schemes, causal explanations of human behaviour and religious injunctions toward meekness and submissiveness are among the many stopping-posts in a waspish itinerary. Despite the author's famed hostility towards psychiatry, only one school of psychiatric thought, the extreme 'organicist' trend which regards all mental illnesses as brain diseases, requiring no understanding of the patient's motives and goals, receives sustained critical attention.[4] The theory and profession of psychoanalysis itself gets off relatively lightly. It is made clear that Szasz's own transactional approach towards psychological disturbances is a development from suggestions formed from within classical psychoanalytical theory (Sullivan, Ferenczi, Fairbairn and Freud himself)[5] and the book as a whole bears something of the character of a neo-Freudian internal document, penned in order to persuade fellow-analysts of the value of a fresh language to encompass their existing practice.

Human action is governed by intentions or motives; these motivations interlock predictably from situation to situation within various bundles of social rules; and behaviour in accordance with such rules may be seen in the light of an analogy with the playing of games of the ordinary and common kind. Such, too briefly it is true, is the explicit content of what Szasz terms 'foundations of a theory of personal conduct'. The game-playing analogue is deployed liberally and with gusto: thus, within the Judaeo-Christian religious tradition, one plays a 'game of "I-am-not-happy" against a partner-opponent', God;[6] a hysteric patient is playing a game of coercion with her or his relatives and even with her or his therapist; modern society is involved in a 'medical game of life' – with prizes for the handsome and healthy winners and penalties for the old, ill and deformed – which has replaced the heaven-bent 'theological game of life' characteristic of the Middle Ages.

Szasz has the capacity to restate the commonplace within a vivid context that heightens the truth value of old truisms. But the apparently radical context can often be discarded as a cover. For example, it is easy to agree with Szasz that the assignation of mental illness undermines the patient's responsibility and actually increases the burden of individual helplessness; the point can be taken as a salutary warning, but does not constitute a theoretical objection to the category of 'mental illness' as such. Where the work engages in a really controversial case – e.g. in its large claim for the virtues of individually conducted and privately paid psychoanalysis – one is likely to find the argument oddly skimped. Such moot points lie embedded in a more graceful and detached discourse which has to do with 'everyday life as a mixture of metagames', 'impersonated roles', 'coercive rules' and similar ironies.

In contrast, the rising curve traced by Szasz's prolific later publications, with its early peak in *The Manufacture of Madness*, amounts to the escalation of a crusade rather than the development of a theory. Every differentiation required by Szasz for the establishment of his initial case is rendered into the sharpest and most unqualified dichotomy. In *The Myth of Mental Illness* it could be admitted that the institution of private psychoanalysis might itself need some suspicious scrutiny,[7] or that psychosomatic illnesses presented some unsolved difficulties for his analysis.[8] Increasingly, however, the practice of psychiatry becomes divided by Szasz into two, and only two, functional types, forming respectively the utmost in totalitarian despotism and the best of all possible therapeutic worlds. The totalitarian pole is termed 'Institutional Psychiatry'; it is characterised by involuntary incarceration in mental hospitals, the use of psychiatric concepts for the extralegal punishment of deviants, and the state's investiture of publicly employed physicians as agents of social order rather than of their patients' welfare.[9] The opposite, benevolent extreme is offered in Contractual Psychiatry: an arrangement founded on an informed consensus between two freely choosing individuals, one a therapist and the other a client, the former providing a service in the unravelling of certain moral problems and the latter, in return, a monetary fee.[10] Neither branch of psychiatry has anything to do with medicine, whose interventions should be limited to cases of 'demonstrably bodily illness'.[11] Szasz has earlier insisted that doctors should even avoid concerning themselves with those social conditions that can precipitate demonstrably bodily illness; it is no part of their job to function as 'attorneys for the poor' since nowadays the poor have enough attorneys and other representatives of their own.[12] But in the latter works social medicine, like social psychiatry, turns into anathema: a simple liberal call from an American public-health administrator asking doctors to join with other community leaders 'to eliminate known producers of stress such as urban slums and rural depressed areas' is enough for Szasz to invoke the spectre of the Psychiatric Purge. 'But who or what might be "producers of stress"? Negroes? Jews? Communists? Fascists?... These possibilities are by no means far-fetched.'[13] An organically defined medical science, blind to the most obvious connections between social environment and personal ailment: an equally individualistic psychoanalytic framework, available only for those patients who are well enough (and well-off enough) to pay cash: such are Szasz's positive therapeutic ideals.

We must now turn to Szasz's negative example of medical misuse, especially to 'Institutional Psychiatry', a phenomenon which he repeatedly states to be the twentieth-century equivalent of witch-burning and the Inquisition.

Medicine is defined by Szasz in terms of an objective subject-matter: the human body and its disorders. Within psychiatry, however, other criteria for definition are employed. Contractual Psychiatry is defined in the terms of an ethic, that of a voluntary exchange between doctor and patient, while Institutional Psychiatry is delimited in terms of a particular procedure, i.e. the certificated delivery of a mental patient into hospital care through a legal process undertaken against his or her will. Involuntary hospitalisation is for Szasz the central paradigm of modern psychiatry – even though it is a minority procedure in Britain (where entry into psychiatric treatment usually presents no greater legal complexities for the patient than admission into any other form of medical care) and of decreasing importance in the United States. Szasz's method is thus to take a particularly disputable type of psychiatric action and define the rest of psychiatry around it. The most indefensible compulsory hospitalisations are presented as though they were typical hospitalisations. And, in order to forestall any possible apologia for an unjustified committal into hospital, the reader's foot is shackled to a chain of linked universal prohibitions and injunctions, so that it can never once be set on the slippery slope that leads from diagnosing a patient to lobotomising him or her; from preventing a suicide to locking up a rich relative; from treating a homosexual who desires potency with women to castrating one who is content with partners of his own sex; from regarding delusions as evidence of illness to interpreting masturbation as evidence of insanity.

All psychiatric concepts are pragmatically re-fashioned by Szasz around the issue of compulsory hospital treatment. Thus, the distinction between neurosis and psychosis which is ordinarily founded on a variety of clinical, behavioural and phenomenological considerations is taken by Szasz simply to represent the difference between voluntary treatment and coercive certification,[14] 'neurosis' being a covert justification for consulting-room psychotherapy and 'psychosis' for forcible retention and punitive treatment in hospital. In actual practice of course, there are a great many psychotics who enter and leave hospital voluntarily, or who live out a mainly out-patient career on mood drugs and professional sympathy, and correspondingly a fair number of neurotics who get detained on compulsory orders, e.g. as serious suicidal risks.

Szasz's theoretical enterprise in anti-psychiatry is thus essentially one of tracing every thread in the web of psychopathological logic which could, under some construction and in some conceivable situation, facilitate the deprivation of the subject's liberty through involuntary hospitalisation. Any unnecessary coercion of psychiatric patients is a scandal which of course deserves whatever public exposure it manages to receive. But Szasz identifies the scandal as *any* compulsory hospitalisation whatsoever, and his remedy – the outright abolition of compulsory procedures in psychiatric hospitalisation and the replacement of public-health psychiatry by fee-paid two-person psychotherapy – is useful more as a provocation than as a programme. The Szaszian case contains both the force and the fragility of any analysis of social evils undertaken from the standpoint of a single absolute moral principle, be it Gandhian non-violence, Cold War parliamentarianism or – as in this case – civil-libertarian individualism. Like all such absolutist standpoints it is capable of moral fervour and narrow sensitivity to certain intolerable wrongs, and a power to demolish more eclectic, more qualified positions: but its absolutism renders it impotent to calculate the complex relations between means and ends, risks and benefits which hold in real life. It seeks legal guarantees against injustice and abuse, and can find them only in the realm of ideas, since history itself contains no possibility of such warranties. By a Contractual Psychiatry, Szasz means a psychiatry which *is* guaranteed, safe, pre-designed to pose no serious ethical problems for therapist or client. It after all consists of a free exchange between approximately equal partners: 'The relationship between contractual psychiatrist and patient is based on contract, freely entered into by both and, in general, freely terminable by both.'[15] Only the mildest mental disorders could possibly be handled within this framework, for one well-known consequence of emotional illness is an extreme dependency that is often manifested towards the therapist. Consequently Szasz is saying that the only defensible psychiatry is that which can be practised with those who need it least.

Towards those who are in most need of psychiatric (as of ordinary medical) treatment – the chronically ill who cannot earn the fee that ignites the engines of Contractual Psychiatry – Szasz offers nothing. Thus Szasz never states how an adequate psycho-geriatrics would be possible within an individualistic fee-paying structure. In the first place, the old and indigent are hardly in a position to compete, in the therapy-purchasing market, with clients who are at their peak of earning capacity. Secondly, the Szaszian market model of free psychiatry assumes that a discrete, specific service – that afforded in the 'analytic hour' – is rendered in return for the client's fee. But intensive, person-to-person analysis is only one of many psychiatric services; one, moreover, which is unlikely to prove useful to the most disabled elderly (who can provide for one another the experience of the 'student of human living' that Szasz claims as the special expertise of the analyst). What old patients in mental difficulties need and want are such services as a supportive residential environment, social stimulation, an easing of such physical burdens as the necessity to cook, help in moving about, and assorted medications which may well be necessary in the psychological as well as in the physical accompaniments of old age. Quite apart from their difficulty in paying for these amenities – an obstacle which could theoretically be by-passed through issuing the aged and other poor vouchers in lieu of money – we have the even greater impediment of supposing that mental patients in a state of emotional distress and lowered attentiveness are going to be able to shop around for a number of psychiatric amenities, picking different items off the shelf of the therapeutic supermart in accordance with their chosen utilities, and presenting themselves to some terminal cashier with a list of purchases which has, through the exercise of a rational consumer sovereignty, fallen within their available budget.

The market model of medical servicing is in general one which fragments the work to be performed along the requirements of a costing system for separate items, whereas the patient's need is for an integrated structure made up of a number of servicing components. The sick person cannot engage in separate contracts with a physician, an anaesthetist, a nurse, a radiographer, a lab technician and a psychoanalyst. In any case, only a few of the therapeutic trades have any tradition of a fee-paying contractual relationship with the patient: nurses and social workers seem content to be part of the salariat, and their aspiration towards 'professional' status does not include any demand for individual-contract methods of payment. The individual chit for services rendered, despatched by one petty-bourgeois to another, is a prerogative claimed only by the more glamorous and status-anxious professionals like doctors and analysts. Thus Szasz's demand that fee-paying practice be made the cornerstone of the therapeutic relationship can only accentuate the already excessive inequalities between different classes of therapist. Whatever the bureaucratic disadvantages of a salaried health service, the employment of doctors and other professional helpers by public agencies does at least provide the foundation for a flexible and integrated delivery of the goods. However, the work-load is arranged – and a much greater variety, with different team-structures, target populations and facilities, is possible with public agency funding than with the individual-contract structure[16] – the public exchequer is there to pick up the tab at the end, up to limits whose extent can be made a matter for social debate and decision. Szasz's 'freedom' amounts to the dissolution of treatment services, atomising the situation of individuals who, whether as therapists or as patients, are already too much atomised.

But then, it is never clear whether Szasz is engaged in a theoretical reconstruction of psychiatric facilities, or in a series of defensive special pleas designed to avoid certain particular barbarities. When we total up all the psychiatric contingencies that he denounces – the evasion of legal responsibility through diagnostic tags, the persecution of homosexuals, and his own central paradigm (in *The Myth of Mental Illness*) of the hysteric, a type of patient who has lost considerable standing from the days when he or she took pride of place in Freud's and Breuer's consulting-rooms and has indeed almost disappeared from the literature – it cannot be said that anything like a comprehensive range of clinical material or psychiatric situations has been given to us. Phobics, depressives, manies, schizophrenics and anxiety-neurotics – in short, the general run of psychiatric patients who, in addition to having 'life-problems', do happen to feel distinctly unwell, rarely if ever enter Dr Szasz's casebook.[17]

In short, despite the voluminousness of Szasz's work, we remain without any sense either of the complex and concrete reality of personal problems that come to the attention of psychiatrists and psychotherapists, or of the nature of the communications from therapist to patient and back that would comprise a valid and effective mode of treatment. Even in unmasking the hypocrisies of the analyst's most intimate ideology of treatment – as he does supremely well in his paper on 'transference'[18] – he is curiously mute on the type of learning that the analysed client undergoes. We are never told what does count for Szasz as a state of affairs where the patient has learned something rather than merely deluded himself or herself. His distinction between 'therapy', which is supposed to be good and libertarian, and 'treatment', which is wickedly coercive, remains a purely verbal solution. All that Szasz's Contractual Psychiatry does is to state some legalistic ground-rules for a psychiatric ethic: and this, in the absence of some detail as to what therapists are supposed to be up to in practice, can only constitute a pious but empty hope. The issue of coercion in therapy, for instance, cannot be resolved without thorough discussion of that much-recorded process in psychoanalysis whereby the patient displays a filial dependency upon the therapist. The immense authority held by psychoanalysts over their patients affords fantastic opportunities for the unequal exercise of power upon or even against the helpless client. At its crudest, this exploitation may be financial in its consequences, as when the analyst goes on milking customers for years, persuading them that enough 'progress' is being made to continue the sessions, while those living nearest to them find their problems as intractable as ever.

Szasz provides neither a convincing paradigm of the psychoanalystic relationship nor even an interior reconstruction of the vicissitudes of the client. His game-playing, behavioural analysis deals only in what the patient does to other people, never in the personal anguish, alienation or stupor which predates the sufferer's communication with others.

Mental illness is a language: but it is also the sick one's miserable inability to use a language. It is, to be sure, a social status: but, before that, it is a private hell. Szasz attains his role as proxy spokesperson for the rights of the mental patient by ignoring, simply, what it is to be a mental patient.

The ideological undercurrents of Thomas Szasz's thinking have never been systematically exposed to the light of day by any of his critics. It may be that the deeper philosophical and political assumptions of his credo are too close to the traditional common sense of the American public to make it easy for a critic stationed in the United States to tease out their full implications. His specifically psychiatric conclusions indeed make sense only within the broader context of conservative political ideology which informs Szasz's work. Seldom are his political values made as obvious as on the occasion when he declared in an interview that 'Man is a predator; everyone knows that. But after World War II, perhaps in the face of the horror of the Nazis, everyone began massively denying that fundamentally we are beasts and that the only things that keep men from murder are moral inhibitions or other people – that is, the sanctions of the law.'[19] The myth of Szasz's radicalism is still pervasive, if perhaps less powerful than on the occasion when a crowd of New Left students went to applaud one of his lectures at the University of Michigan, to be denounced by him from the platform as a pack of Reds who should get back to Moscow.[20] The collection *Radical Psychology*, whose editor calls for 'a people's psychology' to be 'an integrating factor of self-awareness within the revolutionary process', sees Szasz (whom it anthologises along with Marx, Reich, Fanon and sundry other politically left-wing writers) as manifesting a 'contradiction between his political views and his condemnations of psychiatry'.[21] But Szasz's politics are not an aberration, and in no sense contradict the positions he has taken on psychiatric issues. Politically, psychologically and philosophically his beliefs form a unified and consistent whole, a distinct ideological complex which is most succinctly labelled 'libertarian'.

In the contemporary United States the category 'libertarian' has to be understood in a sense distinct from that bequeathed to it by the radical tradition of European anarchism, which attempts to synthesise the demand for individual and social liberty with modes of collective and even communist forms of organisation. The American 'libertarian' is now well-known both in the literature of contemporary ideologies and in the practice of fringe and Republican political movements as a celebrant of competitive business enterprise, a torch-bearer for the arch-bourgeois utopia of capitalist laissez-faire – a stage of economic development whose failure to appear in any determinate form of capitalism known to history has never interfered with its popularity as a model for economists of the right.

Rooted in a venerable intellectual lineage which can be dated at least as far back as Herbert Spencer[22] and possibly to the Thomas Paine of 'Society is produced by our wants and government by our wickedness; society is in every state a blessing – government even in its best state a necessary evil',[23] the conservative libertarianism of America found its most potent expression during the decades of Keynesian consensus through spawning a counter-culture of small societies and publications whose very titles were suggestive: Pennsylvania Society for Individual Liberty; Libertarian Forum; Capitalist Books (a book-club of one such current). For a long time this fringe New Right, with its hippie-style buttons proclaiming 'MYOB – Mind Your Own Business' and its manifestoes on 'The Market for Liberty', seemed to inhabit a wilderness of disestablished anti-politics, bidding for the affections of discontented youth alongside their rivals of the fringe left. But as the post-war consensus on the priorities of welfare spending and economic pump-priming became eroded, this marginal, pro-capitalist libertarianism began to move into the centre of the political stage. The view that economic downswings are only prolonged and amplified into the agony of slump through 'government tampering with market signals' was once the property of the inconspicuous or eccentric right, but has now entered the common sense of Friedman-influenced conventional wisdom. And Szasz's individualist doctrines in the field of therapy can be seen as a parallel strand within this skein of basically neo-Spencerian ideology, the expression within psychiatry and medicine of the anti-statist, bourgeois-libertarian maxims that have become so widely propagated in economics, social philosophy and ethics during the last fifteen or so years.

It may appear paradoxical that an ethos which celebrates the sanctity of unbridled capitalism should be so productive of critics who vehemently denounce the actual policies of an ongoing capitalist social order. But laissez-faire individualism, even in the shape of that Social-Darwinist teaching which glorifies cut-throat economic competition as 'natural selection', has always thrown up passionate spokespeople for particular oppressed minorities. Herbert Spencer, a vociferous opponent of trade-union bargaining, factory legislation, public libraries, municipal wash-houses and increased taxation (to list only a few of the 'measures of coercive rule' which appalled him in 1884)[24] thought of colonial repressions as an unnecessary deviation from the free-enterprise system. He thus joined the radical wing of the London intelligentsia that set out to prosecute Governor Eyre of Jamaica for murder (following his reprisals against a rising); later, Spencer tried to launch an Anti-Aggression League against the extension of the British Empire into India and Egypt.[25] Similarly, America's leading Spencerian and Social Darwinist W.G. Sumner, the moralising prophet of 'a holy war against reformism, protectionism, socialism, and government interventionism' and ruthless advocate of the slogan 'Liberty, Inequality, Survival of the Fittest',[26] drew the fire of mainstream Republicans – who lobbied for his dismissal from the Chair of Political and Social Science at Yale – by opposing Yankee expansionism and the Spanish-American war of 1898.[27] The modern libertarian New Right of the 1970s opposed both state-funded welfare programmes *and* military conscription, antipollution laws *and* dollar imperialism, economic planning *and* police harassment.

Spencer's polemical fury as an intransigent laissez-faire individualist, and the outstanding success of the transplantation of his ideas from Britain to America, arise from the paradoxical chronology of his intellectual life-span, which developed its basic industrialist values within the provincial laissez-faire radicalism of the Anti-Corn Law League in the 1840s, rolled forth its volumes of pacific, evolutionist systematising during the decades of mid-Victorian prosperity, and came into collision with the sharpening of militarism and protectionism, and the parallel vogue of collectivist and statist ideas in the intelligentsia, during England's 'Great Depression' of 1873–96. Increasingly in Britain, Spencer's anti-collectivist ideology could assume the character only of a personal rearguard protest against the military-feudal, despotic structures which he thought to have been supplanted forever by the progress of competitive commerce; but in the United States, the voice that was a mere grace-note on home shores could thunder forth to provide the keynote for the celebration of an ascendant capitalism of laissez-faire which appeared to possess opportunities of unlimited expansion within the frontiers it was still staking out over the ashes of Southern secession and Red Indian rebellion. Spencermania in America reached its apogee in the fall of 1882, when the philosopher made a personal visit culminating in a banquet of fulsome tribute from leaders in business, literature, science, politics and religion. Once back in England he was reduced to the role of a crankish denouncer of contemporary trends, writing in 1884 the sequence of articles on 'The New Toryism' of the Liberals, 'The Coming Slavery' of state administration, 'The Sins of Legislators' and 'The Great Political Superstition' of Parliamentary sovereignty, to be presented in one volume as *The Man versus the State*: a euphemism surely for the lone man Spencer versus the dominant statist capitalism of his own time.

The internal logic of Szasz's psychiatric philosophy matches the positions of Herbert Spencer himself so closely that one might be tempted to suspect a wholesale borrowing of ideas from the Victorian sage. The parallels between Szasz and Spencer that will now be sketched are, more plausibly, to be explained by the fact that both writers start from very simple and very similar first principles: the supreme value of individual competition in a race whose course and progress is to be traced by the record of evolution. Spencer, as an author of exceptionally wide range and productivity, had occasion to touch on many topics in sociology, politics and morals which Szasz also deals with; it may be that the latter author has never read the relevant passages of his predecessor in laissez-faire theory (although at one important point in the argument of *The Myth of Mental Illness* there is sympathetic but critical reference to *The Man versus the State*.[28]) If Szasz appears to shrink from some of the more brutal conclusions of the nakedly capitalistic philosophy propounded by Andrew Carnegie's favourite intellectual, we may be tempted to ask why the laissez-faire lily should have to be gilded by its modern cultivators.

The elements in Szasz's work that need consideration in this comparison are: his development of Social Darwinism; his extreme anti-collectivism: and his legalistic formalism, especially though not exclusively in his proclamation of the contract as the prime paradigm of human freedom.

Although Spencer's philosophy of industrial development explicitly renounced the necessity for coercion and domination – features, as he believed, of an outmoded military organisation of society that was being superseded by the voluntary, pacific arrangements of commerce – his views on the state relief of poverty and disease preached a laissez-fairist refusal to intervene against affliction, a brand of individualism that was not merely rugged but ruthless.

For Szasz also, social life is characterised by the pressure of new demands upon individuals reared in old conditions. It is no longer the single transition from pre-industrial to industrial society which forces change, but rather the ceaseless strain of innovation in an advanced civilisation. All life is game-playing, and 'modern man, if he is at all educated, cannot play the same sorts of games which he played as a youngster, or which his parents played, and remain satisfied with them'. 'The common and pressing problem today is that, as social conditions undergo rapid change, men are called upon to alter their modes of living.' The role of the psychotherapist is a little like the exertions of the philanthropist in Spencer's frame: it is to enable individuals to cope with the inevitable strains of modernity, by teaching them to learn new adaptations. It is futile for people to 'long for the security of stability' since 'stability can be purchased only at the cost of personal enslavement. The other alternative is to rise to the challenge of the unceasing need to learn and re-learn, and to try to meet this challenge successfully.' Szasz warns that 'social conditions make it impossible to survive without greater flexibility in regard to patterns of personal conduct.'[29] There is no possibility in Szasz's work that 'social conditions' may be systematically biased against certain classes, or that these conditions may themselves require to be overturned to make the environment fit human needs rather than *vice versa*.

In order to construct a suitable attitude of stoicism towards the miseries of the disadvantaged, both writers find it necessary to inveigh against ideologies which appear to promise an indiscriminate betterment for mankind. Szasz remarks caustically that:

> there's a Church of America – better known as the National Institute of Mental Health [which] propagates a faith called Psychiatry. It would have us believe that we can lead lives of ambition without anxiety; that we can have success without strife, sociability without conflict, reward without punishment, and pleasure without pain.[30]

Spencer's moralising on painful inevitabilities is similar:

> There is a notion, always more or less prevalent and just now vociferously expressed, that all social suffering is removable, and that it is the duty of somebody or other to remove it. Both these beliefs are false.

For Spencer the primary fault of social reformism is 'to separate pain from ill doing', which is 'to fight against the constitution of things';[31] for Szasz the permanent recurrence of pain is not so much the penalty of evil action as the dialectically linked concomitant of all action, good or evil. Nevertheless, the message is clear from both men's arguments: don't try to change the human lot.

A striking congruence between Szasz and Spencer is to be seen in the fierce opposition that both authors manifest to any generalised sympathy for people in trouble. Both go to great lengths to advocate the cultivation of a calculated indifference towards the sick and needy. Where Spencer fortifies us against the promptings of immediate sympathy by requiring us to calculate the long-term evolutionary risks of supporting the inferior, Szasz armours our conscience by pointing out that the Judaeo-Christian 'ethic of helpfulness' is actually very bad for the persons being helped, since such apparently altruistic notions 'conspire, as it were, to foster man's infantilism and dependence'.[32] Where Spencer sees the risks attendant on 'a retrogression of character' among the assisted,[33] Szasz interprets the social victim's demand for assistance as a 'regression' towards childishness, which is reinforced by orthodox religion's 'endless exhortations commanding man to behave childishly, stupidly and irresponsibly'. This 'unseen ocean of commands to be incompetent, impoverished, and sick' coerces, through a permanent moral blackmail, 'those who exhibit effective, self-reliant behaviour'. Since 'the *rewarding of disability* – though necessary in certain instances – is a potentially dangerous social practice', Szasz urges an incessant propaganda in favour of 'rules emphasising the need for man's striving for mastery, responsibility, self-reliance, and mutually co-operative independence'.[34] The parallel between the Szaszian virtues of self-reliance and the classic individualist sermons of the Industrial Revolution, instructing the masses to be diligent, thrifty, self-supporting and disciplined in collective enterprise, forms a link not only with Spencer but such older nineteenth-century ideologues of capitalism as Andrew Ure and Samuel Smiles.

But what we find altogether missing in Szasz is any tendency towards that nihilistic eugenics (so typical of Spencer at his most eloquent) which bids us to leave society's unfortunates for disposal by the calamities of disease and starvation. Just as carnivorous beasts remove from the herds of their prey 'the sickly, the malformed and the least fleet or powerful', so human society is assisted by 'that same beneficial but severe discipline'. Even though 'it seems hard that... unskillfulness... should entail hunger upon the artisan', or 'that widows and orphans should be left to struggle for life and death... when regarded not separately but in connection with the interests of universal humanity, these harsh fatalities are seen to be full of beneficence – the same beneficence which brings to early graves the children of diseased parents and singles out the low-spirited, the intemperate and the debilitated as the victims of an epidemic'.[35]

The horrors of the National Socialist practice of 'harsh fatalities' inflicted on the allegedly diseased in the name of beneficence have, if nothing else, rendered it impossible for Spencer's eulogies of mass death to be repeated in any modern political theory. Contemporary advocates of non-intervention in the sufferings of the underclasses are unable to enlarge on the benign benefits to be secured in humanity's ultimate future by 'weeding out those of lowest development'.[36] The laissez-faire purists of today find it difficult to announce that the inferior are to die, because the inferior themselves may overhear them saying it. Szasz, for his part, is content to redefine out of existence the structured social problems of the exploited communities of America. Of particular importance here are his views on suicide and narcotics addiction, where Szasz recommends a policy of total non-intervention towards suicide and addiction.[37] The rationale of this stance is clear within the terms of his battle against involuntary psychiatry hospitalisation: the risk of the patient's self-destruction, and the presence in him or her of the self-destructive tendencies manifested in a career of narcotics use, are among the most powerful arguments that can be used to justify forcible detention for care and treatment. Since Szasz has always been so insistent in polemicising against any social principle which would bolster a case for compulsory therapy, it is only logical that he should engage in combating the arguments drawn from addiction and suicide. Indeed, the only surprise is that it took ten years from the publication of *The Myth of Mental Illness* before he reached these advocacies. The physician, according to Szasz, should restrain his lust for life-saving (though the ethically guided psychiatrist can still intervene in cases where the patient displays suicidal urges which have hitherto fallen short of consummation), and society should permit a free trade in dangerous drugs, under restrictions no more compelling than those which prohibit the sale of alcoholic beverages to minors. Indeed, as long as children use narcotics among themselves without experiencing 'pharmacological seduction' by adults, the law should not intervene: 'the use of drugs by and among children (without the direct participation of adults) should be a matter entirely outside the scope of the criminal law.'[38] How Junior is to buy dope without a transaction with an adult pedlar is left as unanswered as unasked: the manufacturer and wholesaler of heroin for the young will, presumably, be used as informers on the retailers (reversing the present tendency of criminal investigation) and the police can collect their hush-money from the small-fry rather than the big-timers of the trade.

It is important to realise that Szasz's approach both to suicide and to addiction reflects an individualisation of social problems which is a necessary tactic in his denial of capitalist social structure. For suicide cannot be sensibly regarded as a personal act, distinct in its quality either from other routes of despair (such as neurosis or unsuccessful suicidal attempts) or from the pressures of large-scale social contradiction. 'Every man's death diminishes me' is a better guide to theory as well as a higher statement of ethics than Szasz's laissez-faire indifferentism. The solitude of the adolescent waiting on the tenth-floor ledge to jump, of the crazed exile in the backroom with a calculated overdose, of the lovesick, the melancholic, the intensely weary – each solitude radiates the social order, incriminates one or more powerful inequalities manifested across segments of collective destiny, shows us who is first, who is fat, who is attached. Szasz's 'fundamental liberty' of suicide is only the obverse of more affluent freedoms, principally those of accumulation and enterprise.

The Social Darwinist of the epoch that preceded our century's mass holocausts could convert the death of others into a good by appealing to the laws of evolutionary progress. The successors to Social Darwinism have no such way with 'nature's failures'. The death of the loser must now be seen as the risk he or she takes in the exercise of freedom, or even as a precious right, threatened by the imperious interference of psychiatry and bureaucracy. The abrupt death of the suicide or the slow death-in-life of a heroin career are matters of individual election, as the older deaths of the defeated were matters, purely, of impersonal natural selection.

Szasz and Spencer differ in their perception and valuation of the fate of the helpless. For any honest observer of nineteenth-century industrial cities, non-intervention in mass misery would have its obvious costs: costs, it is true, which for the Social Darwinist would have to be borne in the main by the victims themselves and by the faceless goddess, Nature. The people's unequal life-chances were visible, so that the existence of affliction could not be gainsaid but only rationalised. There is still, even in a Darwinian lunatic like Spencer, a residue of Christian sentiment over the plight of the misfits. As Hofstadter points out:

> accused of brutality in his application of biological concepts to social principles, Spencer was compelled to insist over and over again that he was not opposed to voluntary private charity to the unfit, since it had an elevating effect on the character of the donors and hastened the development of altruism: he opposed only compulsory poor laws and other state measures.[39]

Szaszian laissez-fairism is that of a post-Christian sensibility. The altruistic imperatives of religion enter the scheme only as causes of the present mess: 'Jewish and Christian teachings abound in rules that reward sickness, malingering, poverty, fearfulness – in brief, disabilities of all sorts' and 'invoke penalties for self-reliance, competence, effectiveness, and pride in health and well-being.'[40] Szasz accepts the code of morals whereby the sight of the drink-sodden is an offence to respectable eyes, and has proposed the extension of police powers to remove the public viewability of junkies.[41] The thrust of his campaign is to remove the squalor of the under-class if not from public sight, then at least from public notice. The oppressed are only noticeable when they can be identified as the scapegoats of the 'Therapeutic State', and the casualties of official and private neglect vanish from an America replete solely with the indignities of official and bureaucratic aggression. Szasz's emphasis on the perils of public action, and collateral omission of the pitfalls of public inertia, amount to a central political prescription: when in doubt, do nothing. He is not a Social Darwinist – though he is an inheritor of Social Darwinism – because the theorists of that description retained, as part of their vision of the struggle between the higher and the inferior, some awareness of the place of the unfit in nature's plan. In Szasz, as in the perspective of millions of traditional Americans before liberal theory discovered 'poverty' in the sixties, any such awareness is strictly off limits. 'It is best that they should die' mentioned what is now unsayable, and we are left with the modern equivalent of 'Let them eat cake': the freedom of the downtrodden to purchase Contractual Psychiatry, as part of the structure of freedom that enables them also to drown, drink, or dope themselves to perdition, or to become President of the United States…

If the affinity between Szasz and Spencer has been so far somewhat circuitous, their parallelism along another major axis of laissez-fairist doctrine is fairly clear: both authors are firm opponents of the collectivist principle in social organisation. The invention of a sharp alternative between 'Individualism' and 'Collectivism' is in itself symptomatic of a special type of rightwing intransigence, a rare species in political theory ever since the movement of the state into the regulation of private enterprise gave nearly all forms of bourgeois ideology – liberal, conservative, fascist or reformist – a markedly collectivist or statist cast. In stating this polarity so forcibly, Szasz and Spencer mark themselves out from the common run of liberal thinking, and annnounce their own close kinship. 'When Collectivism has strengthened itself enough,' warned Spencer darkly, in one of his infrequent uses of the term (for he normally spoke of state-agency, state-superintendence, state-coercion and the like),

> there may come municipal groceries, and so on with other trades, until at length manufacturers and distributors are formed into multitudinous departments, each with its head and its ranks of subordinates and workers – regiments and brigades.[42]

Spencer reads the whole course of social history as a contest between the statist, compulsory, centralising tendency of military societies and the individualistic, voluntary and decentralised structures that are proper to industrial civilisation. Society was advancing 'from the one extreme, where the State is everything and the individual nothing, to the other extreme, in which the individual is everything and the state is nothing':[43] a progression whose failure to ensue in his own highly statised epoch threw Spencer into gloom and indignation, but still formed the basic yardstick for the analysis and critique of social trends.

For Szasz there is no such progression, but a permanent battle of uncertain outcome. Over the nineteenth century,

> the basic value of the individual – as opposed to the interests of the masses or the nation – was emphasised, especially by the upper classes. The professions, medicine foremost among them, espoused the ethical value of individualism. This value gradually became pitted against its antonym, collectivism.[44]

The forces which nowadays impel Western medicine and psychiatry are anti-individualistic and statist:

> Institutional Psychiatry – which always claimed to be a part of medicine and was in its turn always eagerly accepted by it as one of its specialties was created, and always has been, a quasi-totalitarian collectivistic enterprise, in which the physician served the State, not the patient… Institutional Psychiatry has corrupted the individualistic ethic of Western medicine.[45]

The advance of the collectivist model in psychiatry is taken to reinforce the widening powers of the state over and against persons. In a speech in Detroit in May 1970 (which is typical of many of his pronouncements) Szasz called attention to

> the alliance of psychiatry with the police power of the State, which has developed a system of social control paralleling that of criminal law except that it is extra-legal and totalitarian; the logical conclusion of this trend would be a Therapeutic State, much like Plato's Republic, where psychiatrists are philosopher-kings and the rest of the population, called 'patients', are slaves.[46]

Spencer's imagery of state despotism and free individual agency ranges synoptically across the ages and institutions of mankind: Szasz subordinates his many historical-analytical excursions to one propagandist and polemical task, the demolition of collectivist pretensions in psychiatry and medicine. His is a specialised Spencerism, but a Spencerism for all that.

The laissez-faire attack on the state acknowledges no sympathy with the root-and-branch anti-statism of the anarchists. The abolition of government functions is dismissed as a utopia by Spencer, who interprets anarchism as a brainstorm of 'the constitutionally criminal', or of the over-educated, who 'are unable or unwilling to recognise the truth that a governmental organisation of some kind is necessary, and in a measure beneficent'.[47] Szasz's philosophy of the state is likewise one of minimum government rather than no government. Only psychiatric force requires total abolition: the judicial coercions of imprisonment and the seizure of property through fines are to remain, and the intervention of the state through the apparatus of both civil and criminal law is not only presumed but encouraged as the ultimate mode of conflict resolution. In both thinkers the necessity of state organisation arises through the need to check the aggression of one individual against another, but any regulative ordinance which attempts to dictate the moral health of the citizenry has to be resisted.

The threat of the state is usually seen by ordinary liberals as arising from the exercise of its open legal armoury of suppression: the police, the intelligence apparatus, draconian laws and courts, press censorship, and in critical moments the Napoleons of the military. The virtue of all critical social theory is to go beyond liberalism in identifying less obvious forms of civil coercion: for marxists the private monopoly of the means of production, for Weberians the impersonal logic of bureaucratic Organisation, for pluraliste and elitists the great oligarchies of the party machine and the mass institution. The obsessive sweep of Spencer's anti-statism turned over every stone of the contemporary institutional scene, and almost always uncovered the poisonous toad of government. But one particular area of state supervision claimed Spencer's attention over and over again: the guardianship of the physical health of the populace by detailed building laws, publicly constructed drainage and water supply, the compulsory examination of children by school medical officers, and the like. Just as Szasz sees the rise of public psychiatry as the outgrowth of 'the Mental Health Movement' – a totalitarian mass enterprise akin to Fascism and Communism – so Spencer detects a 'sanitary agitation' or 'movement'[48] conducted from the lobbies of the Vaccination Act of 1840 and the New Building Act of 1849 to the Contagious Diseases Act of 1864, the Public Health Act of 1872 and its various successors and corollaries. What 'the Therapeutic State', that repository of totalitarian brainwashing, is for Szasz, 'Sanitary Supervision' is for Spencer; to it he devotes a chapter in *Social Statics*, numerous reflections in *The Man versus the State*, some deeper philosophical musings in *The Principles of Ethics*, an aside or two in his essay on 'Over-Legislation'[49] and a final riposte to the health legislators, 'Sanitation in Theory and Practice',[50] published in 1902 before his death. Spencer is not of course opposed to the cause of the public's health; but he insists that the safety of the people actually suffers through being subjected to Boards of Health and other official inspectorates, and provides many examples of worsening conditions, damage to personal welfare, and even outright loss of life, to be ascribed to the meddling of 'our sanitary agitators'.[51] No good at all for humanity is seen by Spencer to come from the institutions of Sanitary Supervision, any more than it comes for Szasz from the machinations of Institutional Psychiatry, with its forcible lobotomies, compulsory hospitalisations and scapegoatings of the helpless deviant. Spencer's case for 'extending to medical advice the principles of free trade'[52] like Szasz's case for commercial psychiatry as the sole mode of therapy, rests upon a judicious attention to the sufferings of those victimised by the state or public system; and there is no bonus of benefit, no one whose condition (physical or psychological) is restored or even temporarily alleviated, no positive advantage whatsoever from the ministrations of the public agency, to offset the hurt and the tyranny. It is, indeed, not the need of the people which propels the looming Juggernaut of the public-health establishment, but the subjective need of the Juggernaut to perpetuate itself and identify new objects for its concern.

> How is it that beliefs so conspicuously fallacious have been established and are maintained by central and local bodies and their employers? There has developed a bureaucracy which has an interest in keeping up these delusions; and the members of which, individually, have interests in insisting upon these needless expenditures. Every organised body of men… tends to magnify its own importance. (*Facts and Comments*, p. 176)

In like rhetorical vein Szasz writes:

> The massive manpower mobilisation in the Mental Health Movement is best understood as an attempt to increase the number of mental patients 'found' in society… the state and federal governments, their subdivisions, and private and philanthropic organisations are hiring more psychiatrists, psychologists and social

> workers to tear more madmen out of the bowels of society. And for whose good? The answer can only be: for those who hire them, who define their task, and who of course pay them.[53]

In short, both the classical and the modern version of laissez-fairism anti-collectivism are compelled to compress social problems into two varieties: those which are pseudo-problems, artefacts of the 'finding fault' that is necessarily practised by the bureaucratic meddlers; and those genuine problems which can be resolved satisfactorily through the workings of a free enterprise system – as in Spencer's suggestion that the market mechanism would, if left undisturbed, supply the working classes with water closets[54] and in Szasz's elusive hints – he provides no more than these – of a health service organisation based on 'voluntary, mutually competing groups', with 'charity… purged of coercion, and decency of domination'.[55] For the rest, we have no longer a structured configuration of social problem areas, but rather an unconnected series of individual career choices; these range from Szasz's prototype of 'malingering', paralleled by Spencer's 'skilful mendicancy… which induces the simulation of palsy, epilepsy, cholera and no end of diseases',[56] to a whole host of negligences and failings which may either be considered by society within the frame of criminal and civil jurisdiction or else left to run their fatal course.

The picture of society painted so garishly by the laissez-fairist brush would be somewhat deficient in its darkest shading if our artists omitted some portrayal of the veriest abyss of Collectivism – the Socialist State. The various timorous reforms against which they polemicise – reforms usually conducted or advocated by bourgeois philanthropists of decidedly anti-revolutionary views – are understandable, indeed, only as instalments of the despotism to come. 'Western medical ethics', according to Szasz, are being undermined by 'the collectivist ethic of Communism', and for this sad state of things 'we cannot blame an external enemy. The Communists are not imposing their medical ethic by force of arms. The conflict is within our society… Indeed, the erosion… antedates the Russian revolution' and Szasz then approvingly cites the anti-statist alarums raised by the *Journal of the American Medical Association*, that hard core of the hard core right, on the appearance of Lloyd George's modest Insurance Act for health care in 1912.[57] Herbert Spencer, of course, sprinkled the foreboding of Red doom liberally in his texts, writing of the 'Communistic theories, partially indorsed by one Act of Parliament after another, and tacitly… favoured by numerous public men seeking supporters' and of the 'numerous socialistic changes made by Act of Parliament', that would 'by and by be all merged in State-Socialism – swallowed in the vast wave they have little by little raised.'[58]

But then how can Thomas Szasz, in this day and age, really be an anti-collectivist? The media along which he transmits the Individualist gospel are owned by giant conglomerates. The vehicles that transport him from one debonair speech or interview to the next are the property of massive institutional stockholdings, or else are produced by neo-feudal, transnational companies which have long said farewell to laissez-faire and Andrew Carnegie. Even his clients, those of us who can afford to embrace the Contractual Psychiatrist's ethics by giving prompt payment to his invoices, derive their living not from a small entrepreneurial economy, from farmstead or grocery or artisan's trade, but usually from their placement in a stratified hierarchy laid out within some business enterprise, public bureaucracy, or other unmistakably anti-individualistic collective. Even to pose the issues of the present age, as Szasz does, in terms of a contest between Individualism and Collectivism is sadly to misread contemporary history, and to provide what is at best a pious consolation for middle-class status loss, at worst a rhetorical smokescreen that fogs the real social world. The serious contests of our time are not waged between Individualism and Collectivism but between and among the collectives of various sizes, shapes and ideological colourings. Employers' cartel or trade union; Pentagon or National Liberation Front; bureaucratic clique or rank-and-file caucus; liberal capitalist party, conservative capitalist party or workers' party; the pressure group, the multicorporate firm, the welfare office, the association of slum residents, the newspaper or television network, the board of the educational institute, the student strike committee, the workers' picket line, the state itself: such are the terms within which human destinies are being settled. However useful and absorbing the two-person therapy situation may be for its select participants, it is a tiny individualist atoll, fit for the psychoanalystic Crusoe-and-Friday duo, but hardly capable of housing the immense reserves of counter-collectivist firepower that Szasz would wish to be based on it. The invading mechanised divisions of governmental and medical violence are not going to be stopped in their tracks by a barricade of analysts' couches. Politics can be resisted only by politics, institutions by institutions. In Szasz's 'game of life' the stakes have mounted to the level of alternative social orders: the apostles of individualism long ago plumped for a system, a notoriously bad one at that.

The concept of free choice in the name of which Szasz wages his innumerable battles against state coercion is a peculiarly unreal one. At times it seems as if freedom is embodied in all human actions whatsoever, a defining attribute of behaviour whose presence cannot be argued over: 'if by "behaviour" we mean a characteristic of persons, not of bodies, it can strictly speaking never be physiologically determined since it is by definition more or less freely chosen'.[59] On the other hand we are warned that 'voluntary' hospitalisation cannot be taken to express a free choice merely on the patient's say-so, since in most American mental institutions the patient does not have an unqualified right to leave.[60] Against the determinism which his medical training would suggest, Szasz insists that all adults 'are responsible'.[61] He admits of no exceptions whatsoever to this general statement of the capacity of adults to make free and responsible decisions: much of his work indeed consists of a systematic destruction of the claims of psychiatry to impugn the legal responsibility of certain individuals on the grounds of mental incompetence or illness.[62] Whenever possible, the language of personal irresponsibility, with its consequences of the removal of the allegedly incompetent individual from legal to medical auspices, is to be replaced by terms which would endorse the full accountability of the individual in civil and criminal law. Psychiatrists have no expertise which would enable them to declare anyone unfit to stand trial, not guilty by reason of insanity, of diminished responsibility by reason of psychopathy, hallucination or intoxication, or incompetent to manage their own affairs through mental disease or illness. These knotty topics of forensic psychiatry, which have caused so many courtrooms to echo with hectic drama and tortuous logic-chopping, are cut through boldly by Szasz's outright enunciations of principle: there are none unfit to stand trial (unless their incompetence on the stand is so remarkable that the layperson can detect it), none whose mental condition renders them eligible for psychiatric rather than judicial disposal, no mitigating circumstances arising out of diminished responsibility, and (above all) no mental illnesses or diseases which would offer a grounding for any of the above pleas.

The forensic-psychiatric problems of individual capacity or competence occupy, in the pages of Szasz's writings, a proportion of space which enormously outweighs the statistical incidence of such cases in the total population of the 'mentally ill'. There are many psychiatrists of experience who will never have come across one patient whose case-record raises the tangled legal perplexities with which Szasz engages. Such instances are of central importance for Szasz, firstly because the forensic issues of responsibility and non-responsibility pose, like the other deep human issues of suicide and drug addiction, inescapable questions which the absolutist libertarian of psychiatry must face head-on or else concede, dangerously, to his opponents. To allow the possibility that some individuals may display a psychopathology that justifies a compulsory psychiatric intervention is to set the first footstep down the slope of coercive, institutional care. To permit the passage of criminal defendants and civil litigants from the Rule of Law to the extralegal arbitration of medicine is to usher them from a realm where the operations of authority are checked by statute and appeal into a murkier, more sinister terrain where authority enjoys unlimited powers of sentencing, its penalties barbaric, the term set for its 'treatments' utterly uncontrolled. Just as Spencer, in his critique of nineteenth-century prison conditions, pleaded for the consideration of 'equity' towards inmates to be given strict precedence over the criterion of their reformation,[63] so Szasz counterposes the Just State, whose function is 'the maintenance of internal peace through a system of just laws justly administered' to the Therapeutic State whose task is 'the provision of behavioural reform scientifically administered by a scientific elite'.[64] The reinstatement of the total responsibility of the agent is a foremost necessity in Szasz's project of halting the transfer of cases from the secular court to the dispensation of the psychiatric Inquisition.

Szasz's category of responsibility is, peculiarly enough, present only among adults – who are of course alone capable of entering legally binding contractual relationships. It is interesting that, in the one passage I have been able to find where he discusses the position of minors, he is content to leave them 'under the jurisdiction of their parents or guardians'.

> Children do not have the right to drive, drink, vote, marry, make binding contracts, etc; they acquire these rights at various ages, coming into their full possession at maturity (usually between the ages of 18 and 21). The right to self-medication should similarly be withheld until maturity.[65]

(The switch in the last sentence to a normative diction indicates that the earlier catalogue of 'rights' was prescriptive rather than merely informative.) It is significant that Szasz's deeply researched examples of psychiatric coercion always (as far as I have been able to discover) deal in adult material: the whole sphere of juvenile justice, in which pseudo-therapeutic notions of 'treatment' by savage sentencing in corrupt institutions has been so especially pernicious, is characteristically outside his grasp.

The 'positive freedoms' that are a commonplace of left-liberal or radical-democratic political theorising are far removed from Szasz's contractual liberty. For this trend of social thought, our freedom is not something given by definition, attaching to our actions in virtue of some inner logical quality that precedes their effect and their context. Since, in the words of one such theorist, T.H. Green, 'the ideal of true freedom is the maximum of power for all members of human society alike to make the best of themselves'[66] freedom is an achieved, not an inherent condition: it is to be measured by the development of the individual's powers in self-determination, not assumed to exist as an all-or-nothing quality whatever one does. By the standards of this type of positive freedom, the freedom to develop one's own humanity, it is obvious that the pauper begging for pence outside the Ritz is less free than the cultivated upper classes who throng the tables inside. By the standards of contractual freedom, the beggar and the bourgeois are on a par, since both enjoy the same formal legal rights. That aspect of 'positive freedom' deriving from Hegel, which would link human freedom progressively (again as an achievement rather than as a given) to his expanding rationality,[67] is once again foreign to Szaszian contract freedom. By the measure of freedom-as-rationality, structured social inequalities in the distribution of human liberty are again revealed: those deprived of education and culture are unfree when compared with the educationally privileged, the mentally confused are less free than the mentally intact, and the wielders of blind market forces less again than the successful planners of an economy. But under their aspect of potential contractors, litigants and defendants, all these unequals are alike in their freedom. As Szasz claims, contract is the great leveller: it flattens out mountains and raises valleys – but only in the mind's eye of the contractual ideologue. For the rest of us, the rough places remain obdurately rough.

Even those classical liberties of bourgeois theory which are sometimes termed 'negative' because they consist in a freedom *from*, a 'relation of non-interference' or 'non-intrusion' between the individual and some exterior agency,[68] are made by Szasz into a dependency on contract. The violations of Institutional Psychiatry and the bureaucratised evasions of Collectivist Medicine acquire their fullest meaning through a contrast between their ambiguous ethic and the ethic of the open deal between vendor and client in individualist, 'Hippocratic' medicine.[69] The demand for personal privacy, which in its generalised expression constitutes what one commentator has termed 'perhaps the central idea of liberalism',[70] discernible as a key theme in Locke and Mill, Constant and Tocqueville, is renewed in Szasz's context by his selection of *confidentiality* as the prime requisite of all proper therapeutic relationships. And confidentiality in medicine is secured only (it seems) by the private treaty between entrepreneur-therapist and fee-paying client. Szasz maintains that 'The development of privacy as an integral part of the (private) therapeutic situation seems to be closely tied to the capitalist economic system.'[71] Without the clear demarcation of roles and responsibilities that is possible in the private therapeutic arrangement, the doctor or analyst may feel obliged to disclose his patient's confidences to some public agency to which he owes allegiance and possibly employment. Only by contract is the Hippocratic ethic of privacy safeguarded. Unfortunately for the privacy conferred by private practice, the American state's burglary of the office of Dr Daniel Ellsberg's psychiatrist indicates how little the Hippocratic oath is respected by those who have never taken it.

In this discussion of contractual liberty, the resonance between Szasz and Spencer is clearly discernible. The industrial regime of Contract is rhapsodised by Spencer as the conferrer of limitless blessings, affecting the political and social realm no less than the economic. The purely despotic integration of social units tends to vanish. The income differentials demanded by a meritocracy are maintained; personal morality is enriched; contract is the source of economic accumulation and national vigour. Although Szasz indicates that he has read *The Man versus the State* his promotion of contract-as-liberty perhaps follows less from Spencerian influence than from his effort to develop a world-view which generalises and validates his economic role as a privately practising analyst.

The reality of contractual freedom in an industrial society is much more dismal than either Szasz or Spencer can conceive. The formal equality of people as potential makers of economic contract rests on their actual inequality of access to the implements of production, in a society where popular livelihoods are concentrated overwhelmingly around those implements (along with their ancillary services of distribution, transport, educational training of a new work-force etc.). And the formal liberty, which places the two parties to the industrial contract – employer and worker – on the same footing as voluntary signatories, masks the actual subordination of the workers, whose position of permanent empty-handed inferiority to their wealthy monopolisers can be offset not by contractual provision but only by militant combination with their colleagues. That reading of history which measures social progress as a movement from the barbarism of Status to the civilisation of Contract attempts to erase from humanity's collective memory what has long ago been lost to individual memory: the gradual closing off, to the vast majority in the advanced world, of all possible means of livelihood except those which arise from the sale of labour-power to capital. The founders of marxism were able to capture the loss inflicted by capital upon human relationships precisely because they lived in an era when pre-capitalistic social formations based on 'status' still cast their shadow. *In what way does the proletarian differ from the serf?* runs one of the questions in the revolutionary catechism composed by the young Engels in 1847.

> The serf [replies the instructor] has the possession and the use of an instrument of production, a strip of land, in return for which he hands over a portion of the yield or performs work. The proletarian works with instruments of production belonging to another, for this other, in return for a portion of the yield. The serf gives, the proletarian is given… The serf stands outside competition, the proletarian is in it.[72]

The displacement of Status by Contract is seen by Marx and Engels not as the unequivocal linear progress of bourgeois theorists like Spencer and his American descendants, but as a double-column balance-sheet, in which ruin as well as advance is to be marked:

> The bourgeois… has put an end to all feudal, patriarchal, idyllic relations… It has drowned the most heavenly ecstasies of religious fervour, of chivalrous enthusiasm, of philistine sentimentalism, in the icy waters of egotistic calculation. It has resolved personal worth into exchange value, and in place of the numberless indefeasible chartered freedoms, has set up that single, unconscionable freedom – Free Trade.[73]

Szasz, the ideologue of the Free Trade in psychiatry, has said as much. What is Individualism in Szasz's medical ethic? Individualism is the cash-nexus. What is contractual freedom, in Szasz? The freedom of contract is: pay up or perish.

Despite the merits of Szasz's destructive critique of psychiatric institutions, the formalistic, juridical character of his concept of free choice makes it as worthless for the renovation of therapy as it is misleading for the analysis of society. The social liberation conferred by contractual individualism becomes fictive or fatuous as soon as we begin to look outside the capsule of the legal pact between two consenting parties: at the alternatives that are foregone by the conclusion of the contract, and at the latent power, never inscribed in the literal text of the agreement, which may enable one partner to force his or her terms on the other. So too in the micro-politics of psychiatry: Szasz's method of extracting from the flow of decisions and actions in a course of treatment one single element – the patient's expressed intention to seek a service – and then considering this under the sole rubric 'Voluntary/Involuntary' actually does violence to the substantive issues of freedom and subordination which permeate the institutions of therapy. On Szasz's reckoning, compulsory hospitalisation is an irredeemable fall from grace, disqualifying one from any further gradation of virtue or vice in the judgement of what goes on inside any psychiatric facilities that depart from the voluntary-individualistic model. The range of practical alternatives that are offered to patients within either the 'compulsory' world of public hospitalisation or the 'voluntary' space of the analyst's office is now simply excluded from consideration: for contractual libertarianism has no perspective on the field of choices that are available to the chooser. In reifying the patient's act of deciding to enter therapy, in making this moment into the sum of all freedoms, bourgeois libertarianism follows the same logic as that which it displays when it regards a political electorate as 'free' because it delivers its verdict in sealed ballot-boxes, or when it extols the 'consumer sovereignty' of those shoppers who buy goods under the pressures of the hard sell in a market fixed beforehand by giant firms. Any 'voluntary' psychiatric intervention is better, on Szasz's argument, than any 'involuntary' one: and among the involuntary, all are equally bad. But the real scandal of contemporary public psychiatry is not the particular section of the mental-health statutes under which patients get into hospital, but the alternatives offered to these supremely weak members of society by our present social arrangements both inside and outside the mental institution. A voluntary choice to enter psychiatric treatment may simply reflect the patient's confession of an inability to withstand the pressures of an engulfing family or of an alienated work-situation. And, once enclosed within a psychiatric treatment setting, the patient's 'voluntary' stay may reflect no greater freedom than that of a passive despair before the options available either within the institution or outside it. Indeed, Szasz's conception of free psychiatric choice has little ambition for the patient except the desire that he or she should say, preferably in public, 'I will.'

Because its gaze is riveted on the formal exteriors of choice, psychiatric right-libertarianism has nothing to say on the most deadening constraints that are experienced by mental patients (or by common civilians): the internalised shackles of acquiescence, the 'mind-forg'd manacles' that William Blake discerned in the 'marks of weakness, marks of woe' on every passing face as he wandered the 'chartered streets' of free-born England. That unusually horrifying and convincing anti-psychiatric tract of our time, Ken Kesey's novel *One Flew Over the Cuckoo's Nest*, reserves one of its most awesome illuminations on the realities of mental-hospital life for the moment when the compulsorily committed hero McMurphy is left to discover that he, of all the bullied, dosed and degraded inmates of his ward, is almost alone in not being a voluntary patient. In the end, after a rumbunctious mini-rebellion in which McMurphy attacks the persecuting nurse (and is afterwards forcibly lobotomised into an obedient stupor) Harding and several other voluntary patients recover their morale and discharge themselves from the hospital, 'still sick men in lots of ways,' but 'sick *men* now'. The melodrama of Kesey's solution cannot detract from the perceptiveness he brings to the problem of internalised, voluntarised coercion in psychiatric treatment: a problem which Szasz is precluded even from conceiving, owing to the shallowness of his definition of free action.

A kindred formalism is noteworthy in Szasz's discussion of the rival moral framework of physical medicine and the law which he has frequently advocated as replacements for the dictatorial norms of public psychiatry. The ethic of surgery and the practice of the ordinary medical hospital is contrasted with the use of involuntary psychiatric hospitalisation: the surgeon and physician insist on the 'informed consent' of patients before any procedures are set in motion upon their persons, and 'with few exceptions in cases that constitute a public-health hazard', hospital care for physical ailments is provided only for those who express a positive desire for treatment.[74] Similarly, the open pleadings of the law court, with its rules of evidence and its testing of witnesses by cross-examination, are set against the private tribunals conducted by medical bureaucrats who function as prosecution, witness, judge and jury rolled into one, without effective constitutional safeguards for the defendant-patients and for the most part without appeal from verdict or sentence.[75] The contrast between the demands of publicly regulated law and those of behavioural control through therapy has been generalised by Szasz into a polar opposition between two political trends of our age: the Legal State 'in which both ruler and ruled are governed by the Rule of Law', and the Therapeutic State 'in which the citizen-patient's conduct is governed by the "judgement" of the medical despot.'[76] These appeals to alternative models for social conduct are vital and impressive – until one realises that Szasz is not comparing like with like. He does not juxtapose the reality of psychiatry against the reality of law and physical medicine as functioning institutions, or the legal and medical ideals at their noblest against a parallel lofty psychiatric ethic. From medicine and the law, he takes the formal goals and the coded rules: from psychiatry he takes the most dubious, most atrocious actualities. In short, when writing of psychiatrists he tells what they *really* do, especially at their worst; when discussing surgeons and judges he only tells us what they should do. But even a cursory reflection on the actualities of surgery and physical medicine, as well as on the operations of the law courts (especially in the

United States, Szasz's terrain of comparison), will reveal how shoddy in practice are the safeguards of their ideals. The requirement of 'informed consent' in surgery, for example, does not deter a surgeon from over-intervention at the patient's expense. Thus, although both British and American medicine operate a procedure whereby the patient's consent is secured before an operation, the per capita rate for operations in the United States is twice as high as that for England and Wales: a preponderance which is likely to have little to do with any greater incidence of anatomical dysfunctions among American patients, and a great deal to do with the fact that the United States is supplied with twice as many surgeons per head of population (concentrated most intensely in the wealthier communities of the nation) as England and Wales.[77] The coexistence of this maximally active and interventionist fee-paying sector with a dilapidated medical service in public hospitals and general practice for the poorer quarters should make any of Szasz's readers very wary of adopting the existing norms of physical medicine as a substitute for psychiatry's discredited ideals. It is likely that far more unwarranted deaths and ruined lives have resulted from medicine's combination of Informed Consent – or the swaying of patients by surgical zeal – and Uninformed Neglect even than from the worst depredations of public psychiatry.

The proclamation of the Rule of Law as a contestant to psychiatric provision is unlikely to persuade those who have watched the differing angle of tilt that rich and poor can bring to bear on the scales of actual administered justice. Szasz's Legal State would replace the Therapeutic State only by emptying the mental hospitals of the poor, the black and the powerless and filling up the prisons with the same classes of people, who would find little consolation in being found guilty of designated crimes instead of diagnosed maladies. The clause in the American Bill of Rights forbidding 'cruel and unusual punishment' has been impotent against the clubbings and other cruelties imposed, not as vindictive exceptions but as a general method of control, in the worst correctional centres. While there may be little to choose in brutality between the most repressive prisons and the most repressive mental wards, the most humane advances in the devising and running of institutional regimes which minimise damage for their inmates have so far come either from psychiatric hospitals or from penal institutions that, like Grendon Psychiatric Prison in Britain or Herstedvester in Sweden, are managed on a strongly medical, therapy-oriented ideology.

But to stress this point is already to enter too much on Szasz's battleground of the formal ideal which is to enshrine our conduct towards the rejects of the existing social order. It is not in framing the terms of some notional ethical goal, but in the construction of alternative social structures that we will be able to measure progress in the treatment, and even in the toleration of the mentally alienated. The fight against involuntary hospitalisation makes sense not as an absolute, but as part of the fight against hospitalisation itself. The argument over which sort of suicidal patients should be let loose by the doctor to go and kill themselves raises fascinating questions of individual ethics; its resolution, one way or the other, costs nothing except hurt feelings. But the organisation of our social life to enable the dismantling of what we now term the mental hospital, and the provision of substitute-family units in the heart of the community, into which those who have lost their way may find a way, and a way back, is an undertaking which will cost both mobilisation and money. The war on 'mental illness' that Thomas Szasz has been waging is a deflection from a more systematic war over mental illness that is just beginning, and has taken far too long to get started. There are already too many powerful forces of inertia, routinism and plain hostility towards the presence of the mentally ill: forces which can be relied on to set public provision in psychiatry squarely at the back of the queue for resources milked in advance by the well-buckled and comfortably sane. When at the end of 1970, the New York City administration subjected the after-care of the psychiatrically ill to savage financial reductions, it did so as part of the first round of cuts because it knew that all the other possible targets of its measures had a voice and a pull. But, in an action that heralded a long sequence of militancy (which is discussed in Part Two below) mental patients joined with their psychiatrists to charter a subway train on which they rode to lobby City Hall to restore the threatened services. That action, so totally incomprehensible to Szasz, was only one of the forms of struggle which emerged in the seventies for the rights of such patients who generally are in the unenviable position of needing libertarian vigilance and political pressure at a time and in a condition when they are least able to exert any kind of leverage. The forging of an alliance uniting psychiatric patients and the mass agencies of social change is a necessity requiring time and persistence. Only, finally, at the level of the social system itself can the fundamental question behind this, as all other welfare issues be posed: the responsibility of all for the fate of all. It is the politics of a revolutionary, collectivist and democratic socialism which will answer, through irreversible historic shifts in our conception of freedom and care, beleaguered politics of a capitalism that glorifies its indifference.

Part Two:
Psychiatry and Liberation

7. Mental Health Movements and Issues: A Survey and Prospect

In 1975 an industrial region of New Haven, Connecticut, was visited by a research team who proceeded to make an inventory of the mental-health facilities in the area, the types of diagnosis and treatment that were on offer there, and the social composition (including the class composition) of the patients who were receiving the treatments in or out of hospital. One of the main investigators, Dr Fritz Redlich, was no stranger to the target district: 25 years earlier he had been the joint chief investigator, and co-author of the main report,[1] in a pioneering and highly influential study which had engaged in similar sociological and psychiatric probings in exactly the same area of New Haven. The year chosen for the earlier survey had been 1950, just five years short of the all-time peak, in United States history, of the number of inmates in mental institutions. The researchers returning in 1975 found a psychiatric scene that had been transformed, in certain striking ways, by the arrival of the Community Mental Health Centers following the Kennedy Act of 1963, by the great proliferation of tranquillising and neuroleptic drugs as an alternative to long-stay hospital residence, and through the wider movement towards the desegregation of the mentally ill that had proceeded from a host of pressures – medical, administrative, budgetary, political, cultural and judicial – over the intervening decades.[2]

Thus, in 1950 the resident population of the state mental hospital for the region was some 3,000; in 1975 it was 1,000 only. In 1950 the average length of stay for a patient in this hospital was over 20 years: in 1975 it was seven months, with the great majority of patients finishing their spell of asylum in 60 days or less. Admissions for these shorter spells had increased, but readmissions had rocketed upwards, provoking the comment that 'open doors' had become 'revolving doors'. The Community Mental Health Centers in the region now treated more patients in a year than did the state mental institution, and these CMHC treatments were primarily in the form of out-patient care.

The reduced core of inmates in the state mental institution presented a markedly different profile of symptoms compared with their predecessors in the age of the asylum's population-explosion. Then, 45 per cent of all resident mental patients in the region had been listed as schizophrenics, but in 1975 only a fifth were so regarded. As replacements for the schizophrenics who had died, been shunted into nursing homes (the female and the elderly being peculiarly prone to this form of disposal), 'maintained' as out-patients on dosages of phenothiazine drugs, or relabelled through changes in psychiatric nomenclature, there had arrived a new nucleus of permanent or semi-permanent residents: the alcoholics. Appearing in the state mental-hospital census in similar proportions to the old core of schizophrenics, these were principally male, significantly black (30 per cent of all alcoholics on state wards, drawn from a region almost 90 per cent white), with a readmission rate which was, at 75 per cent of all patients with this diagnosis, the highest for any of the mental illness categories.

Absent from the new survey, as the authors acknowledged, was any census of those patients, formerly eligible for mental-hospital treatment, who had been discharged to the 'decentralised back wards' outside the medical system: the rooming-houses, back-street hotels, welfare hostels, Salvation Army shelters, proprietary 'nursing' or 'foster' homes, the jails, the streets themselves.[3] The 'coffin-like room at a deteriorated inner-city hotel or Bowery flop house', or the board-and-care home in which 'there are often three or four ex-patients to a room' and where 'the monthly check which may amount to as much as $230.00 a month for the totally disabled is managed by the home operator, who in return provides board and also a weekly allowance of spending money',[4] is subject to none of the outrage, or even the attention, which have been accorded to the psychiatric institution by novelists, journalists, film-makers, academics and other media practitioners. Their inmates are subject to virtually no registration in statistics, their personnel have experienced little in the way of training and less in public supervision. In the balance-sheet of health care affecting mental patients, who can reckon their measure?

Equally absent from the reckoning is that section of the psychotherapeutic industry which lies outside the strictly medical sector. Primarily in the United States but also in many other countries of the advanced West, the years since 1950 have been those of a long growth-cycle of such forms of counter-neurotic technology as joy therapy, reality therapy, primal scream therapy, transcendental meditation, Gestalt therapy, marathon encounter groups, Reichian massage, co-counselling, psychodrama, Lacan's 'ten-minute psychoanalytic session', rebirthing, 'transactional analysis', bio-energetics, existential therapy, behaviour modification, rational-emotive therapy, postural integration (or 'rolfing') and psychosynthesis.

In an enlightening paper, Joel Kovel has remarked that 'the half-life of therapies now comes to resemble that of schools of art or rock groups'. Such exotic and transient remedies

> have to shout louder and promise more to get a rise out of their increasingly jaded subjects. As a result of these trends – which match on the cultural scale the development in the individual of forms of neurosis which lack clear lines of internal repression and hence lack classical symptoms – there has come to be a gradual coalescence of therapy with other forms of mass culture.[5]

Whatever truth may lie behind these suggestions of a specific cultural and psychic substrate for these forms of Therapy as Spectacle, their economic significance is crudely obvious. Financed on an individual fee-for-service basis, though sometimes underwritten by insurance schemes which may or may not be a burden to the public exchequer, they function to provide skill-intensive and frequent treatments (usually without the controlled trials as to efficacy to which any pharmaceuticals firm marketing a new drug has to make at least some obeisance) for precisely those conditions of emotional or psychological disturbance which are, in the range of psychiatric disorders, among the mildest and the least persistent. The agony of the personal conditions which induces the relatively well-off to seek this sort of help is not to be gainsaid: and there are, of course, neurotic illnesses, for example certain phobias and compulsions, which in any scale of seriousness deserve a high priority in the allocation of skilled therapy. Judged overall, however, the current expansion of private therapeutic practices, although often framed within a non-medical or even anti-medical rationale, amounts to a trend very similar to that contained in privatised, fee-for-service medicine itself; it funnels money, skills and careers away from the severe and the chronic personal problems of the lower socio-economic orders (who cannot foot the bill or speak the language of the more affluent private sector) and into the less chronic, less severe but financially rewarding and culturally voguish difficulties of the well-heeled. 'Alternative therapy' is an alternative not so much to medicine, as to the social organisation of health care according to need.

Such a judgement may, in relation to the dense and uncharted undergrowth of the alternative therapy systems, appear as little more than assertion without evidence. The New Haven researchers have, nonetheless, provided ample documentation of the class inequalities within the formal medical systems of psychiatric care, whether private or public. Indeed, the most obvious continuity between the two psychiatric censuses of the region, separated as they are by a quarter-century replete with practical innovation, lies in the disclosure of a persistent class-related hierarchy in the availability of treatments. Hollingshead and Redlich had devoted some of the most trenchant pages of *Social Class and Mental Illness* to a detailing of the inequalities of treatment accorded to the psychiatrically ill of different classes.[6] In the earlier survey, the patients of 'Class V' – unskilled and semi-skilled workers of poor education – were much more likely than the members of superior social rankings to receive organic treatments (ECT, insulin coma, brain surgery, drugs); if they were given any psychotherapy it would be of the 'brief' or 'directive' kind as distinct from the '50-minute hour', traditional within psychoanalytic piecework, which was prescribed for members of 'Class I' (executive-professional, 'upper') or 'Class II' (managerial-professional, 'upper-middle'). It was a common fate, however, for Class V patients to receive no active treatment, but only custodial care in the state mental institution, and to undergo the longest spells of hospitalisation uninterrupted by discharge and re-admission (that is, if they were psychotic; if they had a neurotic illness, they were likely to be dismissed from treatment much sooner than the members of the upper social classes). When the types of psychiatric treatment were ranked in order of their costliness, Hollingshead and Redlich found that it was the high-status patients who received the most expensive therapies.

The 1975 New Haven study disclosed a number of important changes in the styles of contemporary therapy; in particular, drug treatment had become part of the therapeutic mix for all classes, and the old sharp divide between the 'psychodynamic' school of therapists (engaging in contracts with the disturbed members of the upper social echelons) and the 'organic' and 'custodial' orientations (primarily for the lower orders) had been eroded. Psychoanalysis was rated an important tool only by a minority of resident doctors, and few psychiatrists omitted the prescription of chemical medication from their repertoire of treatments, for whatever class of client. Straight custodial containment of patients (without even an attempt to treat with drugs) had declined dramatically, at least inside the official psychiatric institutions; naturally, it was prevalent in the nursing-home residential complex which formed the new back wards for the intractable and poor.

Nevertheless, the hierarchy of forms of treatment, related to class, remained intact in the new dispensation of Community Mental Health. The medical presence in psychiatry became increasingly diluted as the social level of its clientele moved downwards. Psychiatrists, the accredited high-status profession who provided legitimation for the system as a whole, worked for the most part with middle- or upper-class patients of working age.

> Few psychiatrists or residents reported much contact with the aged, alcoholic, drug-dependent or sociopathic patients... In addition, in 1975 as in 1950, there was almost a complete absence of interest in the mentally retarded and patients with brain disease.

Within the publicly funded system, the doctors devoted less than half their time to direct patient care; this they tended to devolve to a wide variety of subordinate staff, whether psychologists, social workers, nursing aides or clergy. By contrast, almost 90 per cent of the private psychiatrists' hours were spent in direct patient contact; and most of the senior medics in the public hospitals and systems had outside private practices, in which they experienced a large proportion of their contact hours with patients, primarily from the better-off classes. Medical charisma, bestowed on psychologists and social workers to validate their devolved therapeutic role, also brought opportunities for lucrative private practice to these public employees. But the main role of the ancillary staff was to perform as proxies for their medical seniors in the publicly funded facilities, whether inpatient or out-patient.[7]

The social ranking of the patients now correlated closely with the status and accreditation of the particular mental-health professional concerned in therapy: psychiatrists and psychologists treated the middle-to-upper-class neurotic or schizophrenic; nurses and mental-health workers treated the lower-class alcoholic or aged patient; social workers were given the moderately disturbed, middle-class adolescent. 'Not one psychiatrist was involved in the therapeutic care of alcoholics in the state hospital.' However, in the private hospitals, it was the psychiatrists who were the most usual therapists responsible for alcoholics (who here were mostly of high socio-economic status, and nearly always white).

The implications of this remarkable study afford no easy evasions for the citizens of other countries. The special visibility of America's class inequalities in psychiatric treatment does not arise through any United States monopoly in these unequal practices. The combination of privatised medicine for the few with state-sponsored cutbacks in public provision is becoming an increasingly general feature of the Western world in the present period of economic crisis. If we hear little about the concentrated facilities for psychiatric treatment which are available to the very rich in, for example, Britain, it is not because such privileges are absent from their life-style but because no systematic exploration of their nature and importance has been conducted.[8] At the opposite end of the distribution of life-chances, the provision of residential treatment (other than police cells and jails) for the lower-class alcoholic is much less advanced in Britain than in the United States, and even these limited places have been axed first by the Labour and then by the Tory governments.[9] In Britain as in the USA, the reduction in the register of patients resident in mental hospitals – from a peak of 154,000 in 1954 to around two-thirds of this total in recent years – has been achieved through the creation of a rhetoric of 'community care facilities' whose influence over policy in hospital admission and discharge has been particularly remarkable when one considers that they do not, in the actual world, exist. (The private nursing-home solution for the disposal of the elderly and confused has not been a means of reducing the mental-hospital population of the British Isles.) The British Conservative Government announced in Sir Keith Joseph's memorandum of December 1971 that within 15 years all mental hospitals without exception were to be closed down. Chronic patients would be moved to small residential hospitals near their homes, and acute cases would be treated in the short-stay psychiatric wards of the new district general hospitals. Domiciliary social services and large-scale hostel accommodation were to be provided by the local government authorities, who would receive ample grants from the central exchequer for these urgent purposes.[10]

The impulsion behind this onslaught on the mental institution – a cardinal tenet of later social-democratic administrations in Britain no less than with the libertarian wing of Toryism – may have been budgetary as well as ideological. Andrew Scull's analysis of the processes of 'de-carceration', or the evacuation of prison and mental-hospital inmates from institutions into the community, has powerfully argued for the strength of the sheer fiscal constraints that, in Britain as well as America, made the century-old critique of the asylum and the prison a sudden matter of urgent implementation for cost-conscious administrators of the welfare purse, in an era which uniquely combines the pressures of inflation with those of slump.[11] But the drive towards the dismantling of the mental hospital has proven to be markedly ideological in that classic sense of 'ideology' first offered by Marx and Engels in their analysis of the social function of the ruling-class ideas: not to reflect or communicate truths about reality but on the contrary to act as a smokescreen, masking the bitter facts of social oppression in the self-interest of a powerful and articulate minority. In Britain no less than in the United States, 'community care' and 'the replacement of the mental hospital' were slogans which masked the growing depletion of real services for mental patients: the accumulating numbers of impaired, retarded and demented males in the prisons and common lodging-houses; the scarcity not only of local authority residential provision for the mentally disabled but of day centres and skilled social-work resources; the jettisoning of mental patients in their thousands into the isolated, helpless environment of their families of origin, who appealed in vain for hospital admission (even for a temporary period of respite), for counselling or support, and even for basic information and advice about the patient's diagnosis and medication.[12]

By 1975, the Department of Health and Social Services had to confess the failure of the Powell-Joseph plan to decant the mental-hospital population into alternative 'community facilities'. 'A substantial number of the long-stay patients who were in hospital in 1954, the basis for the 1961 projections, are still there.' Indeed, nearly 40 per cent of the patients, who in the 1971 mental-hospital census had been in the institution for more than one year, were inmates of more than 20 years' residence in hospital. 'At the last count in 1974 more than 24,000 patients did not have full personal clothing of their own; many did not have a cupboard in which to hang their clothes.' Outside the hospital, local authority provision of day and residential resources for the mentally ill was in national terms far short of the target set by previous governments, and 'some still have no facilities at all.'[13] Since the publication of these findings both hospital and local authority facilities for psychiatric patients have deteriorated even further, in line with the general run-down of the health and social services through deliberate Labour and Conservative policy.

Any critique of health service provision, whether in psychiatric or in physical medicine, which is addressed primarily to the question of resource allocation remains a seriously incomplete one. Exposure of serious inequalities in the distribution of resources between classes (as in the work of Hollingshead, Redlich and their colleagues) or the revelation of naked scarcity in the provision of basic psychiatric services (as in the British examples) can become such an urgent preoccupation that it is easy to forget the wider and deeper questions of medical politics. The mobilisations necessary to restore budgetary cutbacks or save threatened facilities tend to focus on questions of *how much*: we argue that society should allocate more for health, less for defence, or else we protest at the draining of national resources into the private medical sector while the public services remained under-financed. But in the very act of defining the issues in the terms of 'how much', the question of *what kind* of psychiatric services we need is downgraded in importance. From the work of Hollingshead and Redlich, it would be all too easy to draw the conclusion that injustice would be redressed if the poorer classes were enabled to engage in the face-to-face sessions of psychoanalysis which only the better-off can now afford. But it is wrong to use the standards of the private medical sector, whether of individual counselling by expensive practitioners of doubtful efficacy, or of private bedrooms distinct from other patients and other helpers, as though they were self-evidently the best possible standards of care. The rich parents who buy for their children a private schooling with compulsory chapel, compulsory sports and even, on occasion, compulsory sex, may not be wise consumers of health facilities either. Moreover, the defensive mobilisation in the cause of existing health care resources tends to sanctify the division of labour in the clinical professions, leaving patients as the endlessly demanding recipients of benefit from their betters. The self-help groups which have arisen among different categories of the ill, disabled and otherwise medically eligible (for example, pregnant women), may have originated as a response to failures in provision from the public health service; but the ideals that they subserve, namely the monitoring and control of the individual's own health destiny by himself or herself, form completely valid objectives in their own right.[14] All too often, a demand for medical (including psychiatric) care amounts to a request for some form of tardy and individualised intervention in a problem that should be met in preventive terms implicating the wider social and political system. If the psychological illness of depression is closely bound up in its origins with the onset of early traumatic life-events or with the poor level of intimacy in the patient's personal relationships,[15] then the demand for improved treatments – whether psychotherapeutic or pharmacological – for this condition makes as much or as little sense as a programme for 'treating', purely through individual medication in cases of outstanding disease, these illnesses such as asbestosis or silicosis which arise from the exposure of manual workers to unsafe but profitable industrial processes.

As in the rest of medicine, then, the quality of political consciousness that is involved in a movement for psychiatric reform may run all the way from a simple economism which demands more and more of the same thoroughly bad facilities to a radical questioning of the whole professional-therapeutic enterprise,[16] be it for the disorders of the body or the malfunctions of the psyche. For the most part, the social movements that have criticised the practices of psychiatry – whether from within the ambit of that specialism or else from without, as an 'anti-psychiatry' whose hostile tenor is well-known – have been inspired neither by a medical economism nor by an anti-medical nihilism. To some extent, the concerns of the reformers and radicals in the field of psychiatry present an uncomplicated parallelism with the pressure groups in the rest of medicine. Opponents of a biological, mechanistic model of causation in the psychic illnesses find easy alliances with their opposite numbers in physical medicine, and like them draw certain therapeutic conclusions, tending to a view of the patient as a social role-player rather than primarily as a bearer of pathogenic lesions.[17] The critics of a hierarchical and authoritarian psychiatry, with their demands for power-sharing among other professionals and indeed among patients themselves, are matched nowadays by many contesters of medical prerogative: proponents of the barefoot doctor, of the midwife's legitimacy, or the nurse's sovereignty, of alternative medicines such as acupuncture and homeopathy, or of consumer-controlled forms of health care. It might have been possible some years ago to claim that the surgical and chemical interventions of psychiatry formed an invasion of the subject's freedom not normally encountered in the world of physical medicine; but nowadays scarcely a week goes by without the announcement of some fresh hazard stemming from the application of a zealous medical technology to the body's cell structure. The survivors of that lobby which claims the side-effects of Largactil or neuro-surgery to be a privileged evil, raising questions of an injury necessarily deeper than any experienced by the victims of contraceptive injection or the loss of natural immunogens through antibiotics, are only the latest partisans of an age-old dualism – whose theoretical foundation I have criticised in Chapter 1 – which sees the body and its determinism as separate from the full nature of the person. Even those who dichotomise the public definition of mental and of physical health in terms of the formal and legal provisions for compulsory hospitalisation – rare and generally unused in physical doctoring except in the quarantine of infections and contagions, though universal and traditional in psychiatry – can only maintain this boundary by overlooking the common abuses of 'voluntary' consent procedures in which doctors and their aides, in general hospitals as well as mental institutions, engineer an uninformed compliance from the weak or helpless. The active consumer groups which have sprung up to oppose this manipulation in both spheres of medicine are wiser than these theorists.

The parallelism between the collective movements for the criticism and reform of medicine and the rather earlier ones dealing in psychiatry is by no means an exact one. In what follows I shall attempt to do justice to the specific policies of the various tendencies of reformist or radical change that have grown around the politics of psychiatric provision. But there is one major and obvious element in the militancy of psychiatric politics, as waged in a large number of countries since the end of the second world war, which finds no precise echo in the battles over medical power in general health care. The politicisation of psychiatry has been unique in the degree of attention that it has afforded to *the character of the hospital itself* as an agency for worsening pathology, for manufacturing it where it does not exist, or for operating as an extra-judiciary means of incarceration against those who have scorned official mores. Indeed, for many observers and participants of this sector of struggle, the attack on the residential mental institution forms the principal topic of debate and action in psychiatry. The timing of the various mobilisations against the dominance of the asylum solution for the mentally ill has been staggered over decades from one national culture to another. It is usual to associate the campaign against the mental hospital with intellectual figures from the sixties like Laing, Goffman or Foucault and the practitioners of 'anti-psychiatry' and 'alternative psychiatry' in different countries who have used their work as a medium to win general support among the public. But the first major steps in 'de-hospitalisation' for the mentally ill preceded the arrival of these cultural leaders.

Thus, as we have earlier pointed out, the totals of patients resident in mental hospitals in both Britain and the United States began their rapid descent in the mid-fifties, before Laing, Goffman, Szasz and anti-psychiatry had appeared on the stage of the intellectual media. In certain progressive hospitals in Britain, active attention to rehabilitation and resettlement and the unlocking of closed wards had led to a swift and drastic reduction in the number of in-patients even before the general trend of de-hospitalisation had crystallised, and considerably in advance of the introduction of the phenothiazine drugs and their diffusion through the massive sales efforts of the pharmaceuticals industry.[18] The straightforward 'pharmacological' explanation for the de-segregation of patients – the view that these new medications constitute a collective miracle drug which eradicates the worst psychotic symptoms and enables large-scale discharges into the community to take place as a direct result of their chemical action – is in any case fatally flawed by the relatively late point (1970) at which the in-patient numbers in French mental hospitals began to dip, following a post-war population explosion in the asylums which continued throughout the very period of the fifties and sixties that had been marked by a firm de-hospitalisation in British and

American psychiatry. It should be noted that chlorpromazine (Largactil), the most prominent of the new tranquillisers, had actually been first synthesised in France as early as December 1950, by the pharmaceuticals firm Rhône Poulenc.[19] It is not to be supposed that this lag of 20 years between the availability of the chemical First Cause and its effects on hospital practice was due to inactivity on the part of the merchandisers of Largactil in France. Other countries in the West have shown a trend towards de-segregation occurring as late, or even later, or scarcely at all even now. In Italy the major period of psychiatric reform begins in the sixties, with the therapeutic community organised in the Gorizia asylum by Franco and Franca Basaglia, and the efforts in community psychiatry, replacing hospital places by neighbourhood residences, conducted by Mario Tommasini at Parma (1965–69) and Giovanni Jervis in Reggio Emilia (1969 onwards).[20] Between 1961 and 1971 the number of psychiatric beds in Italy actually increased slightly (from 113,388 to 114,807) mainly through an expansion of private mental hospitals, the public sector having diminished slightly in this period.[21] During the seventies the national organisation *Psichiatria Democratica*, founded by the Basaglias and their co-workers, conducted a series of campaigns against public mental hospitals, whose norms of compulsory admission and custodial restraint at last became recognised as scandalous. Parliamentary legislation over 1978 and 1979 abolished all new admissions to the mental hospitals, and concentrated treatment for acute psychiatric cases in the casualty wards of general hospitals. *Psichiatria Democrática* had by this time waged a number of partially successful battles, particularly in Northern cities, for the funding and public support necessary for the large-scale re-settlement of mental patients from the hospitals into dispersed community dwellings.[22] The dumping of patients from asylums into inadequate neighbourhood facilities remains a horrific prospect, in Italy as elsewhere; but it should be noted that the timing as well as the politico-historical context of psychiatric de-segregation in Italy differs considerably from that in Britain and North America.

The pharmaceuticals industry has, of course, canvassed the merits of the long-acting tranquilliser, whose dosage is released into the bloodstream with an optimally delayed effect. In the Federal Republic of Germany, the homeland of a particularly vigorous and thrusting group of drug firms, the virtues of the tranquilliser have taken a long time indeed to percolate into the creation of any alternative to the mental hospital. In West German medicine generally, out-patient treatment from a hospital base has no standing: the segregative solution has been perfected even for physical illness, so that it is normal for a patient to be hospitalised merely to gain access to testing facilities which his or her private physician does not have at the office.[23] For the psychiatric patients of West Germany in 1972, there were no more than 20 out-patient centres, usually in cities with a university department of psychiatry, across a country of some 60 million inhabitants.[24] At an even severe level of ossified hierarchisation, the Spain of General Franco, despite a bountiful dispensing of psychotropic medicines in the latter years of the regime, had still failed to make any reversal in the institutional incarceration of the mentally ill – nearly always compulsory and conducted to an important degree within the asylums of religious foundation where the patients' average length of stay ran between ten and 20 years. Throughout all the turns in therapeutic fashion which in other countries impelled a timely decline in the hospitalisation of mental patients, the number of inmates of Spain's asylums continued to rise: it was 108 per 100,000 of population in 1960, 180 in 1970 and 239 for 1975. Moreover, the average length of stay for patients – including acute admissions – scarcely declined during those years of the sixties which elsewhere saw great pressure upon hospitals to increase their 'throughput of the treated'.[25] Out-patient facilities, again, were a considerable rarity.

Within the framework of an autocratic and custodial medicine, the addition of further neuroleptic drugs to the repertoire of the psychiatrist does not produce a liberalisation of treatment measures. Depending on the context – social as well as medical – in which it is applied, a particular pharmaceutical discovery may as easily strengthen a tradition of authoritarian containment as challenge it. In Britain today, for example, it is noticeable that the function of a particular medication, such as Largactil or Modecate, varies from that of an out-patient prescription with a specific anti-psychotic action to that of a general purpose bromide, doled out in massive frequency to long-term prison inmates or chronic mental patients as a convenient chemical strait-jacket or liquid cosh. And it should not be assumed that, even when administered on an out-patient basis, the advent of the newer drugs has done all that much positively to enable the sufferers of long-term psychiatric illness to lead a fuller, richer life. Writing in the *British Medical Journal* in 1979, a patient with extensive experience of being treated in a dispensary with a long-acting phenothiazine commented: 'I think that the richness of my pre-injection days, even with brief outbursts of madness, is preferable to the numbed cabbage I have become.' His point was taken up by a psychiatrist of eminence, who coneluded that

> the side effects occasioned by these drugs may be pretty intolerable... There is a danger, as I see it, that the injudicious use (or abuse) of

> psychotropic or tranquillising drugs… we may be edging back to the era of bromides and paraldehyde from which we escaped nearly half a century ago.[26]

To offer these observations is not to try to undermine the role of psychotropic drugs in symptom-relief, but merely to point to some of their limitations.

The movement towards unlocking hospitals and discharging patients cannot be explained, then, in terms of a chemical reductionism. But some cruder attempts to supply a social context for the operations of chemistry, by imputing a direct relation between the economic conjuncture and psychiatric policy, also invite a certain reserve. The two economic models of psychiatric hospitalisation (and de-hospitalisation) that have been recently on offer are those of Andrew Scull and Harvey Brenner. Both of these posit changes in the national economic climate as the main cause of population movements in and out of mental institutions, but their definitions of the relevant economic variables are rather discordant. In Scull's argument, the original impulse during the last century which propagated the asylum (and workhouse) solution of segregation arose from the new dominance of capitalist market relationships, in a crisis of public assistance marked by the failure of traditional forms of parochial help.[27] The subsequent long hegemony of the asylum is ended, during the inflationary years of our own welfare-state epoch, through the growing unavailability of public funds to maintain and improve the fabric of mental institutions now confronted by a rising tide of new admissions.[28]

It is not the therapeutic spirit of Hippocrates, but the capital-accounting ethos denounced by Marx and hymned by Weber, which in different phases of capitalist development herds the multitudes inside asylum walls and expels them again when the operation becomes too costly for a fiscally overextended social order. Brenner's version of the economic propellant for asylum inmates is simpler than this: his book *Mental Illness and the Economy*[29] analyses a series of statistics for mental-hospital admissions in the State of New York from 1841 to 1967 and concludes, by measuring these carefully against indices of economic prosperity for the same years, that (in a large number of comparisons across different ethnic groups, and New York State counties, for both men and women) psychiatric admissions rise with an economic downturn and decrease with an economic revival. The differences between these two authors' arguments stem in large part from the fact that Scull uses total resident numbers in mental hospitals and Brenner calculates only from admission figures. But for the period up to the mid-fifties of this century, admission to an American mental institution was generally the prelude to long-term incarceration. Brenner's case tells us that hospitalisation for the mental deviant is accepted as a necessary cost even in times of economic stringency; whereas Scull's point is that, at least in one epoch of economic decline – our own – the asylum becomes too expensive to maintain. Our less wealthy forebears of the nineteenth century, and our immediate ancestors of the inter-war depression years, could afford to build and maintain an expanding bed provision for the insane, in a manner which (it seems) we cannot emulate.

But, as soon as a broader view of psychiatric policy is taken across different national cultures, it becomes implausible to argue a primarily economic determination of the flow of patients across the boundaries of the hospital. As we have seen in our review of the chemical hypothesis of patient discharge, the dates of commencement for an active policy of desegregating mental patients vary from one country to another. If these critical eras of psychiatry fail to coincide with the timing of pharmaceutical innovation and diffusion, their relationship to the economic conjuncture is even more difficult to generalise. British and American hospitals started running down their numbers in the latter fifties, when the post-war boom was well under way and the 'fiscal crisis of the state' had not been discovered by any economic researcher. This is unfortunate for Scull's thesis, but the subsequent decline in the asylum populations of both countries, continuing into the years of downturn in manufacturing, makes difficulties for Brenner's case. The timing of de-hospitalisation programmes for the mentally ill in Europe, at least in the countries discussed above, provides no obvious support for either of the economically grounded hypotheses. Italy's campaigns against the incarceration of mental patients span some years of relative prosperity as well as the more recent period of spasmodic crisis;[30] whereas the post-war industrial boom in Franco's Spain, with its attendant economic (but hardly political) liberalisation, produced no discernable reforms in the charity madhouses whose tradition of pious containment has continued now over five centuries.

As a general observation, it may be stated that there is no obvious or necessary feedback from the condition of the gross national product into the decisions made by administrators whether to apportion health expenditures into hospitals or into out-patient forms of care. Spiralling health costs have not led to the provision of domiciliary or office services to replace the hegemony of the hospital in West Germany. The visible weakening of the British manufacturing economy did not prevent the foundation or completion of 71 new hospitals in general and physical medicine between 1966 and 1975 – though later on, through deliberate government policy, it wiped out the current-account spending which would have enabled these constructions to be staffed and run at a level of care satisfactory for the patients.[31] And, where mental hospitals are concerned, there is no evidence from European countries, from the period spanning the fifties through the sixties to the recessionary seventies, that the stock of psychiatric beds was run down along the lines that are familiar in the British and the American experience. Some countries even expanded their bed units during these years of growing economic uncertainty. We have already noted the small increase in Italy over the sixties; and the psychiatric bed statistics for those European countries reporting to the WHO over this lengthy period are given in Table 1. In the most sensational case, that of France (which did not report to the WHO) 33,000 mental-hospital beds (around one-third of the present stock) were added between 1960 and 1972.[32]

It would, of course, be quite senseless to deny the part played by wide-ranging economic factors in shaping the course of psychiatric history. But the economic link is at its strongest, not through transmitting the vagaries of the trade cycle, but (as Scull, Rothman and Foucault have pointed out in some sections of their work) via the operations of the different *general systems of public assistance* which come into play in successive economic epochs. The hey-day of the asylum in Britain and America is also the peak era for 'indoor relief', that segregative solution for other forms of deviancy which is witnessed in the construction of workhouses, almshouses, reformatories, orphanages and penitentiaries. As Scull perceptively remarks, any demand for the domiciliary treatment of the mentally afflicted during the nineteenth century would have collided with the insuperable obstacle of a welfare system which insisted, as the precondition of any pauper's being granted social aid, on his or her incorporation within the total institution of the workhouse. 'Outdoor relief', in the form of medication or support for the out-patient lunatic, would have raised awkward questions about the onerous preconditions for relief imposed upon their sane class-sisters and -brothers.[33] In the case of our own epoch, we ought not to overlook the dependency of our recent systems of Bed-stock of Mental Hospitals in European Countries out-patient maintenance upon the prior development of social and health insurance, in the United States since the 1930s, in Britain and France from the years before the first world war, and correspondingly in other welfare states.[34] Without some guarantee by the state of at least a minimal maintenance to the poor living outside the institutions of relief, and without the provision of regular medicines at the public expense, none of the present alternatives to the mental hospital – whether based on short-term admission followed by discharge or on a wholly out-patient style of treatment – could possibly exist.

Austria	1950	9,868
	1962	11,977
	1975	14,314
Belgium	1951	19,841
	1960	27,450
	1974	26,337
Czechoslovakia	1953	13,136
	1963	16,646
	1975	16,598
Denmark	1962	10,648
	1970	10,399
Finland	1951	9,223
	1963[1]	18,803
	1975	19,836
German Democratic Republic	1962	26,976
	1974	32,511
Federal German Republic	1953	86,640
	1962	95,306
	1975	112,791
Italy	1954	88,241
	1961	113,040
Netherlands	1950	25,000
	1962	26,000
	1975	26,259
Norway	1951	6,812
	1962	10,410
	1975	12,495
Spain	1949	25,571
	1963	39,329
	1974	42,493
Sweden	1952	29,110
	1962	33,449
	1974	33,030

1. 11,320 beds in psychiatric hospitals 7,483 beds in hospitals for chronic mental diseases
2. 66,943 beds in psychiatric hospitals 45,848 beds in neuro-psychiatric hospitals
3. includes hospitals for mental deficiency
4. 8,121 beds in mental hospitals 4,374 beds in mental homes
5. 24,127 beds in mental hospitals 8,903 beds in mental homes

Sources: World Health Statistics Annual, 1962, Vol III, Health Personnel and Hospital Establishments, Geneva, 1966; *ibid., 1977,* Geneva, 1977.

Because the provision of a welfare support system has entered the realm of political 'common sense', part of the received conventional wisdom that has been shared by all the major political parties (at least until the revival of laissez-faire liberalism from the camps of Thatcher, Reagan and Friedman), there has been a tendency for the advocates of a more social psychiatry to ignore the structural and political preconditions of the therapies they tend to favour. The entry of political argument into the discussion of alternative possible mental-health systems is seen as an illicit and irrational intrusion, founded primarily in eccentric bias or woolly 'grand theory'.[35] But innovation and reform in psychiatry have always been linked with the arrival of certain *conditions of political possibility*, which have been variously either promoted or blocked by ideological tendencies and social movements. The anti-hospital platform in mental health has always been powerfully assisted by a parallel and connected series of campaigns which challenged the mental institution not solely to replace it by an out-patient treatment modality but also to re-fashion it from within as a veritable 'therapeutic community'. While the practical consequences of the 'therapeutic community' and of the 'de-hospitalising' perspectives may appear to be opposed, these are not so much two divergent arguments, but two strands within a broadly common approach which attempted to avoid the permanent casting of patients into passive roles within a traditional authority structure. The post-war pioneers of rehabilitation and discharge from the institution were often also innovators in the creation of various approximations towards the therapeutic community within the hospital itself. Paradoxically, the military involvement of psychiatrists in the active treatment of psychiatrically disabled service people lent a profound impetus to the de-militarisation of relationships in the civilian hospital after the war. The first therapeutic community of our epoch was set up in Northfield Military Hospital during the war by the influential British group around W.R. Bion; members of the group were convinced of the sweeping political significance of the methods of group therapy among equals that were developed there:

> A wider view will see in it [group treatment] a new method of therapy, investigation, information and education. The widest view will look upon group therapy as an expression of a new attitude towards the study and improvement of human inter-relations in our time... Perhaps someone taking this broad view will see in it the answer in the spirit of a democratic community to the mass and group handling of totalitarian regimes.[36]

In work parallel with the Northfield group, Maxwell Jones also began therapeutic-community work with soldiers at this time, and was to extend the approach into civilian psychiatry first in his post-war re-settlement work with returning prisoners-of-war, and then into a long and impressive sequence of therapeutic democracies in Britain and the United States.[37] In both countries, the psychiatrists returning from service in army rehabilitation units insisted on transferring the lessons of group morale-building with the shell-shocked and battle-fatigued to the ossified civilian hierarchies and institutionalised, dependent patients in the great 'bins' of the post-war period. They had known status, authority and experience of producing results: 'I'd just come out of the British army where I was a captain and I wasn't frightened of being only 25 years old,' remarks one eager-pioneer of social rehabilitation, Ronald Laing, describing his efforts to break through the routines of nursing and medical staff in a Glasgow asylum's 'female refractory ward' in the mid-fifties.[38] Determination was often allied with an enthusiasm specific to its age: ideals of democratic levelling, or at least of open communication across the different ranks, had been diffused widely (often no doubt with little more than lip-service) as an element in the legitimation of the anti-fascist war effort, and continued after the war as part of a widely diffused left-liberal populism on both sides of the Atlantic.

In the United States, mental-hospital reform was slower to follow the promptings of liberal ideology. The basis for a communitarian restructuring of hospital relationships (as also of decision-making in other arenas of administration) had been provided by the influential writings of the experimental social psychologist Kurt Lewin, a passionate advocate of 'democratic' styles of conflict resolution, who made America his home following the rise of Nazism in his native Germany.[39] Lewinian approaches to administrative problems in institutions, founded on a close appreciation of small-group dynamics, helped to inform the scrutiny of the traditional mental hospital that gathered momentum in the academic media by the mid-fifties. A broad social ethic of treatment became popular now among teachers and administrators in American psychiatry, and at this point several important studies of factionalism and immobility in the social structure of asylums were conducted, with evident implications for the assessment and treatment of institutionalised patients.[40] By 1957 the Walter Reed Army Institute of Research could convene a widely-based symposium on social and preventive psychiatry including papers on therapeutic-community experiments in France (by Paul Sivadon) and in US naval and military hospitals (by H.A. Wilmer and K.L. Artiss). It was at this gathering that Erving Goffman offered his now-classical anatomisation of 'Characteristics of Total Institutions', with its harrowing comparisons among mental hospitals, prisons and concentration camps.[41] Of these contributions, Wilmer's proved to have a particular impact: originally introduced in the *US Armed Forces Medical Journal*, as part of a study reporting on the experience of the therapeutic community in a Navy hospital's psychodiagnostic ward over 1955–56, it was extended into a book (H.A. Wilmer, *Social Psychiatry in Action*, Springfield, Illinois, 1958) and a demonstration film popularising the therapeutic-communitarian ideal for audiences well outside the military orbit. During the sixties, further therapeutic communities were established (for example, at Fort Logan, Colorado, and in the mental-health system of Oregon) sometimes with a spill-over into the creation of out-patient community clinics, before these became generally legitimated by the 'Kennedy Act' of 1963.[42] It should be clear from this outline that the chronology of militant social innovation in mental-hospital arrangments fails to match either the onset of economic crisis in the stock-markets or the curve of discovery in the pharmaceutical industry. As the director of Britain's longest-established therapeutic commune, the Henderson Hospital, has observed:

> During the second world war it was both politically and economically expedient to foster the development of the therapeutic community to preserve manpower for the war effort... the objectives and aims of the therapeutic community remained attractive and were in keeping with the new democracy and social aspirations of the post-war era.[43]

A similar link with the progressive anti-fascist mobilisations of the forties (albeit again in a minority current of opinion and action) can be found in the history of innovation in the French psychiatric hospitals. The first liberalisation of the French asylum can be dated to the wartime 'St Alban experiment' in a small hospital in the rural south where the staff, under the leadership of a member of the Communist Party and of a Spanish Republican refugee, were engaged in militancy within the Resistance as well as in the re-structuring of their own institutional hierarchy. Extending after the war into a movement for 'institutional psychotherapy' (very similar to the 'therapeutic community' current in Britain and America), this vanguard grouping, with a strong influence in the professional association of hospital psychiatrists, was to become active in the turn towards 'community psychiatry', shifting the responsibility for these primarily social methods of treatment outside the mental institution and into the clinics of the *secteur* or neighbourhood.[44] The more recent development of a social psychiatry in France is complicated by the involvement of many doctors – including some of the original cadre of *la psychothérapie institutionelle* – in certain psychoanalytic doctrines stemming from Jacques Lacan which, far from assisting in a wider communitarian practice, has tended merely to reinforce a traditional hierarchisation both in hospital and in clinic.[45]

In the different situation of psychiatric change in Italy, which in its own way amounted to a settling of accounts with the institutional legacy of fascism – untouched by decades of Christian Democratic immobility – a similar evolution can be traced in the therapeutic-community movement, from the reform of the hospital to an attempt of its abolition. (And here an anti-fascist struggle had to be waged against the latter-day inheritors of Mussolini's mantle in the furious objections of the neo-fascist MSI to a psychiatric liberalisation). Thus, the example of the Basaglias' conversion of the old asylum at Gorizia into a therapeutic community during the sixties had marked a late transplantation of concepts in social psychiatry that had long been familiar in the Anglo-American literature. The Gorizia team were distinctly conscious of the ancestry of their own endeavour in the earlier programmes of the British and American hospital reformers, although as radicals with a strong allegiance to marxism they expressed some reservations about a mere 'psychiatric reformism'.[46] The turn to a mental-health politics based on neighbourhood collectives and anti-hierarchical work teams gathered a particular momentum from the communitarian politics fostered by 'May events' of 1968 in France and their sequel in Italy over 1968–69. The members of *Psichiatria Democratica* tried to insert their own projects for the de-segregation of the mentally ill into a wider political movement, forging alliances with Communist, Christian-Democratic or Radical sympathisers in local government or central legislature. Nothing in Italy can be achieved without such alliances with one or another political family network; and the result was inevitably to channel the efforts of the mental health militants within the bounds of the very 'psychiatric reformism' which had been the object of their suspicions. According to Giovanni Jervis, one of the founders of *Psichiatria Democratica*:

> The 'new Italian psychiatry', growing in 1968 and 1969 in a climate which involved it with a broader political reality, subsequently became neutralised in a defence – at times rather triumphalist – of *public assistance*; in a practice – frequently generous, but utterly uncritical – of voluntary and paternalistic *relief*; in an 'anti-institutional' struggle which very soon became institutionalised in its own turn; and in an opportunistic and 'democratic' political

> line, which was most often actually conducted to the Right of the Italian CP… Meanwhile, taken as a whole, the situation of psychiatric public welfare in Italy is, almost ten years after the May explosion, hardly very brilliant: on the one hand, 'advanced' therapeutic experiments are still very few in number, and in all probability have produced nothing very new by comparison with the best British experiments of fifteen or twenty years ago; on the other hand, public assistance in psychiatry has become widely extended and touted, while remaining within cultural and organisational limits which are mediocre if not disgraceful.[47]

This report on the Italian situation accurately pinpoints the collision between the two rival psychiatric and political currents which have, between them, produced the present stalemate in the de-segregation of the mentally ill. On the left, the tradition of an active social psychiatry, allied with militant tendencies of social reform varying from marxism to the post-war Keynesian enlightenment, has launched a number of vanguard programmes both in hospitals and in the community. On the right, institutional inertia, conservative political resistance and a cost-cutting budgetary programme have combined to render the field of public mental health into a testing-ground for the ideas of monetarism and Friedmanism even before these anti-collectivist creeds became popularised as solutions for the whole of society. The first British Minister of Health to institute the abolition of the asylum as a foreseeable objective was Enoch Powell, only three years after he had resigned from the Tory Government's Treasury in protest against Harold Macmillan's refusal to countenance a slashing programme of public expenditure cuts.[48]

In the United States, the closure of psychiatric wards and even of whole mental hospitals became a palatable remedy in many localities faced with a crisis of revenue; but nowhere was it prosecuted so vigorously as in the California of Republican affluence, Ronald Reagan and S.I. Hayakawa.[49] At the same time as the psychiatric right has shunted the sick out of asylum beds into the obscure 'community' facilities, it has ensured that in the remaining mental institutions no programme of rehabilitation with any ambition or intensity can expect to receive secure funding. Under-nursed and under-doctored wards depend now on the chemical cure and the pragmatic use of electro-shock rather than on the more social and interpersonal therapies. Such physical methods, within this institutional context of chronic staff scarcity, have a strong tendency to encourage passive patient roles. Schooled into a chemical dependency and the docile view of his or her own condition which society generally trains in its citizens, the sufferer emerges from, perhaps, a brief spell in hospital and may for years later still be content to ingest the routinely prescribed dosages of a medication which has become inappropriate, unnecessary or even hazardous. By a paradox which would hardly have been appreciated by the founders of the social-psychiatry movement, the creation of a community-based psychiatric practice 'has moved the mental health system back into closer juxtaposition with the somatic health system',[50] conceived as the individualistic administration of medicaments by the authoritative and qualified to the powerless and deferential.

The dilapidated asylum structure, which processes the acute patient and warehouses the chronic, has long ago lost any contact with the ideals of open communication and therapeutic democracy which, in a small number of vanguard sectors, stimulated innovation from the forties through the sixties. For the political climate that fostered such idealistic ventures has been replaced by a rightward-moving, depoliticised submissiveness and cynicism. With a pardonable exaggeration, the doctor in charge of the Henderson Hospital (a unit founded originally by Maxwell Jones in 1947) has analysed this sea-change:

> As the 1960s came to an end the freedom of expression and the increased tolerance for deviant behaviour, disinhibition and the general throwing-off of authoritarian controls resulted in a near anarchy in some European countries, and instituted a generalised threat to the stability of many societies. The therapeutic community, with its well-known goals of freedom of expression and replacement of authoritarian direction by democratic process, has come to be seen as a similar threat to the established order of the health services as perhaps never before. The myths of anarchy and loss of control have been resurrected, and there have been instances in both Germany and Holland where links between therapeutic communities and anarchist groups have been alleged and dealt with by police action.[51]

In the German example, the 'police action' encompassed the armed invasion and dispersal of one therapeutic community, the SPK (*Sozialistisches Patienten Kollectiv*) formed in Heidelberg in 1970, and the sentencing of its psychiatrists Wolfgang and Ursula Huber, to four and a half years' imprisonment for their activity in a 'criminal association'.[52]

In France, the nearest equivalent to the therapeutic commune has been the Clinique de la Borde at Cour-Cheverny, a semi-private institution run by Félix Guattari and some Lacanian psychiatrists. La Borde functions also as a mainstream French psychiatric hospital administering chemotherapy, ECT and some individual psychoanalysis; but its public image as the inheritor of the *gauchisme* of May 1968 has attracted a police raid and a search by the local magistracy on suspicion of a link with terrorism.[53]

In the homeland of the therapeutic community, Britain, several such ventures survive as a minority tradition in the face of less blatant but perhaps no less authoritarian pressures. Despite its leading post-war role as the vehicle of social-democratic ideas in psychiatry, the treatment community has 'faded from prominence except in a few isolated centres… occasionally sparking into life but becoming neither fully extinguished nor widely established'.[54] Considerations of cost-effectiveness and the suspicion of traditionally minded, senior managements often render precarious the situation even of a unit which has earned a world-wide reputation in its field and built up a staff complement with irreplaceable social and therapeutic skills: in recent years St Wulstan's Rehabilitation Unit (using industrial and social methods with schizophrenic patients), the Special Unit at Barlinnie Prison in Scotland and even the Henderson Hospital itself have been placed in serious jeopardy, and kept open only with the mobilisation of considerable public and expert pressure on their behalf. The hegemony of the antipsychiatry movement among the liberal and radical intelligentsia during the sixties coincided with the post-welfare state's deliberate dilapidation of the mental-hospital structure: the consequence has been a failure to renew the traditions of social psychiatry outside a very limited sector.

In the world of psychiatry, no less than in the world at large, we are at the end of the Keynesian era. The expectations of full employment and of state responsibility for welfare, fusing with the lingering dreams of a post-war dispensation based on social justice, formed an essential underpinning for left-liberal psychiatry's own disposition to rehabilitate the institutionalised inmates of the asylums into civilian social roles. The later anti-authoritarianism and even libertarianism of the sixties manifested, in countless pressure groups and social movements, what was at first an apparent renewal of the democratic collectivism that had inspired pioneer reformers in various fields of welfare during the post-war consensus on public spending. But in the realm of psychiatric politics, the content of sixties radicalism was highly ambiguous: as prone to demolish the institutions of medical welfare as to enlarge and improve them, as involved in setting the precedents for the burgeoning conservative right as in expressing the protests of a socially conscious left, as much (finally) simon-pure individualist as it was collectivist in any shape or sense. As one surveys the large and heterogeneous range of pressure groups and lobbies in the mental-health field that pushed their way into the headlines during the sixties and seventies, it is striking to observe their almost unanimous abdication from the task of proposing and securing any provision for a humane and continuous form of care for those mental patients who need something rather more than short-term therapy for an acute phase of their illness. Two tendencies are immediately evident in the welter of demands that have sprung from these parties of modern psychiatry: the obsession with legal safeguards and guarantees against the abuse of medical power; and the concentration on rapid or (at the most) short-term modalities of therapeutic technology which reinforce the tendency to discharge sufferers from the institutions of medical care into the grey zones of unsupervised living where in all the proliferation of welfare bureaucracies, no agency will answer to any responsibility for future crises or problems.

The civil-libertarian interest in psychiatry has a long and reputable ancestry stemming from the exposure of scandal and injustice in mental institutions as far back as the eighteenth century, when genteel liberal elements uncovered a series of outrageous confinements and assaults perpetrated on (among others) members of their own class. Proposals for judicial control over admission to mental institutions and for a lay (or mixed medical and civil) invigilation over the conditions in asylums entered the framing of much legislation in Britain and America during the nineteenth century and subsequently. Paradoxically for those who nowadays offer, as an alternative to the medical *fiat*, a formally legalistic framework for the securing of patients' rights, this era of legalistic hegemony in the control of asylum policies was also the epoch in which flourished the worst excesses of the warehousing of the insane and feeble poor, in the multiplication of the totalitarian 'museums of madness' with their scores of thousands of victims who remained utterly ignorant of the advantages conferred on them by the Rule of Law. In our own time, the revival of legalistic redress for the malpractices of psychiatric incarceration has formed an important ideological current in the motivation of public policy. Once again we have a pressure for change stemming from the cultural and ideological environment, whose effects are distinct from the pressures of economics or of pharmacology (though doubtless facilitated by both the latter). In Britain the National Council for Civil Liberties, as far back as 1951, publicised several cases of wrongful detention in mental institutions. The 1955 *Report on Mental Illness and Mental Deficiency Hospitals* from King Edward's Hospital Trust added its own critique of custodial neglect and the mass herding of patients in these institutions; the establishment of a Royal Commission to report on the law in relation both to mental illness and mental handicap, and the embodiment of its liberal proposals (abolishing compulsory admission as the regular mode of hospital admission) in the 1959 Mental Health Act, followed this spate of well documented, public exposures of the conditions in the archaic 'bins' for which the National Health Service had now assumed responsibility.[55]

The continuation of this forceful, civil libertarian tradition of exposure, with its concurrent demand for a legal framework of protection for patients, may be seen in the pattern of campaigning established in the seventies by the National Association for Mental Health (MIND), the main pressure group on psychiatric politics in Great Britain. In 1971 MIND launched a broadly based campaign of publicity covering many aspects of psychiatric abuse, neglect and injustice. The campaign director was David Ennals, later to become minister for health in the Labour government of 1974–79. Under Ennals's leadership, and with the support of the psychiatrists and other professionals on its executive, MIND decided that the safeguarding of mental patients' rights should be its first priority. This task was at first conceived in wide-ranging political and social terms, covering for example housing and community care for discharged patients; but a narrower, more legalistic and more individualist interpretation of human rights for the mentally ill became evident in the work of two key appointees to the MIND office, Tony Smythe (who became Director in 1977 following a period as organising secretary for the National Council for Civil Liberties) and Larry Gostin, an American lawyer who was to head its Legal and Welfare Rights Department. Their legal and libertarian approach has had certain successes: the strengthening of the patient's representation in applying to tribunals for discharge from the institution; the distribution of material (often through MIND's welfare desks in the hospitals themselves) informing patients of their rights; the bringing of class actions to secure the enforcement of these rights in practice (e.g. in obtaining a court declaration that asylum patients should appear on the voters' register for local and national elections). Such achievements, widely implemented through local networks of informed enthusiasts, as well as through the national and regional offices, are deeply creditable, and would not in their own right earn any reproof of the sort that has raged around some of MIND's central activities from conservative sources both in the psychiatric establishment and the House of Commons.[56] The event that triggered the most hostile response from certain British psychiatrists (some of whom concerted a campaign to secure a refusal of funds to the national MIND by local affiliates) was the publication of Gostin's text *A Human Condition*,[57] a triumph of legalistic special pleading which, over its two volumes of closely argued precedents and proposals, managed to avoid any description whatever of the personal or behavioural problems typically experienced, or occasionally inflicted, by the mentally ill. Indeed, in one section displaying great industry in searching the psychopathological literature (but possibly insufficient sophistication in actually reading the articles and books cited) Gostin came very close to stating the Szaszian view that psychiatric diagnosis was in its very nature a sham and a trap.

The British civil-libertarians of MIND were only following a long and copious trail blazed by their ideological colleagues in the United States. In late 1968 the New York Civil Liberties Union began a vast national project of litigation 'to protect and expand the rights of mental patients' through court action at both state and federal level. The director of this project of forensic liberation, which was soon to receive national backing from the American Civil Liberties Union and a number of substantial foundations, has been Bruce J. Ennis, who commenced his campaigning in mental health after qualifying at the University of Chicago Law School and serving in a clerkship to a Federal judge.[58] A vast array of 'rights' have thus apparently been bestowed on the psychiatrically unfortunate by judges and attorneys over the long years of civil-libertarian action in the United States.[59]

If the resources of court action really did represent the high road of hope for the average institutionalised psychiatric patient, one might imagine that the United States would by now possess the finest mental-health system that legal and libertarian reason could invent. The director of the main American litigation project appeared, at one stage, to entertain this as a serious vista:

> It would be cheaper still to shut down mental hospitals and treat all patients in the community. California has come close to doing that... California's new law is far from perfect. But it has shown that most people can be treated in the community, and that the few who must be hospitalized can be quickly returned to the community with no adverse consequences... The goal should be nothing less than the abolition of involuntary hospitalisation. That will not come soon, but it will come. (England, for example, plans to shut down all its large public mental hospitals within 20 years.)[60]

Few, in the eighties, would venture a parallel optimism over the prospect of the mental hospital's demise. It is now agreed by most observers that those communities (like California) which have come nearest to this goal have succeeded only in appeasing the tax-payer at the expense of the needy. After his recent trip to the United States, indeed, Larry Gostin (who has done so much to transplant the Bill of Rights platform into British mental health) has returned somewhat scandalised by the performance of psychiatric legalism in the nation whose libertarian culture trained him:

> Tens of thousands of mental patients have been released in the United States through court suits in the last ten years… It has been a disaster. Institutions have been shut but there has been nowhere for the patients to go. They have ended up in prison, or exploited by private landlords, readmitted to other mental hospitals or just dying… sometimes alone. Courts are unable to plan, budget or build alternative facilities.[61]

The high-water mark of this British mental-health organisation's involvement in legalism may have already been reached. Larry Gostin has become the chairperson of a new organisation, the Advocacy Alliance, set up by five important mental-health charities, and aiming to provide the most vulnerable and forgotten patients in mental-handicap hospitals not simply with advocates for their often denied legal and welfare rights but with befrienders who will be a long-term source of emotional support.[62] Many of the most forceful statements by MIND's officers (including Smythe and Gostin) have emphasised the inadequacies of public funding in the mental-health services and have raised questions of central state policy going far beyond the provision of legal redress for individual mental patients. And, throughout the phase of maximal commitment to the legalistic perspective, the bulk of MIND's work lay in mobilising community and local government support for patients and their families outside as well as inside the hospital system.[63]

The civil-libertarian ethic, in mental health as in other fields where power over the politically weak has manifest capabilities of abuse, has an honourable and indeed essential role. Nevertheless, it has the crucial defect of being unable to focus therapeutic policy on any question other than the misuse of medical power. Consequently, civil-libertarians find themselves cast in the role of a permanent reforming opposition to the main structures of authority and decision in psychiatry. Because their voice is essentially reactive, they depend on medical practitioners to initiate and conduct treatment before they themselves can appear in the next phase of the cycle as protestors and resisters. A further move beyond this partially negative stance is, of course, open to civil libertarians in mental health: that of a complete negation of the legitimacy of any psychiatric intervention whatever. Rather than taking confinement and ill-treatment as the *mis-use* of therapies which are basically sound, we are bidden to see them as the *normal use* of an authoritarian power which is basically evil. Defensive libertarianism in the mental-health field can be pushed, in the absence of a positive programme for valid therapy, into an all-round condemnation of the psychiatric enterprise itself.

It requires, in fact a considerable sophistication to steer one's way among the pitfalls of the two major positions that present themselves in the politics of psychiatric protest. Roughly speaking, when we survey the various follies and crimes of psychiatric power, we have a choice between the language of Abuse and that of Use. The former rests on a distinction between (a) some central core of practice which, when conducted according to certain prescribed norms, is seen as ethically and politically unproblematic, and (b) one or more deviations from the prescribed code which transform the practice into an illicit and unwarranted variation. The vocabulary of 'abuse' generally presupposes (rather than argues) that there is a legitimate 'use' of similar procedures. On the other hand, certain libertarians working in the review of psychiatric practices feel that the critique of (let us say) the involuntary confinement of sane individuals, or of the forcible administration of powerful tranquillisers to Soviet dissidents, calls into question far more than a narrow set of transgressions of an otherwise unproblematic medical code by a particular set of practitioners. 'Involuntary mental hospitalisation,' proclaims Thomas Szasz, 'is like slavery. Refining the standards of commitment is like prettifying the slave plantation. The problem is not how to improve commitment but how to abolish it.'[64] And a similar extension of the libertarian critique, from the campaign against particular maltreatments to a questioning of one or more central elements in treatment itself, has become a leading characteristic of the psychopolitical tendency known as 'anti-psychiatry' in the latter sixties and seventies and still vigorously alive, though less publicised, down to our own time.

Those who reject both the short-sighted denunciation of mere 'abuses' and the wholesale indictment of 'institutional psychiatry' as an enterprise of state-sponsored violence have no easy task in developing a third option to these simplicities. In reviewing the accusations that have been made repeatedly in recent years concerning the use made by the Soviet authorities of compulsory mental hospitalisation, diagnosis and treatment in the handling of dissidents, a leading British psychiatrist has made it clear that, in his view, wider and more searching lessons must be drawn, going well beyond the local complicity between Russian psychiatry and the post-Stalinist police state:

> I have concentrated to some extent on the position in the Soviet Union as the most glaring example of the abuse of psychiatry. Nevertheless, I believe that the situation arose not just because of the Soviet authorities' attitudes but because of the inherent weaknesses in psychiatry. When a branch of medicine deals with intangibles like delusions, when it cannot agree on diagnosis, when treatments are introduced on insufficient evidence, when its relationships with the law are vague and contentious, it is open to manipulation both from within and from without. Psychiatrists, because of the imprecision of their topic compared with other branches of medicine, do not have the means or sometimes the will to resist that exploitation.[65]

The political and ethical problems of modern psychiatry cannot, of course be reduced to the 'imprecision' of its definitions. Such concepts can often reflect, with a relative precision even, moral values and political structures which remain suspect and open to challenge less through the logical difficulties of their subject matter than because of their tendency to express a rather conventional, conversative view of normality and of sanity. All the same, enough has surely been said here to indicate some of the ways in which we can discover a path past the simple and sterile alternatives of the 'use' versus 'abuse' dichotomy in the evaluation of psychiatric practice. The politics of libertarian objection in psychiatry, however, constantly encourages its proponents to engage in a stance of pure resistance or opposition – whether partial or wholesale – which actually blocks the formulation of fresh demands and programmes.

This culture of resistance is assisted by a number of professional and other special interests. In addition to the contribution of a legalistic advocacy, already mentioned, a further source of libertarian pressure has come from social workers. In the words of one member of a British social-work team, who is aware of the conflict that may arise with doctors over compulsory admission to mental hospital:

> Many social workers see their role in terms of restraining doctors from arbitrary exercise of power. Underlying much of social work theory is the belief that problem behaviour is the product not just of a single pathological personality, but of collusion of a group (often a family) to scapegoat a single member for all their difficulties. The social worker, therefore, arrives at a mental health

> emergency to be asked to do something contrary to his normal practice.[66]

Social workers and similar counsellors do not, of course, function merely as attorneys for the defence of their clients against medical power; they make a considerable positive contribution of their own to the mental-health services. Yet the oppositional, libertarian stance, to the extent that it is adopted by social workers, actually helps to limit the challenge to medical monopoly that might be mounted by those helping professions who, like social workers, are at present consigned to a 'para-medical' role (i.e. one subordinate to doctors) in the care of the mentally disabled.

For the development of the mental-health professions from the nineteenth century to the present has taken the form of a strict formal division of labour where superintendence not only of the patients but of all the remaining staff is claimed by one particular occupational class: namely those in possession of a medical degree gained primarily through passing examinations in a knowledge of physical ailments.[67] Whatever departures may exist in practice from these formal routines of staff control (as much through chronic shortages of doctors willing to work in these backward sectors as through any liberalisation of medical power), the processes of referral, institutional placement and discharge, and the ultimate legal responsibility for the sufferer's well-being, remain in the hands of the medical profession. Doctors, moreover, engage in a stubborn and successful corporate resistance to any attempt to wrest from them these areas of decision in favour of, say, psychologists or psychiatric nurses. By an extension of this division of labour, society concentrates in the hands of doctors the responsibility for the most fateful decisions concerning its mental deviants – and then sponsors a whole train of countervailing influences, in the subordinate professions and in the public generally, to moderate and protest this same power. The libertarian posture in mental health shields those who adopt it from demanding and assuming the responsibility for a continuing care for the disabled, whose concentration in other hands forms the target of their obloquy. Some of the most urgent areas of mental-health care involve little or no expertise that is the particular prerogative of a medical or even a psychiatric training: for example, the provision of asylum, in the form of housing or occupation, for the mentally handicapped or other chronically disabled; the estimation of the stress caused by the presence of a disturbed individual to his or her immediate household. There is every reason to suppose that serious and constructive innovations in the care of the mentally ill could be conducted by professionals working, for example, within a social-work ethic, or in the framework provided by social and clinical psychology, or for that matter through a non-professional philanthropy responsive to professional advice. Those who undertake such projects will themselves be liable to scrutiny and criticism from the libertarians who at present have the psychiatric profession and the mental-hospital system as their prime material. But the exchange between the practitioners and the critics, the responsible authorities and the contending pressure groups, the world of psychiatry and the counter-world of anti-psychiatry, has become for some while now routinised and predictable. It is time, surely, for new directions and new roles.

The political and cultural radicalisation of the latter sixties and the seventies, particularly that stemming from the 1968 'May events' in France, laid its principal stress on the self-activity and self-organisation of oppressed and disadvantaged groups in producing alternatives to an authoritarian and bureaucratic system that was blocking the satisfaction of their needs. And there is, of course, a much older heritage of collective self-organisation in the labour movement which, while founded on the trade unions, has often gone beyond day-to-day economic demands in posing substantial policy alternatives to the existing priorities of government and capital. We might, then, expect there to have been some pointers of progress in the mental-health field in the last 20 years or so arising either from the pressure groups and movements founded by mental patients themselves or through trade unions and other groups of mental-health workers expressing a creative dissatisfaction with their conditions of work. From neither of these rank-and-file constituencies, however, can a great deal be reported. Neither the recipients nor the employees of psychiatric care have contributed anything very striking in the development of programmes and examples for future policy.

Mental patients are among the most private of citizens. To the extent that their condition is severe and stressful, it is liable to remove them from the possibilities of common association and organisation. The stigma attaching still to their various disabilities and illnesses usually prevents most of them from asserting a group identity in public, for purposes of demonstration or financial appeal. In this regard, the psychiatric patient, even when recovered or in remission, is in distinct contrast with the physically handicapped. The occupation of Stoke Mandeville Hospital by paraplegics in early 1980, or the repeated wheelchair demonstrations in France by the *Comités de Lutte des Handicapés* in the cause of state aid rather than charity,[68] have little parallel among the psychiatrically ill. Among certain diagnostic groups in psychiatry, a self-help movement to provide support among people with a similar disability has become widely established. In my own medium-sized town of West Yorkshire, for example, there are local groups of depressives, agoraphobics, alcoholics and compulsive gamblers. (I omit from consideration, at present, those organisations which cater principally for the relatives or befrienders of persons with a mental illness.) Such peer-groups of patients or ex-patients are often extremely effective in providing morale and insight to sufferers, and form the healthiest possible consequence of the do-it-yourself populism which has become such a general political mood within the last decade or so. On the whole, they are not equipped to work as a strong public lobby within their field of disability. Their relationship with the orthodox psychiatric services is loose enough not to form a serious challenge or pressure in relation to the defects of public provision; in the case of mutual-aid groups like Synanon or Depressives Associated, the grouping's own ethos, formed from a mixture of compassion, common sense and (sometimes) religion, represents a move in the direction of self-sufficiency, away from a primarily medical framework.[69]

During the late sixties and early seventies, several much more ambitious attempts were made to constitute an 'alternative therapy' of self-help networks and groups, available to all the mentally ill without regard to diagnosis, and owing nothing to the official facilities, public or private, based on a medical model and a medical personnel. The identity and the viability of such movements tend to be fragile and transient: at one extreme of severity, their precarious resources of housing, counselling and support can become loaded to breaking-point by a high proportion of very disturbed 'heavy cases', the rejects and failures of the entire mainstream psychiatric system;[70] at the more moderate end of the spectrum of emotional miseries, they shade into the terrain of 'alternative therapies' which are marketed for the nearly normal. Take for example, the problem presented by one participant in a Red Therapy Group:

> D. was feeling agitated and not-present in the group because she was aware of all her pressing commitments. She had promised to sew up some bags for the Abortion Campaign – having a sewing machine she felt she ought to really. She had not realised how time-consuming it would be – was feeling guilty about not having finished them – and was rather wishing that she'd never agreed to sew them.[71]

It should be clear that at some point the term 'therapy' changes its meaning from that belonging to a specialised form of care for people in unusual and definable sorts of distress to a loose label covering virtually any kind of chat about even the most transient and everyday problem of conflict. There is obviously a range of serious personal and emotional problems where the services offered by 'alternative' therapy facilities are at least as good as in a medically based, psychiatric centre.[72] On the whole, though, it seems evident that 'alternative therapy' does not constitute a true alternative to the public sector in psychiatric care, since it soaks up a clientele that overlaps only partially with the state system.

It is also doubtful whether the more thoroughgoing 'alternative' networks really represent very much that is genuine in the way of self-organisation by patients themsleves. Each network possesses a theoretical rationale and a code of practice – sometimes based on psychoanalysis, sometimes on communication theory, sometimes on transcendental religion – that incorporates a claim to expertise as well as, more often than not, a professional contract sustained by a fee passing from the user to the provider of the service.[73] The situation of the 'alternative' therapy movement in relation to the dominant structures of psychiatric medicine is hardly that of 'dual power', the uneasy and temporary co-existence of an antiquated authority system with new and contrary power-forms that aim to displace the old regime. It is much more like the situation of 'the second economy' in communist states: a bootlegging private market assisting (at best) in the humanisation of an inflexible bureaucratic order, and (at its most suspicious) rendering therapy into a sector of small-scale commodity production, with its own brands of mystification, inequality and rip-off.

More militant and adversary attempts at self-organisation among the mentally ill have come from a series of activist groups in Britain, Western Europe and the United States. In New York the Mental Patients' Liberation Project,[74] in San Francisco the Network Against Psychiatric Assault, organising patients and ex-patients nationally through its journal *Madness Network News*,[75] have been active since the early seventies. Both associations have been instruments of consumer complaint in psychiatry, raising issues of maltreatment or compulsory hospitalisation within an ideology roughly corresponding to the civil-libertarian framework described above. NAPA is an enthusiastic proponent of the laissez-fairist ideas of Thomas S. Szasz, objecting on principle to any involuntary confinement in a mental institution and proclaiming its opposition to the Therapeutic State. The Liberation Project has sometimes had more radical affiliates: the socialist-feminist writer Marge

Piercy has worked for its causes, and acknowledges some help from the Project's activists in devising the brilliant scenarios of her novel *Woman on the Edge of Time*, in which a Puerto Rican working-class woman is projected, through visions and voices which are treated by psychiatrists as hallucinatory (and therefore, as eligible for forcible and squalid 'treatment'), into a number of telling episodes within a liberated communal society of the future. All the same, on first viewing, the founding perspectives of the Project seem to rest on an apple-pie Americanism which invokes the Declaration of Independence, the Federal Constitution, and a series of proposed rights for mental patients covering such demands as the removal of censorship, the refusal of compulsory labour and compulsory treatment, and the retention of personal property from confiscation 'no matter what reason is given'.

Nevertheless, the Mental Patients' Liberation Project does include (within its Bill of Rights) some demands – the right to 'decent medical attention' and to 'decent living conditions' – that stem (however vaguely they are put) from a welfare-collectivist tradition which is sharply at odds with the pay-or-perish market philosophy of the liberal right. Its single concrete proposal for newly founded facilities in the care of patients consisted of 'neighbourhood crisis centres as alternatives to incarceration and voluntary and involuntary commitment to hospitals'.[76] Crisis centres for out-patients in acute forms of distress, usually offering 'walk-in' clinics with either no residential facility or only short-stay beds, had in fact been pioneered within the community mental-health centre movement, organised by psychiatrists and their associates, from the early sixties onwards. The 'neighbourhood crisis centre' was offered by socially minded medics, as an alternative to hospitalisation for a sizeable proportion of patients, some years before it became proposed by patients and ex-patients as an alternative to psychiatry itself. It is not in fact immediately obvious that a 'crisis centre' which contains beds is a different sort of institution from the acute ward of a mental hospital, or that one which has no beds is any different, intrinsically, from a psychiatric day hospital.[77]

Some short-stay or out-patient psychiatric units catering for emergencies do operate with doctors and social workers in conventional clinical roles; other have a role-sharing or team approach working from a socially based 'crisis intervention' theory rather than a medical model of illnesses. But, while it is obviously useful for further facilities to be added at the less conventional end of this spectrum (such as those suggested in the New York mental patients' project), there cannot be any pretension on the part of crisis-centre practitioners that they offer more than a partial and selective range of services affecting a minority of prospective patients. 'Those that keep statistics find that about half their work involves comparatively young, single (or separated) persons, often unemployed or with alcohol problems, and often coming back repeatedly after acts of selfpoisoning'.[78] The problem of securing continuing care for people in recurrent or chronic difficulty, who can soon silt up a facility with few residential places, remains on the whole unresolved in the crisis-centre. In such difficult cases, the centre may have to act as a feeder for more orthodox mental-hospital processing.

Still, the importance of crisis-intervention ideas in psychiatry goes well beyond the question of the numbers of 'patients', 'clients' or 'guests' – their exact nomenclature is varied – who can fit such centres. We have here an attempt to move away not only from the segregative solution of the traditional asylum but also from the pill-pushing options that plague the usual medical model of care whether in hospitals or in general practice. The activities of the crisis centre offer a model of therapy and care, which to a large extent, does not need to draw on the roles offered by medical training; and the very language of 'crisis' offers different implications for the causes of an individual's problems than does the vocabulary of 'illness'. This is one point at which libertarian lobbying has coincided with good therapeutic sense.

The news from the mental patients' movements in Europe is harder to track down. Because of their connection with ideologically formed traditions of the far left, such groupings are likely to augment the difficulties of mental patients with the further problems of survival experienced by revolutionary and radical organisations in a hostile world. We have already noted the fate of the *Sozialistisches Patientenkollectiv* of Heidelberg in the early seventies. Had this group disbanded from its *foco* in the University Clinic and dispersed itself into a propaganda or pressure-group role within a wider public, there can be little doubt that it would have escaped the annihilation visited upon it by the official terrorism of West Germany's police and judiciary. In France, the mobilisations of May 1968 soon produced a spate of patient groups having intellectual links with situationists, structural-marxists, trotskyists, anarchists and maoists. Several *Groupes Information Asiles* (GIAs), stimulated initially by young psychiatrists, got going from 1972 to 1978, as a parallel to the GIP movement (*Groupes Information sur les Prisons*) animated for oppositionists in the prison system by Michel Foucault. Transplanted to a university campus atmosphere, the GIAs revelled in debates on psychoanalysis and madness, mass meetings and public campaigns against arbitrary internments and specific grievances in mental hospitals. GIAs were formed in various Paris districts and a number of provincial cities, but within a couple of years most of these had disappeared as a result of 'the battles between political groups, the shrinking of the political base, and dogmatism',[79] and the field was taken by a group of patient-based GIAs instigated by a group from the 17th *arrondissement* of Paris who organised nationally around the journal *Psychiatrisés en lutte* and its charter of mental patients' rights (*Charte de psychiatrisés*). The founding platform of the patients' GIA focussed upon the increasing use, even by 'progressive' psychiatrists and 'progressive' hospitals such as the Clinique de la Borde, of powerful psychotropic drugs, without regard to side-effects (such as tremor following anti-hallucinants) or the social context of the patient's symptoms.

> It is not a matter of abandoning our treatment from one day to the next, nor of breaking with psychiatry in a single stroke; but rather, in the first place, of submitting it to control; for which purpose it seems indispensable that we should re-group ourselves.

The fruits of this re-grouping by *les psychiatrisés* have been seen not only in a large number of published exposures of outrage and insult inside mental institutions but in a series of projects that attempt to draft detailed and serious safeguards over both the preconditions for hospitalising patients and the circumstances of their treatment once hospitalised: these programmes of control have taken the form either of Patients' Charters (like the 36 demands of the French *Charte des Internés* elaborated over 1975–76[80] for the control of mental-hospital life), or of a critical review of the relevant national legislation governing mental-illness matters. Such a review has for example been conducted by the Clientelbond, a 1,500 strong group of patients and ex-patients in the Netherlands[81] and by Belgium's own GIA, which has proposed a control of all compulsory hospitalisations by the country's judiciary, with a formal adversary procedure embodying legal representation for the patient.[82] We must note again that the dismal record of judicial control over psychiatric committals in the United States and Britain, during the most horrendous epochs of the mass incarceration of inmates in the asylums of both countries, never seems to deter libertarians from demanding more of it.

The continental patient-groups have found particular inspiration in the work of the Mental Patients' Union in Britain, a federation of the psychiatrised which began in March 1973 (preceded by an embryonic group formed in Scotland two years earlier) through a meeting held in London at the Paddington Day Hospital, an 'official' therapeutic community sympathetic to group work by and among patients. A serious battle had to be waged by the MPU branch at Hackney Hospital to secure permission for its meetings there; most hospitals and staff find the idea of independent and collective patient action threatening to their own status. In these years of the maximal ascendancy of the British left's 'rank-and-file' politicking, the MPU engaged in squats, the shopstewardly representation of patient interests and the drafting of a 'Declaration of Intent' which became a model for some of the European movements.[83] The MPU in its charter and activities placed particular emphasis on an informed-consent ethic of psychiatric care, producing a Directory of Psychiatric Drugs (complete with their undesirable side-effects) so that patients could regulate their chemical intake in as full a knowledge as possible of what the consequences might be.

Despite the precariousness of those forms of organisation (the MPU cadre, for example, nowadays making only a sporadic and unpredictable appearance in the far-left press to argue particular cases of oppression), some long-term lessons seem to be possible. The authenticity of these demands and programmes, as expressing grievances widely felt among large groups of psychiatric patients, can hardly be in doubt. It would be wrong to dismiss these manifestoes simply because some of their commonest demands, such as the appeal for the end of compulsory hospitalisation and compulsory treatment, simply evade such vexed questions as what would constitute 'informed consent' during a psychotic condition, or what would be a legitimate or an illegitimate intervention to prevent suicide. Some of the campaigns waged by mental-patient movements in both Europe and America have corresponded closely with issues already in play within the debates of legislators and professionals on matters of psychiatric controversy. As aspiring organs of consumer representation, the patients' groupings have little choice but to scan the trade journals of those who manufacture and dispense psychiatric wares, so that there is some danger of a mental-patient activism that concentrates on issues in active practice which are already spotlighted (like the adverse effects of psychotropic drugs) and says little or nothing about the crimes of psychiatric omission and neglect such as those affecting mental handicap and the care of the old. The gravest disappointment of virtually all these movements is their shortage of ideas about what to put in place of the traditional bin. The 'bill of rights' which they traditionally offer for public attention is full of demands insisting for example, that nursing staff should stop censoring patients' correspondence, or that hospitals should pay patients properly for worked performed in them, all of which assume the existence of mental institutions and inmate roles. A few 'alternative' centres on a self-governing basis were set up as residences by some of the patient groups;[84] their character and outcome remains uncertain. Instead of putting their weight behind programmes for housing and support outside the traditional mental hospital, the patients' groups condemned themselves to a permanently defensive role within the framework of the institution. In an age when the vast mental institutions constructed in the last century were concentrating their services on acute treatment of short-stay or medium-stay clientele, leaving their deteriorating chronic wards with a minimal staffing and no rehabilitative programme, the patients' unions limited themselves to demanding control over existing forms of care.

Even more limited objectives – and not all of them by any means progressive – have characterised the attitudes of organised health workers within the mental-hospital system. The most articulate sections of the mental-health employee rank-and-file have had to establish trade union organisation (often in the face of disciplinary action and victimisation by hospital managements) by opposing the 'service ethic' which elevated the individual employee's sense of vocation and self-sacrifice at the expense of the workers' advancement as a combined pressure group.[85] The actual scope for collective industrial struggle by mental-hospital staff (as with hospital staff in physical medicine) is in any case limited by a serious reckoning of the damage or even death that would be wrought among patients if these workers engaged in serious strike action. When it comes to strike action in hospitals, employees of whatever grade nearly always take a 'professional' rather than 'trade union' view of their responsibilities and will not leave wards unstaffed even though, arguably, some shock action which places patients in jeopardy would be preferable, as a means of securing adequate resources for health care, to continued collaboration with a system which, daily and quietly, harms and kills the sick through routine under-staffing and neglect. Attempts to devise forms of 'imaginative industrial action' which will put pressure on hospital health authorities without endangering patients are still fairly rare, it seems. Faced with a savage cut-back in staffing, the trade-union activists in one Lancashire mental-handicap hospital occupied a chronic ward and conducted a work-in at a high level of service for the patients and with considerable support from the local community – action which was however defeated in the end.[86]

The fight against the closure of particular mental institutions has, especially in recent years, attracted great resources of energy and ingenuity from nursing and other staff. On such issues, trade-union and professional identities experience less contradiction, and wide public support can be attracted, which is important in reinforcing the morale of a group of workers usually inexperienced in any form of direct action. As an example of one such campaign, we may cite the case of Etwall Hospital, a geriatric unit in Derbyshire, where the trade unions NUPE (National Union of Public Employees) and COHSE (Confederation of Health Service Employees), with the support of the doctors and the patients, set up a 24-hour picket in early 1980 against attempts by the local Health Authority to remove the patients and close the hospital down. The protest was successful for four months, but was broken by the deployment of non-union labour, as well as large numbers of police, who sealed off the hospital approaches against picketing trade unionists, supervised the forcible transfer of the patients and arrested the local COHSE official present for obstruction.[87]

And yet, on other occasions, workers in the mental-health service have been concerned to defend particular jobs and conditions by proposing authoritarian and anti-therapeutic models of care. During the California programme of mental-hospital closures over 1973–74, the California State Employees' Association mounted a defence of the threatened facilities by orchestrating a campaign in the media against the violence and squalor which they claimed would be spread into the community by ex-patients.[88] Basaglia's phased replacement of the Trieste asylum by district mental-health centres and group apartments for long-stay patients was fiercely resisted by a large section of hospital workers:

> During 1972 and 1973 there was a series of strikes by nursing staff who objected to the closing of wards and the presence of student and graduate volunteers. In the end, the nurses' resistance was overcome and their small administrative hierarchy disbanded.[89]

In Trieste – contrary to the position in other parts of Italy, where the psychiatric-reform movement has received considerable help from the majority trade-union federation, the CGIL – most of the mental nurses belonged to the Christian-Democratic or even the fascist trade union. The fascist militancy was particularly troublesome, engaging in strike action against the liberalising 'bosses' of the medical administration in order to keep wards locked and nursing prerogatives untouched. This right-wing syndicalism was superimposed on the more general trade-union initiatives of these years, affecting nurses as a whole in their struggles for improved conditions and wages.[90] Such definite identification of a nursing staff's conservative-authoritarian tendency with outright fascism is of course rare. More usually, the nurses' and orderlies' opposition to the changes initiated by more middle-class professionals stems from their own institutionalisation into custodial or physical-servicing roles which are less threatening, in terms both of personal identity and of professional responsibility, than the behaviours expected in a more social and even 'alternative' psychiatry. When a British psychiatric nurse was sacked from his hospital through allowing a situation to arise in which a man and a woman patient were found cuddling in bed on a mixed-sex ward, the trade-union representative of COHSE who appeared for him (unsuccessfully, as it happens) at a tribunal did not defend the right of the patients to enjoy sexual affection, or of the staff to take risks in the cause of a more normal life for their charges. Rather, he stated that 'it was because of such situations that the union had tried to have mixed wards discontinued' (*Guardian*, 1 August, 1980). And a similar disposition towards a crude and conservative interpretation of social order can be seen in the repeated bannings and blackings organised by different union branches in Britain against the operation of facilities for mental patients who have been before the courts.

Such negative actions by psychiatric nursing staff have not been confined to the reasonable instance of an under-staffed personnel refusing the admission to their hospital of a particular dangerous or disruptive patient – although one might hope that such decisions on exclusion would be shared by the nursing staff in discussion with doctors and the other patients affected. Banning of admissions has been targeted instead towards any patient, even of the most harmless and docile description, whom a court wishes to settle in a psychiatric unit rather than in a prison. Thus in one case in October 1975 which received particular publicity, a man who had pleaded guilty to the manslaughter of his wife in an episode of jealousy but who was certified by a psychiatrist as not in any way dangerous, had to be given a sentence of life imprisonment – described by the judge as 'wholly inappropriate' – because COHSE threatened to strike at one Bristol mental hospital if he was admitted there as the court intended; two other hospitals fell into line in refusing him admission. Fortunately, the staff at another psychiatric hospital in Cornwall displayed more sympathy and acceptance: the sentence of imprisonment was replaced judicially by a hospital order with restriction, and the man was subsequently reported to have settled there as a 'model patient'.[91]

It has sometimes been argued by the defenders of this form of psychiatric blacking that we have here only the usual type of industrial action by service workers. Any stoppage involving service is bound to cause suffering or discomfort to the innocent, but cannot be opposed on principle except by conceding an oppressive power to management (who could then act unchecked by the possibility of any collective retaliation by the work force). In the case of the mental-health blackings in Britain, it was sometimes suggested that the bans on court-referred patients were operated only as a means of pressurising administrations to hasten the building of Regional Secure Units. Such units would be properly equipped to accommodate difficult or dangerous patients in a manner impossible in the lax and under-staffed wards of the normal mental hospital. It appears, though, that some union branches do not wish to be associated with the secure facilities that may be necessary to house these patients. Thus, the membership of the Rainhill Hospital, Liverpool, branch of the National Union of Public Employees added their own threats of strike action to the local press scare whipped up in 1976 against the introduction of 'potentially violent criminals' through the building of an interim secure facility there. A similar interim unit, at Prestwich Hospital near Manchester, was refused co-operation in the daily chores of staffing by NUPE, apparently in their capacity as outraged local residents.[92]

The trade-union refusal to operate secure hospitals or admit court-referred patients is of course an important contributory cause in keeping the prisons and the criminal mental institutions full of psychiatrically disabled offenders, many of them working people themselves and in any case, for the most part, posing no threat to the safety of nursing or other staff. The plea heard on some sections of the left that such industrial action represents 'workers' control over the conditions of work'[93] simply ignores the repressive labelling of whole categories of patients as 'dangerous' as well as the law-and-order populism that has been inherent in some of these bans. Sometimes it appears as if certain nursing trade unionists actually prefer a custodial role to one that involves a professional responsibility shared with psychiatrists. For example, the COHSE shop steward at one mental hospital in Kent was asked why his branch, operating a blanket ban on all judicially-referred admissions, did not favour the arrangement that had been made with the same union in Scotland (whereby COHSE members have an equal say with the doctors on the admission of possibly difficult patients). He replied:

> Medical staff and the authorities decide individual admissions. We didn't want to get involved in examining each individual case to see if the nursing staff could cope with such and such an individual.[94]

Where trade-union attitudes among mental-hospital workers extend thus far in their refusal of 'managerial' responsibility, they simply reinforce the older custodial tendencies inherent in the time-worn stance of the asylum attendant, the turnkey whose social distance from the patients is only the obverse of his own lowly position in relation to the medical hierarchy. While the psychiatric nurse usually aspires to something more than a custodial role, the under-staffing of mental institutions often makes it impossible for him or her to perform more than the basic maintenance functions of grooming, feeding and monitoring patients whose interests would be better served by some encourgagement to perform as many as possible of these functions for themselves to the very limit of their capabilities. Institutionalised into the routines of ward life (as much as the long-stay patients but on the giving rather than the receiving side of the traditional services of the attendant), the mental-nursing profession resists its own incorporation into a menial and unskilled role by stressing its link with the medical experience of its superiors; and this borrowed status, a moonlight over the inmate beds reflected from the imputed magnificence of the consultant (who is usually absent somewhere well below the horizon), draws its glory from the most mechanical, organic and unsocial traditions of medicine itself.

To take one extreme but perhaps telling example, an attempt has been made in some British mental hospitals to involve nurses in the care of discharged patients by visiting them in their homes on a regular basis. This move to 'community psychiatric nursing' has some obvious advantages: the administration of drugs with checking for dosage and side-effects; continuity with the original therapeutic staff; the knowledge the visiting nurse may have about key aspects of the patient's condition – a knowledge, incidentally, often absent among modern social workers, who may compound gaps in their training on medical matters by a tendency to dissolve all biologically founded deviancies into the flux of interaction within the family. Evidence suggests, however, that roving mental nurses may take with them into the community the organic-individualist attitudes and perceptions they have acquired in the institution. For example, on commencing to give anti-psychotic injections to the patients, they may stop chatting with them on a person-to-person basis; or else the problems in the household may be seen exclusively through the course of one individual's 'condition', at the expense of the support or orientation other family members may need quite desperately.[95]

This is only one example of the way in which caring institutions – and not merely in the psychiatric sphere – tend to encapsulate a division of labour among grades of personnel, each category of which becomes professionally committed to a highly partial vantage-point on the needs of the client. (The doctors who complain about the 'restrictive practices' of the different groups of subordinate staff were, of course, historically just about the first professional group to hog certain kinds of caring work for themselves and insist that nobody else could do it either their way – unless medically certificated – or any other way.) The mental-health services now comprise a constellation of partial staff interests, whose trade-union representation runs along the lines of this alienated institutional order, sharpening the boundaries between the fragments rather than offering any opportunity for joint work in the wider goals of therapy. In this era of psychiatric monetarism, when health-service resources are continually stretched and depleted, the mental-health worker is forced into a defensive and often ungenerous stance because of a fear that a more adventurous approach will further worsen his or her conditions. While there is no reason (in principle) why the health trade unions could not aspire to a vanguard role in developing creative forms of intervention by their membership, this has not historically been their function.

It falls, therefore, to a different sort of health-workers' movement to construct forms of action and education to overcome sectional boundaries and promote a therapeutic consciousness. The years after 1968 in France saw a very large number of strikes and other revolts in psychiatric hospitals, involving doctors, nurses and inmates over contentious questions of admission and regimen.[96] From 1974 to 1978 the organisation *Gardes Fous* (with a nationally circulated journal of the same name) attempted to group the lowest, subordinate ranks of mental-hospital personnel within the same action groups as the patients themselves, in the hope of avoiding a solidarity among the most exploited staff which would direct itself against the patients' interests.[97] We have already noted the crusading work in Italy of *Psichiatria Democratica*, an association which has united psychiatrists, nurses, administrators and other professionals in a far-reaching campaign of local and national reforms. Post-Franco Spain has also seen the emergence of a *Psiquiatria Democratica* founded on a similar cross-professional alliance, though the lack of a structure of public assistance outside the asylum itself has rendered its operations, so far, much more tentative.[98] Paradoxically, in those countries like Britain and the United States where a community psychiatry movement was established in the forties and fifties with official sponsorship from the socially sensitive wing of mental medicine, the development of a voluntary, radical reformist movement such as *Psichiatria Democratica* seems to be inconceivable. The therapeutic community innovations of the post-war period never gathered the evangelistic momentum of their continental counterparts, and neither in Britain nor the United States did there exist the broad, civic movement, such as that offered by the Communist Party or even the Christian-Democracy of

Italy, which could transmit the professional concerns of the psychiatric reformers into a more popular mobilisation.

The task of integrating the diverse demands of mental-health workers, patients and the public has never been undertaken by the organised left, despite its pretension to possess a reasoned and principled overview of the social order and its problems. Issues and partial vantage-points have come and gone over the years, to be taken up by one or more marxist faction, or else by a professional element within it. Radical social workers have taken a roughly Laingian standpoint, endorsing disorder in patients as a social protest. Radical nurses have defended their own right to exclude disorderly patients from wards. When it was fashionable to blame the family, the category of 'hyperactive child' was declared to be a myth, the product of repressive labelling by schoolteacher and paediatrician.[99] But the very same label was employed for the purposes of political critique by the ecology lobbyists, who have variously blamed adulterated food, or lead pollution from petrol fumes, for the slow learning or behavioural misdemeanours of schoolchildren.[100] At one point, again, schizophrenia is declared to be a non-disease, or artefact of 'clinical conspiracy'; a few years later, it becomes preferable to complain that its cure, as a disease, is being blocked by the shortage of state funds for research into its biochemical causes.

One particularly important set of cross-currents in the politicisation of mental illness has been provided by feminism. Thus, it has sometimes been argued that the role of the mental patient is one which is specifically and substantially the woman's lot: according to Phyllis Chesler, 'women of all classes and races constitute the majority of the psychiatrically involved population of America, Britain, Sweden and Canada.'[101] Alternatively, particular feminine sex-roles (and more especially those involved in being a married woman)[102] have been incriminated as predisposing to an unusual vulnerability towards mental breakdown, at least in its diagnosed forms. Further to this, Chesler suggests that psychiatry has a woman-hating bias, a double standard of mental health which, in its proclamation of masculine norms as the sole virtue, ensures that 'women, by definition… are viewed as psychiatrically impaired.'[103] Other feminist critiques of diagnostic bias in psychiatry suggest that it is those women particularly at odds with the male's stereotype of female propriety who get assigned to a psychopathological category, more especially that of 'neurosis.'[104] The shift in feminist arguments from a stress-related explanation of woman's vulnerability to one which dissolves the diagnosis into a patriarchal label is typical of the ambivalence with which politically committed radicals view the attribution of mental illness. One the one hand, calling someone mad or mentally disturbed is often seen as a nasty demeaning insult, on a par with the foulest of racial slurs. On this showing, if a particular social group gets more than its fair share of psychiatric labels, it is being singled out specially for insult, as well as for assignation to the mental patient's horrible 'career'. Yet, on another radical view, the labels of psychopathology are (like some of the labels of physical pathology) indicators of the stress inflicted by our social order and its arrangements upon those who lack power. In this case, to label a social group, in more than usual proportion, as mentally ill is to indict not them but the social system and the helplessness of their ranking within it. One cannot easily adopt both perspectives on the same labels of mental disorder and the same groupings of the labelled. Yet, commonly, the stance of psychiatric radicalism has been that of having one's cake in the form of stress-theory as well as eating it in the substance of labelling or anti-psychiatry theory. More significantly: both of these radical analyses involve the casting of the psychiatrised in the role of victims, in the one case as victimised by psychiatric prejudice, in the other as casualties of the larger social order. There seems to have been little or no mileage for radicals in viewing a distressed person who seeks psychiatric care as having exerted a greater control over his or her destiny than those who continue to suffer, without therapeutic intervention, perhaps expressing their sorrows via whiskey or ulcers.[105] Women may have, in certain situations, entered the statistics of mental treatment more often than men because they are more willing to recognise certain of their problems and ask for help with them.

The politicisation of mental-health problems by radicals or left-wingers is, then, very often of a considerable crudity. The psychiatric patient tends to be slotted into the general case offered by a certain radical ideology, at the expense of the specifics that hold good for a particular pattern of illness or of care. An extraordinary burden is placed on the psychiatric sufferer, in that he or she is expected to be a cadre in the assemblage of counter-forces and counter-structures constructed in antagonism to our present oppressive society. Thus, from an American account of Basaglia's work in Italy:

> Ideally, therapy is a political act; and it becomes so to the degree that it tends to integrate an ongoing crisis back into the roots from which the crisis sprang, giving the individual an awareness of the personal and social conditions which provoked his crisis... the therapeutic community must be only a transitional step toward the full assumption of political awareness and personal responsibility.[106]

'Only a transitional step' – the theme is repeated in another American contribution to psychiatric politics:

> the struggle against psychiatric intervention cannot be directed purely and simply against the psychiatric system, given that the power of psychiatry and the techniques of normalisation have invaded all the levels of our life, waking and sleeping. Commitment to the fight against normalisation must go beyond the struggle against psychiatric atrocities (though this is an essential sector); in their place there must be created denormalising, de-psychiatrising, joyous actions and passions, and work-relationships which completely change the function of work, into an intense, un-alienated activity of struggle towards social change.[107]

Such generalised manifestoes were not uncommon in the psychiatric radicalisation of the latter sixties and the seventies. It is obvious from such texts that a social and political movement in the area of mental-health policy is here being asked to take on an extraordinarily ambitious range of goals, which would tax the resources even of a well organised and widely supported mass radical party. As well as the danger of over-burdening, mental-health professionals and (even more) mental patients with this daunting series of tasks, there exists also the risk of fracturing the precarious unity of the various projects for psychiatric change by asking them to agree on matters which are both contentious and without much possibility of a common adjudication. When the *Sozialistisches Patientenkollectiv* of Heidelberg present a sophisticated case stating that 'illness is the condition and the result of the capitalist relations of production' or when the Mental Patients' Union argues that 'psychiatry is one of the weapons used by capitalism to make sure that frustration and anger are internalised rather than expressed against the system of repression,'[108] they are making points which are suggestive and, perhaps, in a wider project of social understanding, helpful – even though the well-known existence of both illness and mental illness, and of both medicine and psychiatry, in pre-capitalist epochs would prevent any sensible person from accepting either statement literally. But it is hardly plausible to attempt to organise large masses of sufferers, or of sympathetic helpers and professionals, around such propositions.

Programmes for radical action in mental health do need a long-term and structural political awareness as well as the correct demands for immediate change. But these deeper sources for the framing of strategy must come, above all, from the realisation that some of the most basic needs of the mentally disabled – above all, the needs for housing, for occupation, and for community – are not satisfied by the market system of resource allocation which operates under capitalism. These needs are at present not even satisfied, systematically and appropriately, for normal people who labour without the further disadvantage of a mental or other disability. The crisis of mental-health provision, outside the problems of acute care which often reflect dilemmas of an intensive, dependency-producing medical technology, is simply the crisis of the normal social order in relation to any of its members who lack the wage-based ticket of entry into its palace of commodities.

The pitfalls of an acute and intensive medical-psychiatric technology are already widely canvassed both in the popular and the professional media: a pragmatic de-medicalisation is visible already on several fronts, as evidenced (to take a couple of instances) in the large psychiatric literature on 'tardive dyskinesia' as an unwanted effect of anti-psychotic medication, or in the refusal of British paediatricians to follow their North American colleagues in the routine prescription of stimulant drugs for troublesome children. This partial retreat from an over-biologised, bureaucratic model of medical care will be blocked, if not thwarted altogether, by powerful interests in the private sector (such as the pharmaceuticals industry) and the professional world of medicine itself. The training of doctors and their servitors, auxilliary or administrative, runs counter to any serious move in the direction of real power to patients. Nevertheless, the current of de-medicalisation is unmistakable. As well as displaying a progressive and emancipatory dynamic, it also chimes in well with the major ideological themes of right-wing libertarianism in the field of social policy in the eighties: *self-help* and *consumer choice*. Better individual choices and a reduced dependency on collective provision have become serious perspectives which are being offered to the psychiatrised masses in lieu of the indiscriminate medication which hits the tax-payer's purse in an age of recession, squeeze and arms race.

The de-medicalisation of acute therapy does nothing, however, to switch resources towards the funding of new institutions of continuing care which, for the tens of thousands of the poor, disabled and old, must replace the horrors of the asylum. The denunciation of asylum conditions, which has formed the staple subject of a large number of publicity campaigns from the late eighteenth century to the present era, has produced a highly paradoxical effect. For, by arousing an immense guilt in the collective unconscious of the public, it has harnessed the most effective means of coping with guilt that is available to the human psyche: denial, or refusal to admit the existence of the problems and processes, traumas and crimes, which trigger the shame and the horror. The repressed truth of the asylum, like the truth of the holocaust repressed in Germany, the truth about Ireland repressed by the British people, the truth about slavery and the bloody defeat of militant labour repressed in America, the truth of the gulag so long repressed in Russia, has a habit of returning now and again into the conscious imagery of different successive generations and publics. The ancestral spectre, bloodstained and foul, stalks the corridors of memory and the newly opened spaces of sensibility. Then – unless it is embraced and released by the spirit of a new transformative purpose – it is pushed back again, to lodge disruptively in the nether-world of the political process. Unacknowledged and yet latently active, it reveals itself on the surface of the citizens' and the rulers' behaviour, in a thousand dishonest, deflected initiatives of timid restitution or of yet further infamy. Our corner of the late twentieth century has become the battlement on which these spectres walk; and, unless we face these demanding, questioning ghosts, on open terms of action, liberation and final exorcism, they will drag us with them into new gulags, new enslavements, new worlds of madness and control, and new holocausts.

In the preceding argument, a number of examples of sectoral struggle in psychiatry were reviewed, with a critical and even negative conclusion. If such partial endeavours are seen as essentially flawed or wanting, what sense does it make even to begin to pose the wider questions of political and social reconstruction which have just been presented? One has to answer that the partial, sectoral campaigns that have been discussed were selected as examples of the ritualistic evasion of the serious questions of long-term psychiatric care. The civil-libertarian stance, the corporate trade-union response, the hyper-politicised annexation of anti-psychiatry by the far left, the 'alternative therapies' which cater only for the milder and the acuter forms of distress all stand as glib, guilt-discharging displacements of the central problem of the asylum: how to create the economic means of employment, the material apparatus of housing, the ethical structures of fellowship and solidarity, for those who through various forms of mental disability cannot purchase these benefits as commodities in the market-place. It will not suffice to reverse the long historical process of hospitalising the mentally disabled by despatching them back to their families. It is curious to note the tone of enthusiastic approval with which David Cooper, the well-known critic both of psychiatry and of the family, has greeted one such attempt at 'community care' in Italy: 'People in the villages in the hills came down to recover their own people from the psychiatric institutions.'[109] In the first place, there are getting to be fewer and fewer villages in the hills, and fewer and fewer people in them. Secondly, there can be little doubt that such attempts to purge the asylum by evacuating its inmates into their homes of origin are increasingly doomed as the expectations of men and women (and particularly of women) move towards an independent social and economic role for themselves. 'Community care', in this form at least, means tying down women in traditional servicing roles for their disabled kinsfolk. To loosen the tyranny of the mental institution by reinforcing an archaic sexual division of labour is a solution which may appeal to some sections of the right: it should have no currency elsewhere.[110]

In some countries the relatives of mental patients have, in fact, formed one of the most serious sources of political pressure in demanding the construction of fresh alternatives of residential care which will neither lock their vulnerable offspring, parents, siblings or grandparents in the warehouses of degradation nor force them into the intense, isolated nexus of the immediate family circle. Doubtless the civil libertarians have had a strong case in pointing to the conflicts of interest that may arise between a psychiatric patient and his or her relatives, especially in matters where a pecuniary or material asset is at stake. But the libertarian critics of the family's role in mental illness have been slow to recognise the community of interest that may bind the sufferer with his or her kinsfolk or with other befrienders, both lay and professional. Special organisations of support for the relatives of people with severe psychiatric disabilities are becoming an increasingly common element in mental-health politics in a number of countries: for example, the Association of Relatives and Friends of the Mentally Ill in both Australia and Canada, Japan's National Federation of Families with the Mentally Handicapped, Austria's HPE (Hilfe für Psychisch. Erkrankte). Britain has a particularly rich legacy of interest groups covering different diagnostic lobbies: the National Society for Mentally Handicapped Children and its local branches, the Alzheimer's Disease Society – organised for the victims of 'pre-senile' and 'senile' dementias who may number three-quarters of a million in the United Kingdom, the NSF or National Schizophrenia Fellowship (which has stimulated collateral bodies in Ireland, New Zealand and the United States). Despite the extreme difficulty of securing a stable self-organisation among relatives prone to intermittent family crises of a consuming intensity, these groups (often with the support of sympathetic professionals but also with some resistance from those elements of the medical profession who have no interest in the plight of their patients' families) have shown a fierceness and a continuity of assertion which have often been lacking in the more publicised – and more transient – faddisms of the anti-psychiatric counter-culture. Far more psychotic patients, for example, must have participated in the work of the British NSF (with its 90 local groups) alongside relatives and other sympathisers, than have ever been seen in the 'patients' union' networks of more politicised repute.[111]

The elements of a cross-sectional alliance, which will struggle for the replacement of the asylum system by genuine, socially funded resources of community care, are in fact already appearing on the historical stage. Doctors, nurses, patients, social workers, researchers, relatives: in each sphere of interest a 'minority movement' is assembling, determined to meet the challenge of the asylum with that vow which unites all those of liberal and radical conscience who have witnessed, or passed through, an inhuman and totalitarian experience: *Never Again*! The movement has small and confused beginnings: it needs, undoubtedly, more recruits from each of the serious constituencies of psychiatric change; above all, it needs to add fresh contingents from the untried reserves of organised labour, of political parties, and of the diffuse but vocal strata among the intelligentsia. As a revolutionary-socialist writer and teacher, trained in the earliest and the most recent battles of the post-war New Left, I here make my own appeal, for sympathy and solidarity from honest revolutionaries and radicals everywhere. It is wrong, comrades, to dismiss these real beginnings of contestation and construction in mental-health policy as being – what? – 'reformist', 'recuperative', 'collaborators of the Therapeutic State', 'agents of social control', or worse. For a general justification of the strategy of radical change in this as in other fields, I cannot improve on this statement from two experienced left-wing publicists:

> While committed to the primacy of extra-parliamentary action, we believe that it is necessary to work within the system as well. First, the platform provided by that system cannot be ignored: while it does not inspire much commitment from ordinary people, it does relate to the population in a way that fringe groups do not…
>
> Second, although 'revolutionary' and 'reformist' strategies are often posed as contradictory… most self-styled revolutionary parties engage in struggles which have as their *immediate* objective demands that can be accommodated within the system – for example, most strikes. If they did not engage in such struggles, these groups would not relate in any way to ordinary people. It is the political perspective within which these struggles are waged, rather than the actual demands themselves, which makes them revolutionary. We need to start where we are – not where we would like to be; and this means fighting on those issues which are in the hearts and minds of working people and posing a series

> of transitional demands, not embarking on a grand design with impeccable theoretical credentials but no practical relevance to day-to-day life.
>
> To refuse to work within the system means a rejection of short-term changes, which we find morally and politically unacceptable… A serious socialist strategy must alleviate deprivation and misery *now,* and simultaneously prepare for the basic changes that can eliminate the structure and the conditions which create deprivation.[112]

This outline of course begs the question: what *is* 'the system' within which even the most intransigent revolutionary is obliged to work? I personally do not believe that it is encompassed in any particular party of reform, as these authors have argued, first for the Liberal Party and then for the Labour Party in Britain. But regardless of the more general revolutionary-socialist argument about the nature of reformist parties (a debate which cannot be pursued here), there should be little doubt that, for radicals and reformers within the politics of mental health, 'working within the system' means working *within the publicly funded system of health and social-welfare provision.* The argument for a practical orientation within *this* system seems to me to be overwhelmingly justified within the terms used by Peter Hain and Simon Hebditch in the passage just quoted. Those psychiatric reformers or 'anti-psychiatric' revolutionaries, whether from the ranks of the psycho-professionals, from the psychiatrised themselves, or from other interested publics, who have turned to 'alternative' sectors of treatment and care outside the public-welfare system condemn themselves to the marginality and irrealism so sternly (and, I believe, rightly) denounced by Hain and Hebditch. In the realm of chronic disability and handicap – which now encompasses the preponderant bulk of serious psychiatric misery, particularly among the elderly and ageing – it has been demonstrated over and over again, in a large number of sectors, institutions and countries, that privately based facilities – whether funded by individual consumers' fees or through more charitable and philanthropic initiatives – are totally incapable of meeting the actual extent and specificity of need. The public system of social assistance and insurance, grotesquely inadequate as it is, is the only framework which relates to the mass of the population. Almost every pressure group and campaign in the modern era which works seriously towards the goals of betterment in health and social welfare has to pose its objectives in terms of demands upon the state. The exceptions are in areas where the state has historically never made any provision at all, such as refuges for battered women and hospices for those dying of terminal illnesses. In areas where an inadequate state-funded facility coexists with forms of private and voluntary care, the logic of the market dictates that the latter must become marginalised as a ghetto, and sometimes a gilded ghetto.

In entering and confronting the system of public maintenance and assistance, radicals, reformers and consumers in the psychiatric arena (as on other fronts of welfare politics) will find themselves juxtaposed awkwardly between the paternalistic, parsimonious inheritance of socially funded institutions bequeathed from the Keynesian era of the second world war (and its sequels in the different national post-war settlements) and the advancing counter-revolution of welfare cutbacks and other dilapidations decreed by rightward-moving governments in the present period of recession and militarisation. The dilemma of all innovators for whom the present state-run facilities offer little in the way of a model, and even less in the way of inspiration, is that of engineering a voluntary alternative mode of care which will not abdicate from the broader responsibility of posing more general and long-term demands.

For socialists and allied radicals attempting to acquire a perspective in the present-day crisis of health care there is an added ambiguity. There is a widespread and sharpening discontent among thousands of left-wing people because the models of political intervention proposed both by leninism and by social democracy involve the endless postponement of any personal sense of satisfaction in the achievement of socialist objectives. Social-democratic (and, in a more ruthless way, Stalinist) governments deprive the idealist left of satisfaction by reneging on their parties' programmes for an egalitarian reconstruction of society. After all the promises and hopes, we are always landed by these governments with some version of capitalism, or with a bureaucratic despotism, or with some hybrid of the two which combines, apparently, the least palatable features both of private ownership and of state control. Revolutionary groupings and parties that spring up in opposition to these betrayals also demand an endless deferment of gratification. Outside those exciting, transforming interludes where a full-scale revolution seems to be almost around the next corner (although usually in some other country than one's own), there are no instalments of the future liberated society that any militant can hope to see in his or her own lifetime: and all the current fronts of active commitment – in the newer personal and sexual politics no less than in more traditional militancies – seem to spawn an infinity of permanently frustrated goals, none of which can be abandoned without the risk of surrender to the existing conservative and hegemonic power structures. Against the continual futility and frustration that is engendered by these various experiences of political action on the left, socialists have become attuned to the possibilities of constructing institutions and relationships in the here-and-now which already embody the values of a liberated alternative society. Often these attempts are seen in terms of a 'prefigurative' politics: that is, they are intended to prefigure, or herald, the forms that will be characteristic of a society of advanced socialism. This is not to say that the construction of such here-and-now forms will alone suffice to usher in the socialist succession to the existing unequal order. The establishment of, for example, producers' co-operatives, or of communal networks of child care, are meant primarily to set an example, and to work out some of the practical problems of the full implementation which must be achieved by further means.

In the history of mental-health politics, the idea that radical and dramatic reforms in patient care might be of a more general emancipatory significance is not a new one. The liberation of asylum patients from their chains and fetters, allegedly conducted in 1792 by the eminent physician Philippe Pinel but actually carried out by a senior attendant working without medical instructions, became a much publicised tableau in the idealised imagery that was harvested from the scenes of the French Revolution.[113] The example of socially progressive therapy attributed to Pinel was drawn on also by the anarchist theoretician Prince Peter Kropotkin – who was the most brilliant discoverer and populariser of prefigurative examples of 'mutual aid' in all stages of history – during his lecture of 1877 on 'Prisons and Their Moral Influence on Prisoners', delivered in Paris before a workers' audience and later widely distributed and reprinted.[114] A passionate opponent of incarceration and confinement in the psychiatric no less than in the criminal sphere, Kropotkin sought inspiration, and an alternative model of care for mental illness that would become the norm of a future free society, not only in the Pinelian replacement of constraint by moral appeal within the hospital but also in the more thorough communitarian precedent offered in the Belgian farming village of Geel, whose inhabitants have for centuries opened their homes and their fields for the lodging and occupation of severely disturbed mental patients:

> And liberty worked a miracle. The insane became cured… They cried that it was a miracle. The cures were attributed to a saint and a virgin. But this virgin was liberty and the saint was work in the fields and fraternal treatment.

For Kropotkin, the search for communitarian examples of mutual aid would often involve a reference back to the precapitalist, anti-individualist epoch of medieval Christendom: 'not only many aspirations of our modern radicals were already realised in the middle ages, but much of what is described now as Utopian was accepted then as a matter of fact.'[115] And it is striking to notice the dearth of contemporary examples he could quote from his own era for the communal provision of welfare and health services, outside such semi-charitable voluntary bodies as the Lifeboat Institution of Britain and the International societies of the Red Cross.[116] This despite his incessant combing of news sources for those pre-figurative exemplars of mutual aid which were to be found in

> those associations, societies, brotherhoods, alliances, institutes and so on, which must now be counted by the ten thousand in Europe alone, and each of which represents an immense amount of voluntary, unambitious, and unpaid or underpaid work.[117]

The nineteenth century, from which he surveyed both the past and (as he hoped) the emancipated future, was of course precisely the epoch of impersonal and institutional segregation for the destitute, disabled and deviant. New forms of community care, whether in mental disability or for other handicaps, were hardly in evidence for him to cite.

But a modern Kropotkin of the latter twentieth century, reviewing the rise of modern community approaches to treatment and care in mental illness, would – provided that she or he avoided his predecessor's somewhat aristocratic preference for private philanthropy over state-funded provision – find many examples of a warm and imaginative 'mutual aid and support' which – as a libertarian socialist today would argue – require multiplication, extension and (above all) reliable material funding to serve as a reasonable pointer to the forms of assistance that a progressive, humane and responsible society would tender to its mentally infirm. The modesty of these enterprises usually debars them from offering themselves as prefigurative samples of a utopia in welfare. Still, for the case of Britain (a country on which there is a ready mass of published material),[118] a contemporary Kropotkinist would be able to produce the following critical guide:

1. THE MENTAL AFTER-CARE ASSOCIATION

Begun in Kropotkin's own day, in 1879, by the chaplain of one of Britain's largest asylums (Colney Hatch, now Friern Barnet Hospital), the MACA had over the next hundred years expanded to a grand total of eight long-stay hostels giving permanent homes – sometimes in sea-side resorts – to nearly 250 former mental-hospital patients, nearly all with a diagnosis of schizophrenia. None of them was expected ever to gain an independent livelihood or to live outside some form of sheltered housing. The hostels are staffed by experienced wardens and other helpers, who try to encourage the residents to overcome the combined effects of their institutionalisation and their illness. 'One old lady, for example, had initially many eccentric mannerisms, and almost no capacity to look after herself. After a year's stay, she could wash and dress herself, do her own washing, and go to town for shopping or to collect her pension'. The MACA operates only in London and the South East of England.

2. GROUP HOMES

There are now a fairly large number of households in Britain occupied solely by smallish groups of mental patients: usually there are three to five residents, but sometimes larger communes have been established. Thus, the Cherries Group Home established in Slough in 1973 (by the local Society for Mentally Handicapped Children) has provided a home for 12 mentally disabled adults of low IQ (sometimes as low as 41–45) who live without a warden, though with frequent visits from social workers, and who contribute towards the costs of the household, wherever possible, from their earnings. The Cherries is unusual in having accommodation for married couples; in fact, during one period covered by a study of the home, two of the residents got married to one another.[119] But it is far from untypical of the many initiatives of the group-home movement: local Associations of Mental Health run well over 150 communal households; many mental hospitals have outlying unstaffed group homes or (as in the case of the Maudsley Hospital) more supervised high-dependency hostel facilities within their grounds; housing associations have also been formed in many areas for the needs of the mentally disabled; and charities like the Richmond Fellowship and the St Mungo Community (the latter working with destitute and handicapped vagrants) have also been in the vanguard of voluntary residential provision.

The internal organisation of these small communities is of extremely varied character, from a benignly autocratic wardenship to experiments in communal decision-making. The expectations of residents themselves vary, even concerning the simplest outside occupation or social activity. In group homes that receive visits from a supervising professional worker, much depends on the experience and outlook of the supervisor (whether from a nursing or social work background) and on the support given her or him by the residents or by the sponsoring organisation: both quarters can be unsupportive or over-demanding. Nevertheless, the general record of these communities is quite impressive: very few of their residents wish to enter or re-enter mental hospital, and conditions in them do not seem to have replicated the more chilling features of asylum back-ward life, as might have been reasonably feared.[120]

3. THE CAMPUS CONCEPT

The principal drawback affecting all these schemes of community placement for mental patients is the inflexibility of their arrangements for the many possible changes of fortune and misfortune that may crop up in a patient's lifetime. To opt for one particular category of sheltered housing (staff-free group home, say, or the semi-independent villa on or near the hospital terrain) risks a severe disruption of the resident's regimen on each occasion when his or her condition shifts in the direction of a greater or less dependency, or of an improved or lessened sociability. Of particular (but not sole) importance here are the conditions characterised by interludes of fluctuating lucidity and confusion (some of the schizophrenias), by catastrophic mood-swings, or by broader progression and plateaus in a generally deteriorating direction (Alzheimer's, Huntingdon's and the other dementias, including multiple sclerosis). Such circumstances suggest the construction of a multi-purpose psychiatric housing community, with dwellings along the whole gamut of independent apartments, common households, supervised hostels and highly staffed villas (for both the episodically and the long-term disabled), along with day centres for meaningful, properly paid work and for occupational and social rehabilitation. In the absence of such an estate, or 'campus', uniting the several varieties of residential care, the fate of any person suffering from a condition or situation with variable nursing and social needs will inevitably be one of eviction from one address or location to another, probably with a significant disruption of social contacts of whatever order. No such integrated community exists anywhere at present.

Dr Donal Early has for many years mounted a forceful campaign for the building of such an estate – with special attention to the needs of new long-stay mental patients – on land adjacent to a Bristol hospital. Despite wide support, including endorsement from the hospital trade unions, the plan has faltered owing to apathy or buck-passing from national and local financial agencies. The National Schizophrenia Fellowship has also argued for the establishment of a residential campus with mixed levels of housing under the same management, as a model to be tested for more general application;[121] the fate of this project will be of interest to lobbyists for different disabilities outside the diagnosis of schizophrenia.

4. THE ANTI-THERAPEUTIC STATE

In one aspect, Kropotkin's suspicions about the limitations of publicly-financed avenues of care have been amply justified. Inveighing against the development of a state-inspired welfare-collectivism in his own day – exemplified for Britain in the Fabian doctrines of municipal and central government socialisation – Kropotkin warned that 'in proportion as the obligations to the state grew in numbers the citizens were evidently relieved of their obligations towards each other.' Instead of personally watching over the illness of a sick colleague – as the medieval guildsmen were obliged to do – 'it would be sufficient to give one's neighbour the address of the next paupers' hospital'; and, far from sharing all available food with those in need, according to the example even of the 'savage' Hottentots of Africa, 'all that a respectable citizen has to do now is to pay the poor tax and to let the starving starve.'[122] The bureaucratic administration of welfare would thus poison the well-springs of a genuine communitarian help.

Whatever may be true for other countries – and in Italy (for instance) elected local administrations have at times been attentive to the demands of a creative psychiatric reform – the record of the British state authorities in mental-health after-care has been little short of abysmal. After seven decades of social insurance, and more than a quarter-century of a supposedly comprehensive national health service, a government White Paper of 1975 had to report, as if confessing to the indictment mounted by the author of *Mutual Aid*, that 'by and large, the non-hospital community resources are still minimal' for psychiatric patients, and deplored 'the failure, for which central as much as local government is responsible, to develop anything approaching adequate social services.' For the financial year 1973–74, £6.5 million was spent on residential and day-care services for the mentally ill, compared with £300 millions for their care in hospital institutions.[123] Spending on residential facilities for the mentally ill by local authorities – who in Britain have the major responsibility for public housing – amounted to only 0.04 per cent of their total expenditure. According to a latter Consultative Document from the same department, 'a good many' local authorities 'could point to mental illness schemes' (for housing and day care in the community) 'for which they had requested loan sanction in the last few years but which the central government of the day had felt unable to approve.'[124]

Even greater blasts of disapproval were to be visited by Whitehall and Westminster upon the housing of mental patients: future governmental edicts (both Labour and Conservative) would launch ruthless attacks upon welfare and social-service funding, in the cause of billionfold nuclear weapons budgets, the colossal expansion of police technology and pay, and monetarist dogma about the evils of public expenditure. But, even where the national government did earmark substantial sums for collaborative projects between hospitals and the local authorities – as with the centrally allocated 'joint funding' millions available for this vital interface over many years – little of it was channelled towards the provision of community living space for the mentally ill.[125] It was not simply the lack of money, but a shortage of imagination and will, that crippled the Fabian programme of care decreed from city hall, government department and medical think-tank.

The bankruptcy and dishonour of our modern welfare-collectivism have more specific political, economic and historical causes than its mere collision with the ethical outlook of 'mutual aid'. But Kropotkin's insistence on the countervailing power of voluntary social initiative, outside the bureaucratic compass of the state, holds good for our time also. His prime example of the benefits to be gained from a communitarian, mutual-aid approach in psychiatry, i.e. the centuries-old therapeutic activity of the Belgian villagers at Geel, repays a closer examination – especially as the work of the Geel neighbourhood for insane and mentally handicapped boarders continues down to the present day. Kropotkin's astuteness in singling out this experiment as the most complete available embodiment of a liberated, non-segregative solution to the housing and treatment of the mentally disturbed is all the more extraordinary because, since the time of his own citation of its importance, none of the theoreticians or publicists of 'radical psychiatry', 'alternative psychiatry' or 'anti-psychiatry' has even mentioned it. There have been brief allusions to Geel in some of the literature of social and transcultural medicine during the sixties; and from 1969 to 1974, a distinguished international research project for the description and analysis of the communal therapeutic processes at work in Geel was conducting field studies there with the backing of large scholarly and financial resources from the United States and Belgium itself. With the recent appearance of the first publication in English from this project, Eugeen Roosens' book *Mental Patients in Town Life*,[126] Geel and its inhabitants can at last be given the recognition which their tradition of care deserves, originating as it does from the year 1250.

The references by Kropotkin to the Geel experiment were somewhat over-idealised. In his version, the peasants of this 'little Belgian village' said to their citizenry

> 'Send us your insane. We will give them absolute freedom.' They adopted them into their families, they gave them places at their tables, chance alongside them to cultivate their fields and a place among their country balls. 'Eat, drink and dance with us. Work, run about the fields, and be free.' That was all the system, all the science the Belgian peasant had. (I am speaking of the early days. Today the treatment of the insane at Geel has become a profession, and where it is a profession for profit, what significance can there be in it?)[127]

The facts about Geel's past and current practice are different, but scarcely less impressive. From its medieval beginnings in the thirteenth century, Geel functioned as a centre of pilgrimage and settlement for the mentally afflicted, who came to be exorcised at the church of St Dympna, their special patron. These ceremonies continued, along with the hospitality afforded by local families under the supervision of the Church, until 1797, when the cult was closed down by the occupying authorities of revolutionary France. Soon afterwards, in a remarkable anticipation of the more modern shift from asylum placement to 'community care', Brussels evacuated the hundred inmates of its mental institution and boarded them out in Geel; by 1850 over 900 patients had settled there, drawn from asylums all over Belgium. The Geel family-care system separated from the Church (which, however, continued the annual pageant of the patient-boarders, in honour of St Dympna, until quite recent years). The conditions in which patients were kept were, in the first period of nineteenth-century secular control, characteristically harsh, with the chaining and fettering of the disruptive who were sent there along with the docile. Nowadays the policy of settlement at Geel operates under strict selection by the medical authorities, who keep aggressive or very difficult patients well away from host homes.

Despite these exclusions from Geel, and the stricter screening of the families who apply to receive boarders, there were, by 1938, 3,736 patients in the colony. The number is now smaller (1,600 or so); but since Geel – a township rather than an idyllic 'village' – has a population of thirty thousand, the saturation of the community by severely disabled patients (who include a large proportion of retarded as well as the psychotic) is considerable indeed. In 1945, 11.4 per cent of the population of Belgium's mental institutions lived at Geel; in 1975 the proportion was 5.8 per cent. (All the above details are taken from Roosens, who reports them as a background to his social-anthropological study of current life in Geel.)

The system of family placement enjoys a well developed supportive structure provided by the psychiatric hospital of the town. The hospital screens candidate-boarders, accepts troublesome or sick patients from the community, and tags each boarder with precise instructions for her or his host-household, e.g. as to whether she or he can be allowed to walk in the town unaccompanied. The medical centre also organises sporting, fishing and vacation outings for the patients, as well as work and hobby activities. There is a strict prohibition of sexual contact. That, and the rather extensive limiting of unaccompanied excursions into the town itself (affecting some two-thirds of these patients), constitutes the entire extent of formal, bureaucratic regulation of the patients' freedom of movement.

Roosens' careful study of the interactions between the boarders and the Geelian citizenry reveals a surpassing ordinariness in the flow of public life. Forty per cent of the patient-guests did the shopping regularly for their host families. Of the 400 patients whose circulation in the town was unrestricted, he reports an almost complete lack of incidents affecting public order. They are not stared at. Oddities or breaches of decorum are tolerated by the public or else 'managed' with great tact in the community's long tradition of under-reaction. There has been over the years an almost total absence of spectacular crimes or traffic accidents involving patients. Discrimination on the grounds of mental status is practised on a fairly wide scale in bars and other public settings where the 'people from the Kolonie' and the straight citizenry may potentially mix: but often such distinction takes place as a 'joking relationship' between normals and boarders, with a great deal of comradely and friendly interaction across this line, which is decidedly not one of taboo.

Kropotkin's dismissal of the developments at Geel in his own time, as being linked with economic reward and therefore without significance, accords ill with the realities of life there. The remuneration of the host-households from public sources of support is of course a *sine qua non* of any family-care boarding system for the disabled. Aside from a certain degree of economic exploitation as cheap farming or domestic labour (extremely difficult to check where members of the family are involved in such labour as a matter of normal expectation), the patients are received into care at Geel in a spirit which transcends any attribution of either selfishness or of altruism to their hosts. The research team established that the motive of compassion or Christian charity is not dominant in the hearts of Geelians who elect to take a mentally sick person into their household. Economic reasons are decisive, since fostering is traditionally regarded as a normal business there, but the economic component alone cannot account for the strength of the boarding-out tradition in host families. It is usual for a patient who has entered a household to pass into the care of its younger members when their parents die or become too infirm for fostering:

> The personal tie between patient and family cannot be broken without serious reason. Legally, of course, one is free; morally, one is not. Anyone who does not observe this code is criticised by his peers… Age-old tradition has proved that 'normal people' can establish personal relationships with the mentally ill and with all kinds of 'deranged' persons and that the tie is such that it seems immoral to break it. We may perhaps speak of some kind of 'structural' built-in humanity or brotherly love.[128]

It is here that the example of Geel and the Geelians is so particularly significant for the whole future of mental-health care. Geel is not simply a 'family care system' comprised of all individual households who take boarders. The care-giver at Geel is not alone and isolated in times of crisis or difficulty, as is the member of a 'normal' individualist household in the atomised consumer societies of the more 'advanced' parts of the West. On the contrary: she or he is only one element in a web of care and consideration with countless threads running across a much wider community. (Problems and worries about a boarder's conduct or well-being, for instance, would be shared among listening neighbours, and be taken as a responsibility by all bystanders whenever the patient become disturbed in a public place.) This dramatic and total contrast with even the most adventurous attempts at community care within our less sensitive public environments (at once more individualistic and more impersonal) derives, of course, from the inheritance by Geel of the norms of one of history's few great social orders which offers a thoroughgoing alternative to the capitalist way of life: that of medieval society. The Middle Ages will never be reconstituted: the tasks of care for the weak and the poor today pose the construction of yet another total alternative to the inhumanity of capitalism.

In one respect, Kropotkin's vision of Geel was completely accurate: its care-givers, then as now, know no science. The family hosts and the general public of the town are not instructed in the medical details of schizophrenia or mental handicap. Their triumph does not depend even on a knowledge of Freud, Lacan, Laing or Wilhelm Reich. Still less are they indebted to the miraculous products of the pharmaceuticals empire: many patients have not seen a doctor in years, and have largely discontinued all medication. The work of Geel is indeed the victory of humanity: but not simply via the actions of individual humanitarians, in the liberal or philanthropic model of welfare. Rather it expresses the practice, voluntarily conceived and materially implemented, of a *socialised* and *organised* humanity.

The achievement of this kindly and efficacious condition, for all patients and all societies, is the central problem of psychiatric care. It is also the central problem of social liberation.

References

New Introduction

1. Gary Greenberg, *The Book of Woe: The DSM and the Unmaking of Psychiatry* (New York: Blue Rider Press, 2013).
2. Allan V. Horwitz, *DSM: A History of Psychiatry's Bible* (Baltimore: Johns Hopkins Press, 2021).
3. Gary Greenberg, *Manufacturing Depression: The Secret History of a Modern Disease* (New York: Simon & Schuster, 2010); Gerald L. Klerman, 'Mental Illness, the Medical Model, and Psychiatry', *Journal of Medicine and Philosophy*, Vol. 2, No. 3, 1977; Peter Sedgwick, 'The Fate of Psychiatry in the New Populism', *Psychiatric Bulletin*, Vol. 7, No. 2, 1983.
4. Tad Tietze, 'Peter Sedgwick: Mental Health as Radical Politics', *Critical and Radical Social Work*, Vol. 3, No. 1, 2015.
5. *PsychoPolitics*, p. 20.
6. *ibid.* p. 33.
7. *ibid.* p. 10 (emphasis in original).
8. *ibid.* p. 28.
9. *ibid.* p. 26.
10. *ibid,* p. 26 (emphasis in original).
11. *ibid.* p. 28.
12. For a detailed account see Wilbur J. Scott, *Vietnam Veterans Since the War: The Politics of PTSD, Agent Orange, and the National Memorial* (Norman: University of Oklahoma Press, 2004), pp. 27–73.
13. Derek Summerfield, 'The Invention of Post-Traumatic Stress Disorder and the Social Usefulness of a Psychiatric Category', *British Medical Journal*, Vol. 322, No. 7278, 2001.
14. *PsychoPolitics*, pp. 31–33.
15. Peter Sedgwick, 'Medical Individualism', *Studies – Hastings Center*, Vol. 2, No. 3, 1974, p. 77.
16. Ben Goldacre, *Bad Pharma: How Medicine is Broken, And How We Can Fix It* (London: Fourth Estate, 2012).
17. Vinayak K. Prasad and Adam S. Cifu, *Ending Medical Reversal: Improving Outcomes, Saving Lives* (Baltimore: Johns Hopkins University Press, 2015).
18. Stefan Leucht, Sandra Hierl, Werner Kissling, Markus Dold and John M. Davis, 'Putting the Efficacy of Psychiatric and General Medicine Medication into Perspective: Review of Meta-Analyses', *British Journal of Psychiatry*, Vol. 200, No. 2, 2012, pp. 97–106.
19. Tietze, 'Peter Sedgwick', p. 112.

20. John P.A. Ioannidis, Sally Cripps and Martin A. Tanner, 'Forecasting for COVID-19 Has Failed', *International Journal of Forecasting*, Vol. 38, No. 2, 2022.
21. Celia Blanco Jimenez, 'Why Didn't Pandemic Planning Anticipate the Need for Lockdowns?' LSE COVID-19 Blog, 17 Mar 2021. https://blogs.lse.ac.uk/covid19/2021/03/17/why-didnt-pandemic-planning-anticipate-the-need-for-lockdowns/ (last accessed 2 April 2022).
22. *PsychoPolitics*, p. 36.
23. Mark Cresswell and Helen Spandler, 'PsychoPolitics: Peter Sedgwick's Legacy for the Politics of Mental Health', *Social Theory & Health*, No. 7, 2009, p. 133 (emphasis in original).
24. Sedgwick, 'The Fate of Psychiatry'.
25. Athena Helen McLean, 'From ex-Patient Alternatives to Consumer Options: Consequences of Consumerism for Psychiatric Consumers and the Ex-Patient Movement', *International Journal of Health Services*, Vol. 30, No. 4, 2000.
26. *PsychoPolitics*, p. 210.
27. *ibid.* p. 34 (emphasis in original).
28. Peter Conrad, *The Medicalization of Society: On the Transformation of Human Conditions into Treatable Disorders* (Baltimore: Johns Hopkins University Press, 2007).

Part One: Anti-Psychiatry

1. Anti-Psychiatry, Illness and the Mentally Ill pages 7–35

1. J.C. Maleval, in an enlightening paper (*Schizophrénie et folie hystérique, L'Information Psychiatrique*, vol. 54, 1978, pp. 743–65), has complained that the modern framework for the diagnosis of schizophrenia has excluded the possibility of observing a psychosis which is hysterical in nature: 'the introduction of the concept of schizophrenia authorises not so much the disappearance of the hysterical delirium… as the expulsion of hysteria from the terrain of madness.' Hysterical psychosis, he argues, has every right to be observed – and he cites the case of Mary Barnes as one such instance. The British diagnostician of schizophrenia, J.K. Wing, also argues that Mary Barnes's manifestations of disorder indicated hysteria rather than schizophrenia (*Reasoning About Madness*, Oxford, 1978, p. 162).

2. The following discussion will assume that the concepts of 'disease' and 'illness' raise roughly similar problems in the debates over anti-psychiatry. Christopher Boorse (On the Distinction between Disease and Illness', *Philosophy and Public Affairs*, vol. 5, 1975, pp. 49–68) has argued for the separateness of the concepts; Robert Brown ('Physical Illness and Mental Health', *Philosophy and Public Affairs*, vol. 7, 1977. pp. 17–38) finds Boorse's distinction too finicky for purposes of useful discussion, and I tend to concur.

3. F. Kraüpl Taylor, 'The Medical Model of the Disease Concept', *British Journal of Psychiatry*, vol. 128, 1976, pp. 588–94.
4. Georges Cangouilhem, *Le normal et le pathologique* (Paris, 1966, pp. 40 *et seq.*) offers a lively review of the failures of the various quantitative criteria devised by experimentalists for separating the abnormal from the normal.
5. R.E. Kendell, 'The Concept of Disease and Its Implications for Psychiatry', *British Journal of Psychiatry*, vol. 127, 1975, pp. 305–15.
6. J.G. Scadding, *Lancet*, 1967.
7. Letter dated 10 November 1975. I am grateful to Professor Kendell for permission to quote from this letter.
8. See E. Rubington and M. Weinberg, *The Study of Social Problems: Five Perspectives*, New York, 1971, especially chapters 6 and 7, for a good presentation on the different vantage points on deviancy problems.
9. T. Szasz, 'The Myth of Mental Illness', *The American Psychologist*, vol. 15, February 1960, pp. 113–18.
10. *The Second Sin*, New York, 1974, p. 99. This quotation is well discussed by Ronald Pies in his notable paper, 'On Myths and Countermyths: More on Szaszian Fallacies' (*Archives of General Psychiatry*, vol. 36, 1979, pp. 139–44), a particularly trenchant and scholarly discussion of disease concepts in medicine and psychiatry.
11. R. Leifer, *In the Name of Mental Health*, New York, 1969, p. 35. Leifer is a systematic expounder of Szaszian doctrine with a much more extensive use of sociological theory than his mentor.
12. *Stigma*, New York, 1961; *Asylums*, New York, 1961, pp. 125–70.
13. E. Goffman, *Asylums*, Harmondsworth, 1968, p. 317.
14. In the Appendix, 'The Insanity of Place', to *Relations in Public*, Harmondsworth, 1972, pp. 389–450.
15. *ibid.* pp. 345, 346.
16. See e.g. *The Politics of Experience*, London, 1967, pp. 17–18, 41–44; *The Divided Self*, London, 1960, pp. 19–25; *Interpersonal Perception*, London, 1966, pp. 6–7, 40–41.
17. *Psychiatry and Anti-Psychiatry*, New York, 1971 edition, pp. 7–14.
18. See e.g. his *Intervention in Social Situations*, London, 1969, p. 17.
19. David Cooper, 'The Anti-Hospital: An Experiment in Social Psychiatry', *New Society*, 11 March 1965.
20. *The Myth of Mental Illness*, New York, 1961, pp. 143–45; *Ideology and Insanity*, New York, 1970, pp. 234, 210–11.
21. Interestingly, Foucault has allowed this work to go out of print and tried to eliminate it from the English translations of his work. The reasons for this remain obscure. See Alan Sheridan, *Michel Foucault: The Will to Truth*, London, 1980, p. 8.
22. *Maladie Mentale et Psychologie*, Paris, 1966 edition, p. 101.
23. Sheridan (*loc. cit.*) has a translation and useful commentary on this striking passage.
24. From the editorial text contributed to the 'Sanity-Insanity: Madness: Violence' issue of *Peace News*, 19 May 1967.

25. There are several different descriptions of what 'positivism' is, referring to quite separate philosophical tendencies. David Ingleby, for example, in the first chapter, 'Understanding Mental Illness', of his collection *Critical Psychiatry: The Politics of Mental Health* (Harmondsworth, 1981, pp. 28–45) appears to use it as a denunciatory term against any theory or method depending on empirical evidence except Freudian theory, which he exempts from the charge. My short definition above is somewhat indebted to L. Kolakowski, *The Alienation of Reason: A History of Positivist Thought* (New York, 1968), but has been invented mainly in order to contrast the 'immanent' sociological descriptions of mental illness with alternative, more medically based frameworks of analysis. It is not intended to provide clues as to what 'positivism' might be in other controversies or other fields.

26. E.g. C.J. Klett and D.M. McNair, *Syndromes of Psychosis*, New York, 1963; R.R. Sokal and P.A. Sneath, *Principles of Numerical Taxonomy*, London, 1963; and, in a refreshingly incisive vein, R.E. Kendell, *The Classification of the Depressive Illnesses*, London, 1968, and 'The Classification of the Depressions: A Review of Contemporary Confusion', *British Journal of Psychiatry*, vol. 129, 1976, pp. 15–28.

27. This observation is not intended as a dismissal of these studies, whose method is often compatible with the valuational outlook on mental illness that will be developed later in this chapter.

28. R. Dingwall, *Aspects of Illness*, London, 1976, p. 49.

29. Dingwall, *loc. cit.*

30. Talcott Parsons's well known discussion of 'the sick role', in Chapter 10 of *The Social System* (Glencoe, 1951), referred not to the social status of 'being ill' but to the situation of *being a patient*, within a system of medical facilities; his conflation of the sick and the patient identity bears an odd resemblance to the similar blurring of the two concepts offered (and criticised earlier in this chapter) by Kraüpl Taylor. David Mechanic's specification of what constitutes disease ('some deviation from normal functioning which has undesirable consequences, because it produces personal discomfort or adversely affects the individual's future health status', given in *Medical Sociology*, New York, 1978, p. 26) is far too general. It would not be possible on this definition to distinguish illness from fatigue or bereavement, since both these deviations from 'normal functioning' indubitably produce 'discomfort'. The literature on the definition of illness has now become considerable, both among sociologists and among philosophically-inclined clinicians.

31. *Social Science and Social Pathology*, London, 1959, p. 225.

32. J. Zubin, 'A Cross-Cultural Approach to Psychopathology and Its Implications for Diagnostic Classifications', in L.D. Eron (ed.), *The Classification of Behavior Disorders*, Chicago, 1966, pp. 43–82.

32. The above discussion is heavily indebted to René Dubos' masterly *The Mirage of Health*, New York, especially pp. 30–128.

34. See the excellent account of Homeric medicine in P. Lain Entralgo, *The Therapy of the Word in Classical Antiquity*, New Haven, 1970.

35. This observation is taken from a contribution by Dr L. Robbins in the symposium edited by Eron, *op. cit.* above.
36. Cited by A.L. Knudsen, *The Individual, Society and Health Behavior*, New York, 1965, p. 49.
37. Cited by Mechanic, *op. cit.* p. 26.
38. Knudsen (*op. cit.* p. 48) quotes one New York study showing lower-class indifference to the need for medical attention for such conditions as ankle swelling and backache. This finding does not, however, imply that the respondents refused to view these inconveniences as illnesses: they could merely have had sound reasons of their own (such as lack of cash) for avoiding self-referral to a doctor.
39. There is now some doubt among dental experts as to whether 'caries' is a genuine disease entity or an artefact of diagnostic labelling.
40. See M. Foucault, *Madness and Civilization*, New York, 1965, pp. 119, 121, 123, 129 and 151 *ff.* for examples of these. Lain Entralgo's work on the ancient Greeks' approach to therapy (see note 32 above) has similar explanations collected from Hippocratic medicine.
41. M. Siegler and H. Osmond, 'Models of Madness', *British Journal of Psychiatry*, vol. 112, 1966, pp. 1193–1203; and the same authors' 'Models of Drug Addiction', *International Journal of the Addictions*, vol. 3, no. 1, 1968, pp. 3–24.

2. Psycho-Medical Dualism: The Case of Erving Goffman pages 38–57

1. Erving Goffman, 'The Insanity of Place', p. 449, reference in 3, below.
2. *Asylums*, Harmondsworth, 1968, p. 317.
3. *Behavior in Public Places*, Glencoe, Illinois, 1963; 'Mental Symptoms and Public Order', in *Interaction Ritual*, New York, 1967, pp. 137–48; 'The Insanity of Place', in *Relations in Public*, Harmondsworth, 1972, pp. 389–450.
4. 'Mental Symptoms and Public Order', *loc. cit.*, p. 147 and pp. 146, 148 for the argument summarised in the text.
5. 'The Insanity of Place', p.420. This paper lays particular emphasis on manic disorders and paranoid actings-out within a family setting, which constitute highly visible infringements of a person's imputed 'place' within the terminology used by Goffman. The article makes passing reference (p. 420) to 'withdrawals – depressions and regressions', but the analysis is not worked out for these. Nor does Goffman provide any discussion of schizophrenic symptomatology within his situational-disruption framework. Indeed it is difficult to conceive how he could have extended his argument since most psychiatric syndromes are defined in terms other than those of face-to-face situational disturbance, e.g. by a fragmented or alienated subjective, experiential state or by other failures of public functioning such as inability to work. See the rest of my text for a development of this case.

6. The example is revealing in several ways. A doctor may prescribe some form of minor tranquilliser to relieve some of the effects of a bereavement, even though depression of activity and feeling following the death of a close relative would scarcely be regarded as constituting a 'mental illness'. Bereavement has, however, also been reported as a significant precipitating event in the onset of actual psychiatric illnesses. In one British study the widowed were found to have higher rates of entry into psychiatric care than the married, for all categories of psychosis and behaviour disorder (though not for the neuroses). See Z. Steiner and M.W. Susser, 'Bereavement as a Precipitating Event in Mental Illness', in E.H. Hare and J.K. Wing (eds.), *Psychiatric Epidemiology*, Oxford, 1970, pp. 327–33. The line of division between a bereavement and a 'psychiatric illness following bereavement' would seem to depend on our culturally derived expectations about how to mourn properly.
7. 'The Insanity of Place', p. 411. See also 'Mental Symptoms and Public Order', p. 147.
8. 'The Insanity of Place', pp. 406–07. Goffman does qualify this pronouncement, adding some riders about types of physical patients who are socially disruptive (for instance, persons with a visible face deformity), but the distinction of etiquette, of 'keeping one's place', remains the cardinal one in distinguishing medical from psychiatric complaints.
9. D.P. Ausubel, 'Personality Disorder *Is* Disease', in Thomas Scheff (ed.), *Mental Illness and Social Processes*, New York, 1967, pp. 259–62.
10. For a good demonstration of the psychosomatic features of coronary illness, see 'Socio-Economic Aspects of Heart Diseases', in *Historical Sociology: The Selected Papers of Bernard J. Stern*, New York, 1969, pp. 401–11: e.g. death rates for cardiovascular disease are consistently higher for blacks (both female and male) than for whites in the United States, and a study of juvenile rheumatism in Britain implicates 'the whole life of the underprivileged child' in its high incidence within slum areas.
11. From J. Ralph Audy, 'Measurement and Diagnosis of Health', in P. Shepard and D. McKinley, *ENVIRON/MENTAL: Essays on the Planet as a Home*, Boston, 1971, pp. 153, 160.
12. 'Mental Symptoms and Public Order', p. 146.
13. I am not arguing here for the primacy of a neurological, 'brain damage' model of mental illness over the various psychiatric (or psychoanalytic) models. But the existence of 'organic' psychiatric cases with a known brain lesion is sufficient to dispose of Goffman's argument that mental patients are no more than the rejects of small-scale society, labelled in pseudo-medical terms because of their infractions of due decorum.
14. *Stigma*, pp. 145–55.
15. *op. cit.* p. 145.
16. *Asylums*, p. 320.
17. *Encounters*, New York, 1961.
18. D. Matza, *Becoming Deviant*, Englewood Cliffs, 1969, chapters 2 and 3.

19. *op. cit.* pp. 49–66, 70–85.
20. Frank Cioffi has even argued that Goffman's *oeuvre* is only accidentally factual in content, since it functions, much as does the sober moralising of a storyteller like Shakespeare, to arrange our emotions rather than the facts of social life. This persuasive case is made out in Cioffi's 'Information, Contemplation and Social Life', Royal Institute of Philosophy *Lectures,* 4, 1969–70, pp. 105–31.
21. Walter R. Gove, 'Societal Reaction as an Explanation of Mental Illness,' *American Sociological Review*, vol. 35, 1970, pp. 873–84. Goves cites the study of Harold Sampson, Sheldon Messinger and Robert Towne, *Schizophrenic Women: Studies in Marital Crisis*, New York, 1964.
22. Kathleen Jones, in 'The Twenty-Four Steps: An Analysis of Institutional Admission Procedures', *Sociology*, vol. 6, 1972, pp. 405–15.
23. *Asylums*, p. 124.
24. *ibid.* p. 384.
25. Roger Barker, *One Boy's Day*, Hamden, Connecticut, 1966; *The Stream of Behavior*, New York, 1963.
26. For a summary of the literature on methodological individualism, see Steven Lukes, *Individualism*, Oxford, 1973, pp. 110–22.
27. In *Interaction Ritual*, pp. 149–270.
28. Frame Analysis: *An Essay on the Organization of Experience*, New York, pp. 13, 14.

3. R.D. Laing: The Radical Trip pages 59–87

1. M. Siegler, H. Osmond, H. Mann, 'Laing's Models of Madness', *British Journal of Psychiatry*. vol. 115, 1969, pp. 947–58; reprinted in R. Boyers and R. Orrill, (eds.), *R.D. Laing and Anti-Psychiatry*, New York, 1971. It may be noted that two of these authors have no medical qualification themselves.
2. Roger Brown, Chapter 13 in R. Brown and R.J. Herrnstein, *Psychology*, London, 1975, pp. 686–89.
3. See D. Cooper, *The Death of the Family*, London, 1971; *The Grammar of Living*, London 1974; *The Language of Madness*, London, 1978.
The year of maximum collaboration between Laing, Esterson and Cooper was 1965, when they were co-authors of a report on the 'Villa 21' project run at the Shenley Hospital, Hertfordshire (A. Esterson, D.G. Cooper, R.D. Laing, 'Results of Family-Orientated Therapy with Hospitalised Schizophrenics', *British Medical Journal* 2, 1965, pp. 1462–65. In the following year Esterson left both the Philadelphia Association and the Kingsley Hall community founded by himself, Laing and Cooper. He did not join in the establishment of the Institute for Phenomenological Studies, with Cooper, Laing, Joseph Berke and Leon Redler, which sponsored the 'Dialectics of Liberation' conference at the Round House, London, in 1967. Berke and another psychiatrist who had worked at Kingsley Hall, Morton Schatzman,

in their turn broke away from Laing, leaving the Philadelphia Association to found in 1971 another residential crisis centre for mental patients in North London, the Arbours Association. Hints as to the nature of what are still, to the public, rather mysterious splits between Laingians are conveyed in Laing's interview 'An end to fashionable madness', *The Times*, 4 October 1972 (with some oblique repudiations both of the Arbours project and of Cooper's position) and in the interview-review by Ann Grant, 'Come Fly With Me…', *Guardian* 11 November 1977 (on Joseph Berke's work). It remains as both a tribute to Laing and an irritation for researchers that neither Cooper nor Esterson nor any of the Arbours group have publicly stated in any detail why they have been unable to continue as his collaborators; indeed, several of them have gone publicly on record in his defence long after their breach with him.

4. R.D. Laing and A. Esterson, *Sanity, Madness and the Family*, London, 1964.
5. A. Esterson, *The Leaves of Spring: Schizophrenia, Family and Sacrifice*, London, 1971; 'Families, Breakdown and Psychiatry: Towards a Science of Persons', *New Universities Quarterly*, no. 30, Summer 1976, pp. 285–312; see also his 'Whither Psychiatry?' *Scottish International*, vol. 6, no. 5, May-June-July 1973.
6. 'Schizophrenia in Santa Monica', interview with S.S. Mahan in the *Los Angeles Free Press*, 10 December 1972.
7. Except where otherwise stated, the details in this account have been compiled from the data in Martin Howarth-Williams' *R.D. Laing: His Work and Its Relevance for Sociology*, London, 1977; the autobiographical sections of Laing's *The Facts of Life*, New York, 1976; the interview with Peter Mezan ('After Freud and Jung, Now Comes R.D. Laing…') in *Esquire*, vol. 77, January 1972, pp. 92–97, 160–78; Laing's radio talk on 'Religious Sensibility', published in *The Listener*, 23 April 1970; the December 1972 interview in the *Los Angeles Free Press* (see note 6 above); the interview article by James S. Gordon, 'Who is Mad? Who is Sane? R.D. Laing: In Search of a New Psychiatry', *The Atlantic Monthly*, vol. 227, January 1971, pp. 50–66; and from the data provided on the dust-jackets and introductory pages of Laing's other books as well as from passages in the writings themselves.
8. Peter Mezan, 'R.D. Laing: Portrait of a Twentieth-Century Skeptic', in R.I. Evans (ed.) *R.D. Laing: The Man and His Ideas*, New York, 1976, pp. lix–lxii. Laing remarks at the end of this disquisition: 'I haven't met anyone with a mind quite like mine. It's somewhat original.', p. lxii.
9. M. Esslin, *Artaud*, London, 1976, p. 61. The information comes from Laing's own conversation with Esslin. Artaud is listed as a cultural hero in *The Politics of Experience* but not mentioned in Laing's earlier works.
10. Interview with Max Charlesworth in M. Charlesworth, *The Existentialists and Jean-Paul Sartre*, London, 1976, p. 49; Interview with *Los Angeles Free Press*, p. 11.
11. *The Facts of Life* pp. 110–15.

12. Laing's graphic story of this relationship is given in the Mezan interview published in early 1972, reference in note 7 above.

13. 'Patient and Nurse: Effects of Environmental Changes in the Care of Chronic Schizophrenics', J.L. Cameron, R.D. Laing and A. McGhie, *The Lancet*, vol. 2, 1955, pp. 1384–86. The development of the project after Laing left the hospital is described in T. Freeman, J.L. Cameron and A. McGhie, *Chronic Schizophrenia,* London, 1958, chapters 4, 10 and 11. The theory of schizophrenia as a breakdown of 'ego boundaries', outlined in this work, has some resemblance to the framework used by Laing in *The Divided Self.*

14. According to the Mezan interview; the Gordon interview and *The Facts of Life* (pp. 120–23) also go over this formative early work of Laing's.

15. The point was first made in a paper by G.W. Brown, G.M. Carstairs and G.G. Topping, 'The Post-Hospital Adjustment of Chronic Schizophrenic Patients', *The Lancet*, vol. 2, 1958, pp. 685–87; several papers from this team and its successors have shown that a high degree of emotional involvement with patients from parents or spouses was the largest single factor that could indicate a poor outcome for discharged schizophrenic patients, and that a subdued and isolated social environment in lodgings was a far more suitable reception-setting for discharge. See G.W. Brown, 'Experiences of Discharged Chronic Schizophrenic Mental Hospital Patients in Various Types of Living Group', *Millbank Memorial Fund Quarterly,* vol. 37, 1959, pp. 105–31; G.W. Brown, E.M. Monck, G.M. Carstairs, and J.K. Wing, 'The Influence of Family Life on the Course of Schizophrenic Illness,' *British Journal of Preventive and Social Medicine*, vol. 16, 1962, pp. 55–75; G.W. Brown, J.L.T. Birley and J.K. Wing, 'Influence of Family Life on the Course of Schizophrenic Disorder: A Replication', *British Journal of Psychiatry,* vol. 121, 1972, pp. 241–58; and, more recently, C.E. Vaughn and J.P. Leff, 'The Influence of Family and Social Factors on the Course of Psychiatric Illness: A Comparison of Schizophrenic and Depressed Neurotic Patients', *British Journal of Psychiatry*, vol. 129, 1976, pp. 125–37, a study which, using the somewhat crude index of the number of derogatory comments made by relatives against the patient, again establishes the unique explanatory value of hostile involvement within the family as a factor in breakdown. I cite this section of studies to indicate the existence of a sociological tradition in psychiatry, alternative to that of Laing and his collaborators, which in its own way was focusing on the ambivalent embrace of the close-knit family, and which has continued work in this vein when Laing had largely forsaken his interest in the patient's immediate household.

16. *New Left Review* May-June 1962, No. 15.

17. 'The Collusive Function of Pairing in Analytic Groups', *British Journal of Medical Psychology,* vol. 31, 1958, pp. 117–23.

18. A summary of the findings of this research tradition (which produced fewer and fewer studies from the late sixties through to the seventies) is provided by J.H. Liem, 'Family Studies of Schizophrenia: An Update and Commentary', *Schizophrenia Bulletin*, vol. 6, 1980, pp. 429–55.

Laing had visited the United States in 1962 to discuss his own family researches with Bateson and Wynne, and with other experts on social signalling in small groups like Ray Birdwhistell, Albert Scheflen and Erving Goffman.

19. Such at least is Laing's concept of 'process'; see *Sanity, Madness and the Family,* 1970 edition., p. 22. Sartre however uses process to designate a type of group action (as that of workers on an assembly-line) where the purpose of the group is exterior to its members: *Critique de la Raison Dialectique,* 1960, pp. 541–52. For a critique of Laing's use of 'process into praxis' as a paradigm of therapy, see Andrew Collier, *R.D. Laing: The Philosophy and Politics of Psychotherapy,* Hassocks, 1977, pp. 55–62, 76–82.
20. G. Bateson, D. Jackson, J. Haley and J. Weakland, 'Toward a Theory of Schizophrenia', *Behavioral Science,* vol. 1, 1956, pp. 251–64.
21. Lee has extended this method of analysis to the schizophrenic's family, while departing from the precise techniques used in the 1966 book. A. Russell Lee, 'Levels of Imperviousness in the Schizophrenic's Family', *Psychiatry,* vol. 38, 1975, pp. 124–31.
22. These quotes are from 'Series and Nexus in the Family', *New Left Review,* May-June 1962, no. 15.
23. It has been persuasively suggested that the moral norm of reciprocity is a universal component of human ethical codes, and a logical prerequisite of any attribution of either exploitation or stability within a social system: Alvin Gouldner, 'The Norm of Reciprocity', *American Sociological Review,* vol. 25, 1960, pp. 161–78.
24. According to Laing, this research has not been published partly because 'I didn't have the mathematics of groups – quite advanced mathematics' which would have resolved 'major methodological difficulties in making comparisons between group processes.' He cites only one example of the observations drawn from this sample of 'ordinary families in London', that of a 16-year-old apparently being intimidated and double-bound by her father and mother in connection with her romantic life. No 'schizophrenogenic' outcome is recorded by Laing in this case of distorted family communication. Mathematical difficulties can hardly be held to blame for this failure to report research which even at an obvious descriptive level makes significant comparisons with the material in *Sanity, Madness and the Family.* The report is on pp. 30–31 of Evans, *op. cit.,* reference 8 above.
25. In Bateson's introduction to *Perceval's Narrative: A Patient's Account of his Psychosis,* Stanford, 1961.
26. *The Politics of Experience and The Bird of Paradise* (hence *PE*), Harmondsworth, 1967, p. 129.
27. *PE,* p. 106.
28. For Laing's association with 'sigma', a London-based avant-garde precursor of the counter-cultural underground, see Jeff Nuttall, *Bomb Culture,* London, 1968. The project was launched by Alexander Trocchi's brochure, 'The Invisible Insurrection of a Million Minds', to which Laing contributed an enthusiastic note of sponsorship.

29. *PE*, p. 101.
30. An informed critic pointed out that Laing withdrew the preface in one reissue of *The Divided Self*, and speculates that this may signal 'some theoretical or ideological backtracking': Alan Tyson, 'Homage to Catatonia', *New York Review of Books*, 11 February 1971.
31. In D. Cooper, (ed.), *The Dialectics of Liberation*, (hence *DL*), Harmondsworth, 1968, pp. 21–25.
32. From a BBC Radio 3 programme, 'The Politics of the Imagination', broadcast in March 1972, on the theme of Laing's influence on contemporary literature.
33. For an account of this political tendency see my 'Varieties of Socialist Thought,' in B. Crick and W. A. Robson (eds.), *Protest and Discontent*, London, 1970, pp. 49–54, and 'The Two New Lefts', in D. Widgery, *The Left in Britain*, 1956–68, Harmondsworth, 1976, pp. 131–53. Laing's name appears on p. 45 of the 1967 New Left *May Day Manifesto*, published in London.
34. The British edition (Harmondsworth, 1967) speaks of the 'heartland of a senescent capitalism' in which the author and his readers live. The American version (New York, 1967) reads 'heartland of a senescent civilisation' (p.11 in both editions), but goes on, in a slightly longer text, to endorse the neo-marxist analysis of the world economic system 'undertaken by Paul Baran and Paul Sweezy in *Monopoly Capital*.
35. David Martin, 'R.D. Laing: Psychiatry and Apocalypse', in M. Cranston (ed.), *The New Left*, London, p. 179.
36. *Pensiamento Critico* no. 5, June 1967.
37. Nuttall, *op. cit.* p. 227.
38. From the BBC programme, 'The Politics of the Imagination' (see note 32 above).
39. *PE.*, pp 136, 117; *DL*, pp. 32–33.
40. 'Transcendental Experience in Relation to Religion and and Psychosis', *Psychedelic Review*, no. 6, 1965 (reprinted in modified text in *PE*, p. 108); *PE*, p. 114. A similar statement by Laing likening psychosis to a religious state of mind and invoking the interest of priests is his preface to Morag Coate, *Beyond All Reason*, Philadelphia, 1964: this, even though the author of this outstanding memoir of a schizophrenic career repudiates the religious content of her old psychotic fantasies.
41. *PE*, p. 114, and *Psychedelic Review*, *loc. cit.*
42. *PE*, pp. 113, 103, 50.
43. *PE*, pp. 104, 106, 137; 'What is Schizophrenia?', *New Left Review*, 28, November-December 1964, p. 68 (reprinted in modified text in *PE*, p. 107). Daniel Aaron has pointed out to me the resemblance between Laing's voyage backward into evolution and Walt Whitman's cosmic journey in *Song of Myself*, where he returns to 'plutonic rocks', gneiss and coal-forests.
44. *PE*, p. 119.
45. *PE*, pp. 113, 114, 116.

4. R.D. Laing: The Return to Psychiatry pages 89–108

1. Andrew Collier's book on Laing, published in 1977, states that his own marxist perspective on capitalist society 'appears to be shared by Laing and his collaborators' (*R.D. Laing: The Philosophy and Politics of Psychotherapy*, Hassocks, 1977, p. x) but ends his account with Laing's arrival at a position of 'Gnosticism or nihilistic mysticism' (pp. 184–94, 203). Thomas S. Szasz's attack on Laing in *The New Review* for August 1976 (vol. 3, no. 29) termed him 'a preacher of and for the "soft" underbelly of the New Left' and accused him with his co-thinkers of being 'all self-declared Socialists, Communists or at least anti-capitalists and collectivists'. Edgar Z. Friedenberg, on the other hand, (*Laing*, London, 1974, pp. 118–19) while acknowledging Laing's exit from leftism still sees his connection with mystic self-cultivation as his most lasting heritage: 'the thrust of Ronald Laing's work, as well as much of its substance, has been the very stuff of the counter-culture's vision. The old friend of Baba Ram Dass and Timothy Leary has never betrayed their joint ideal.'
2. *PE*, p. 101
3. R.I. Evans, *R.D. Laing: The Man and His Ideas,* New York, 1976, pp. 62–63.
4. 'Paradox of the Dissidents', *Guardian,* 21 July 1977. The 'research and development' urged upon the Presidency in the last sentence is presumably military, unless it represents a cryptic plea to the United States to engage in a psycho-technical effort paralleling that of Soviet psychiatry.
5. See the interview with Laing in Charlesworth, *loc. cit.* (see note 10 of chapter 3), pp. 49–50. At a discussion at G.M. Carstairs' house following a lecture at York University in May 1974, Laing remarked that he had never been a marxist. When I reminded him that he had signed the New Left *May Day Manifesto*, he said: 'Which one was that?'
6. *Los Angeles Free Press, loc. cit.* in note 6 of chapter 3.
7. In Evans, *op. cit.* p. 63.
8. *DL*, p. 28.
9. *PE*, p. 76.
10. *DL*, p. 32.
11. Martin Howarth-Williams, *R.D. Laing: His Work and Its Relevance for Sociology*, London, 1977, pp. 33, 120–21, 124, 159–64. The limitation is seen in Laing's application of Sartrean group-theory rather than in the theory itself.
12. *The Politics of the Family*, Toronto, 1969, p. 49. The later British edition (London, 1971) contained some substantial revision of this text, e.g. in changing a chapter title from 'The Family, Invalidation and the Clinical Conspiracy' to 'The Family and Invalidation', but still retains the passage cited (pp. 123, 124).
13. Vernon Reynolds, 'Don't Shoot the Family', broadcast on BBC Radio 3, 16 September 1971.

14. 'An end to fashionable madness', interview with Victoria Brittain in *The Times*, 4 October 1972: 'It suited people to be able to pin me out there in that ideological position.'
15. *PE*, p. 156.
16. Timothy Leary, *The Politics of Ecstasy*, London, 1970, p. 95.
17. From a recording of a talk given in August 1969 by Dass, transcribed in Mezan, *op. cit.* reference in note 7 of chapter 3.
18. *Howarth-Williams, op. cit.* pp. 74–76.
19. Gordon, *op. cit.* p. 59, reference in note 7 of chapter 3.
20. In the interview with *Los Angeles Free Press, loc. cit.*, reference in note 6 of chapter 3, where Laing goes on to observe, somewhat disingenuously, 'It was by no means meant to be and I didn't realise at the time that it would be taken as sort of a slogan for psychedelic turning-on.'
21. 'Religious Sensibility', *The Listener*, 23 April 1970. In a long discussion of this talk, Howarth-Williams points to its repeated refusal to take any explicit position on the truth or falsity of religious statements (*op. cit.* pp. 94–97).
22. Mezan, *op. cit.* p. 164 and *passim*.
23. Dr Ageha Bharati, Chairman of the Anthropology Department of Syracuse University, New York, in a letter to me in November 1971. Dr Bharati's informant on Laing's mystical expertise was the senior monk at the Kandubodda monastery.
24. 'Busman's Holiday', interview given to Oliver Gillie, *Sunday Times Magazine*, 17 September 1972.
25. 'Qui est fou?' *L'Express*, 23 July 1973 (cited from the translation in Howarth-Williams, *op. cit.* p. 103). Laing went on to admit here that life in Sri Lanka at the time was not so tranquil 'for those who live there. Whilst I was there, there was an uprising and 6,000 people were killed with 12,000 imprisoned in detention camps.' We can observe Laing's extraordinary state of dissociation from the left which enabled him to sit meditating in a monastery which was part of Sri Lanka's landowning Establishment while peasants, students and trade unionists were being slaughtered and rounded up by the government's forces of repression.
26. Mezan in Evans, *op. cit.* p. lxi.
27. *The Times*, interview, 4 October 1972.
28. *ibid.*
29. *PE*, p. 149.
30. Quoted in David Cohen, 'R.D. Laing: the Divided Prophet', in *New Society*, 5 May 1977. Laing told Cohen: 'I'm not anything like that politically. My position is one of extreme scepticism on all sides of the question.'
31. Laing seems to have begun systematically with his new theorisation of birth experience following his return from Sri Lanka and India. His talk of 10 October 1972, given before an audience at the Friends Meeting House, London, offered the hypothesis of 'umbilical shock' at the moment of cord-cutting, when 'a few seconds then can make a profound difference for the rest of one's

life, I think' (from a transcript of the speech very kindly provided to me by Dr Laing). The theme is repeated in the Mezan interview of November 1972 (Evans, *op. cit.* pp. xxxviii, xxii) and in *The Facts of Life* (pp. 59–62, 64–65).

32. I have outlined this radical-rationalist critique of Laing in 'Laing's Clangs', *New Society,* 15 January 1970; 'Doctor for an Age', BBC Radio 3 talk published in *The Listener,* 18 May 1972; and in 'Who is Mad – You or the System?', a review of the Laingian film *Family Life,* in *Socialist Worker,* 5 February 1972. Such was the vogue of Laing on the left in that period that, immediately after this last review article, the journal concerned received its hitherto-largest volume of protest letters, rallying to the defence of Laing.

33. See Peter Sedgwick, 'The Social Analysis of Schizophrenia', in H.M. van Praag, (ed.) *On the Origin of Schizophrenic Psychoses,* Amsterdam, 1975, pp. 183–208, which extracts a social paradigm from the work of Laing and Cooper and pits this against two alternative paradigms of schizophrenia with a more medical logic. It must be admitted, though, that this exercise, constructed for an audience of biologically orientated psychiatrists, attributes more consistency and sense to Laing and Cooper than their works actually possess.

34. I have attempted an account of positivism in psychiatry in chapter 1 above.

35. 'I see myself in the skeptical tradition of Western thought… That's a discipline in the spirit of Keat's negative capacity – what he calls the capacity for uncertainty, mystery, and doubt, rather than certainty, objectification, and having arrived at the answers.' Laing in Evans, *op. cit.* p. 90.

36. I am particularly indebted for this discussion to Russell Jacoby, *Social Amnesia: A Critique of Conformist Psychology from Adler to Laing,* Boston, 1975; and to Juliet Mitchell, *Psychoanalysis and Feminism,* London, 1974. I do not share the confidence of these two authors in Freudian instinct-theory, but their grounding in classical psychoanalysis gives their interpretation of Laing and other 'revisionist' writers in psychiatry a vigour and lucidity for which one can only be grateful.

37. Howarth-Williams (*op. cit.* pp. 17–31) concurs in grouping *Self and Others* and the work on the IPM as instances of a common moment in Laing's development, and makes an interesting comparison with some passages on the dialectic between Self and Other in Hegel.

38. From Sigal's novel, *Zone of the Interior,* New York, 1976, p. 162. The prefatory author's note makes it clear that this is 'fiction, a work of imagination' in which 'Any similarity to persons living or dead is accidental.' The novel's reconstruction of a Laingian network, outside and inside the British National Health Service, is stupendously (if, doubtless, accidentally) accurate and insightful.

39. *PE,* p. 33. The whole of this essay ('The Mystification of Experience') develops the pre-social vision of personhood. Collier's discussion is useful here (*op. cit.* pp. 31, 39–40).

40. Jacoby, *op. cit.* pp. 67, 68.

41. *PE,* pp. 61, 62, 57.

42. *PE,* p. 106.

43. *PE*, p. 63.
44. See Mitchell, *op. cit.* p. 291.
45. *Los Angeles Free Press. op. cit.* This observation is preceded by a highly perceptive set of comments by Laing on the abnormal stresses induced within the two-generation nuclear family from which grandparents, and all other extended kin, are absent.
46. Howarth-Williams, *op. cit.* p. 33; Collier, *op. cit.* pp. 81 *ff.*
47. *The Politics of The Family*, 1971 edition, p. 49. *DL*, p. 15.
48. Jacoby's observations, pp. 135–40, are particularly valuable here. For reference see note 36 above.
49. *DL*, p. 16.
50. Laing in Evans, *op. cit.* p. 52.
51. See note 2 above.
52. From Laing's introduction to *PE*, p. 2. The name of Marx is included among the theorists of 'alienation' along with Kierkegaard, Nietzsche, Freud, Heidegger, Tillich and Sartre.
53. David Cooper, 'The Anti-Hospital: An Experiment in Psychiatry', *New Society*, 11 March 1965. Cooper's book – *Psychiatry and Anti-Psychiatry* (London, 1967) provides a further rationale for the unit. I visited 'Villa 21' in 1964 and learned much from attending a community meeting there, as well as from conversations with the charge-nurse, Frank Atkins, whose paper 'Villa 21: An Approach to Schizophrenia' provides a first-hand summary of the ward's approach. The chapters in Sigal's *Zone of the Interior* dealing with 'Conolly House', an entirely fictitious therapeutic community for the Laingian treatment of schizophrenics within a British NHS hospital, provide a satisfying analogue of the Villa 21 experience.
54. Appendix B, 'Philadelphia Association, 1964–1974', pp. 157–59 in Evans, *op. cit.; Pulman's Weekly News*, Yeovil, 29 November 1977.
55. For the Arbours group's experience, see Joseph H. Berke, *Butterfly Man: Madness, Degradation and Redemption*, London, 1977. This group has run a small, primarily brief-stay crisis-centre without any use of medications, along with an associated network of households comprising some 40 people. Depressions and anxiety-states, rather than schizophrenias, appear to be its main subject matters.
56. Quoted in Gordon, *op. cit.* p. 57.
57. Cooper, 1965, 1967, references in note 53 above. The book *Psychiatry and Anti-Psychiatry* includes as an appendix the paper 'Results of Family-orientated Therapy with Hospitalised Schizophrenics' which Esterson, Cooper and Laing wrote as a report on the project for the *British Medical Journal* in December 1965.
58. This old-fashioned piece of straitjacketing is recorded in G. Jervis, *Le mythe de l'antipsychiatrie*, Paris, 1977, pp. 31–32. For Jervis, the Laingian communities were not 'anti-psychiatric' but simply 'continue, in an unprejudiced and creative fashion, the principles and methods of therapeutic

communities.' As to method, neither Laing nor Cooper has ever provided an account of any type of family therapy that would correspond to a reversal of the distorted communication patterns characteristic of their families. Esterson appears to have pursued this line of treatment more deliberately; the reports cited in note 5, chapter 3, are illuminating on his methods, and he gave a moving and telling lecture on the 'clarification and undoing' process with a double-binding parent and her schizophrenic daughter (illustrated with tape-recordings from the case) at a conference I attended in Edinburgh in 1974. His work is, of course, explicitly structured within a psychoanalytic repertoire of roles and skills.

59. From a patient quoted in Morton Schatzman's account of Kingsley Hall, 'Madness and Morals', in R. Boyers and R. Orrill (eds), *Laing and Anti-Psychiatry*, Harmondsworth, 1972, pp. 181–208.

60. Mary Barnes, in particular, insisted on a medical definition of her situation at Kingsley Hall; see Mary Barnes and Joseph Berke, *Mary Barnes: Two Accounts of a Journey through Madness*, London, 1971, pp. 233–35, 254–57. In one spectacular episode, she refused to accept food from two therapists who were medically unqualified until Esterson openly exercised a doctor's authority by ordering her to eat.

61. Michael Barnett, *People Not Psychiatry*, London, 1973, pp. 179, 180. The witness's recollection of this commune and this therapist is very favourable, however.

62. Leon Redler, writing on behalf of the Philadelphia Association to *The New Review*, vol. 3, no. 32, 1976.

63. For an evaluation of a trial withholding all drugs from schizophrenic patients, see W.T. Carpenter, T.H. McGlashan and J.S. Strauss, 'The Treatment of Acute Schizophrenia without Drugs: an Investigation of Some Current Assumptions,' *America Journal of Psychiatry*, 1977, vol. 134, pp. 14–20. The authors here attempt to distinguish between those patients who can benefit from a withdrawal of medication and its replacement by structured group-therapy meetings and those for whom the anguish consequent on withdrawal is too much since 'their psychosis was destructive and their attempt to understand it of no value.' A preliminary report, distinctly favourable, has also been published on Soteria House, an intensive residence for up to six schizophrenic patients staying between two and four months, usually without phenothiazine drugs: L.R. Mosher, A. Menn, S.M. Matthews, 'Soteria: Evaluation of a Home-Based Treatment for Schizophrenia', *American Journal of Orthopsychiatry*, vol. 45, 1975, pp. 455–67.

64. For a historical resumé of occupational treatments in psychiatry see my *St Wulstan's and the Battle for Rehabilitation*, National Schizophrenia Fellowship, 1977.

65. Laing's expression in 'Metanoia: Some Experiences at Kingsley Hall, London', in Hendrik M. Ruitenbeek (ed.), *Going Crazy*, New York, 1972, p. 15.

66. Barnes and Berke, *op. cit.* p. 66. Mary Barnes almost always describes her personal project as one of 'going down' (and 'up' into recovery) rather than as a 'going back' or 'return' in the Laingian sense of regression to an original oneness.

67. Evans, *op. cit.* p. liv. Berke (1977, pp. 92–95, 106–08, 121–22) has recorded two or three further cases of self-limiting psychosis, none of them very similar to Mary Barnes's voyage.

68. David Reed, *Anna*, London, 1976, p. 84.

69. A Esterson, D.G. Cooper and R.D. Laing, 'Results of Family-Orientated Therapy with Hospitalised Schizophrenics', *British Medical Journal*, 18 December 1965, pp. 462–65.

70. G.M. Carstairs, letter, *British Medical Journal*, 1 January 1966, p. 49. The Edinburgh study cited (which used social and psychological measures of the patients' welfare as well as the re-admission index) was: C.A Renton, J.W. Affleck, G.M. Carstairs and A.D. Forrest, 'A Follow-up of Schizophrenic Patients in Edinburgh', *Acta Psychiatrica Scandinavica*, vol. 39, 1963, pp. 548–600.

71. A further follow-up performed over a decade later with the same Edinburgh sample revealed that while the re-admission rate was still comparable with the earlier study (19 per cent in 1972; 18 per cent, including two suicides, in 1961–62), the death rate had gone up to 26.2 per cent; of the males who could be traced, nearly a third (28 out of 86) had died: J.W. Affleck, J. Burns and A.D. Forrest, 'Long-term Follow-up of Schizophrenic Patients in Edinburgh', *Acta Psychiatrica Scandinavica*, vol. 53, 1976, pp. 227–37. It might be noted that death from unnatural causes (suicide, neglect etc.) never figures as a risk or an actuality in the reports on schizophrenic careers offered in the various Laingian testimonies.

72. From Appendix B to Evans, *op. cit.* pp. 158–59.

73. *ibid.* p. 157.

74. Dr Leon Redler, one of the Association's directors, has emphatically refuted the charge levelled by Thomas Szasz to the effect that the PA was an expense on public revenue: 'over half the residents pay out of private funds' for their stay in the households as well as for any extra therapeutic or educational facilities that they use there (letter to *The New Review*, reference in note 62 above). 'Half the residents' by no means necessarily implies the same proportion of patients, given the mixed character of the households. The Association's attachment to a contractual model of servicing for its residents is likely, however, to bias its intake of patients both upward socially and away from schizophrenia as the prime source of referral. Few schizophrenics have any cash at their disposal.

75. While Laing himself has added nothing to his theories of the latter sixties – except to allow the reprinting of his books containing this theme without amendment or retraction – David Cooper has re-asserted the case: 'Madness is the destructuring of the alienated structures of an existence and the restructuring of a less alienated way of being. The less alienated way of being is a more responsible way of being… In the destructuring moment of madness there is a paradoxical union of ecstatic joy and total

despair… the restructuring is never towards normality but always towards sanity.' D. Cooper, *The Language of Madness*, London, 1978, pp. 40, 41, 52.

76. Manfred Bleuler, the most eminent psychiatrist of schizophrenia of recent times, has stated that the number of benign schizophrenic episodes with complete and lifelong recovery after the first attack has not, to a statistically significant extent, been raised by modern treatment. See J.K. Wing, *Reasoning about Madness*, Oxford, 1978, p. 123.

77. A parallel distinction between the socially innocent acute phase of schizophrenia and the historically contingent course of the chronic form has been tentatively put by workers from the World Health Organisation's international comparative study of schizophrenic symptomatology: A. Jablensky and N. Sartorius, 'Culture and Schizophrenia', in H.M. van Praag (ed.), *On the Origin of the Schizophrenic Psychoses*, Amsterdam, 1975, pp. 99–124; and J. Cooper and N. Sartorius, 'Cultural and Temporal Variations in Schizophrenia: A Speculation on the Importance of Industrialization,' *British Journal of Psychiatry*, vol. 130, 1977, pp. 50–55. Their case is historically and anthropologically better anchored than Laing's, but oddly similar to his, in that the acute syndrome is seen as passing through a natural termination, without consequences for the sufferer's later life, given a suitably supporting social environment. The local rural community with its extended kinship structures and the integrating amenities of magic or religion here play the role suggested by Laing for Kingsley Hall. The case is more complex than this, and is worth examining.

78. As I write this paragraph, the morning's newspaper reveals that Mary Barnes, whose case has been widely advertised by Laingian enthusiasts as a vindication of Kingsley Hall methods, has undergone several more periods of traumatic 'going down'. These are presented in the report as more akin to an intermittent acute depression than to a psychotic breakdown; but in essence seem to me to be quite similar to the problems of managing a recurrent illness faced by most of those with a chronic and severe psychiatric difficulty. See 'Inside Story' (interview of Mary Barnes with Angela Neustatter), *Guardian*, 5 January 1979; and (for some accounts of coping with relapse and daily living by schizophrenic patients) J.K. Wing (ed.), *Schizophrenia from Within*, London, National Schizophrenia Fellowship, 1975.

79. J.K. Wing, *Schizophrenia and Its Management in the Community*, London, National Schizophrenia Fellowship, 1978, pp. 23–24. I am indebted to this paper, as well as to Chapter 4 ('Schizophrenia'), in the same author's *Reasoning about Madness*, for valuable orientation in drafting this section.

80. *PE*, p. 103; and cf. 'perfectly natural and necessary process' (p. 106); 'a natural sequence of experiential stepping stones' (p. 107); 'a natural way of healing' (p. 136). The parallel between the Laing of the sixties and the propagandist for the LeBoyer method of child-birth should now be obvious.

81. *Reasoning about Madness*, p. 136.

5. Michel Foucault: The Anti-History of Psychiatry pages 110–128

1. A fascinating resumé of psychiatric classification schemes, from ancient times through to recent centuries, can be found in the Appendix: Attest and Exhibits, to K. Menninger, M. Mayman and P. Pruyser, *The Vital Balance*, New York, 1967, pp. 419–89.
2. Richard Hunter and Ida MacAlpine, *Three Hundred Years of Psychiatry, 1535–1860*, London, 1963, p. 603.
3. Valerie Sinason, 'Return to Ancient Wisdom: The History of Psychiatry, Part XIII', *New Psychiatry*, 5 June 1975.
4. Richard Hunter, 'Psychiatry and Neurology – Psychosyndrome or Brain Disease', *Proceedings of the Royal Society of Medicine*, vol. 66, 1973, pp. 359–64. The same perspective is maintained, from the nineteenth-century material, in R. Hunter and I. MacAlpine, *Psychiatry for the Poor*, London, 1974, pp. 217–20.
5. R. Neugebauer, 'Treatment of the Mentally Ill in Medieval and Early Modern England: A Reappraisal', *Journal of the History of the Behavioral Sciences*, 1978, vol. 14, pp. 158–69; 'Medieval and Early Modern Theories of Mental Illness', *Archives of General Psychiatry*, vol. 36, pp. 477–83.
6. G. Rosen, *Madness in Society: Chapters in the Historical Sociology of Mental Illness*, New York, 1969, pp. 14–16, 239–41.
7. Quoted in Hunter and MacAlpine, 1963, p, 49, reference in note 2 above.
8. Editorial lead to Valerie Sinason, 'Medieval Magic and the Witch Hunt: The History of Psychiatry, Part V', *New Psychiatry*, 30 January 1975.
9. E.g. Denis Leigh, *The Historical Development of British Psychiatry, Vol I, 18th and 19th Centuries*, Oxford, 1961, p. xiii; E. Fuller Torrey, *The Death of Psychiatry*, New York, 1975, p. 8; Menninger, Mayman and Pruyser, *op. cit.* pp. 16–17, 52.
10. *The Manufacture of Madness*, New York, 1970, p. 278.
11. *ibid.* p. 288.
12. *ibid.* p. 285.
13. *Ideology and Insanity*, London, 1973, pp. 198–216,
14. R.D. Laing, *The Politics of the Family*, London, 1971, pp. 91, 101.
15. *op. cit.* pp. 123–24.
16. *Histoire de la Folie*, Paris, 1961; shortened English translation, *Madness and Civilization*, London, 1965, from which quotations are taken here unless otherwise indicated. The full text has many important passages but these are not crucial to Foucault's argument.
17. *Naissance de la Clinique*, Paris, 1963; English translation, *The Birth of the Clinic*, London, 1973. The case is summarised in chapter 7, 'The Invention and Elimination of Disease', in Ivan Illich, *Medical Nemesis*, London, 1975.
18. *L'Archéologie du Savoir*, Paris, 1969; English translation, *The Archaeology of Knowledge*, London, 1972.

19. *Surveiller et Punir,* Paris, 1975. English translation, *Discipline and Punish,* London 1978. See also 'Michel Foucault on Attica: An Interview', *Telos,* no. 19, Spring 1974.

20. A. Megill, 'Foucault, Structuralism and the Ends of History', *Journal of Modern History,* vol. 51, 1979, pp. 451–503.

21. C. Gordon, 'Other Inquisitions', *Ideology and Consciousness,* no. 6, 1979, pp. 23–46.

22. A brilliant analysis of Foucault's empirical deficiencies, using the full French edition and citing important Dutch and German sources, has now appeared. H.C. Erik Midelfort, 'Madness and Civilization in Early Modern Europe: A Reappraisal of Michel Foucault', pp. 247–65 in B.C. Malament, (ed.), *After the Reformation: Essays in Honor of J.H. Hexter,* Pennsylvania, 1980.

23. E.g. in E. Fuller Torrey, *loc. cit.*; and in Phil Brown, *Towards a Marxist Psychology*, New York, 1974, p. 39.

24. David J. Rothman, *The Discovery of the Asylum: Social Order and Disorder in the New Republic*, Boston, 1971, is a major work in social history outlining the early development of mental and other institutions in the United States; the details of the earlier uses of mental institutions in Europe are taken from Pliny Earle's study of 1853, cited in Rothman, pp. 135–36.

25. Brown, *op. cit.* p. 40.

26. Judith Haig, 'Capitalism and Insanity, Part One: Moral treatment', *Workers Press*, 20 July 1974.

27. For sixteenth-century Germany especially, see the examples of mental institutionalisation in H.C. Erik Midelfort, 'Madness and the Problems of Psychological History in the Sixteenth Century', *Sixteenth Century Journal*, vol. 12, 1981, pp. 5–12. The medieval evidence for treatment of the mentally ill is summarised for England by P. Allderidge, 'Hospitals, Madhouses and Asylums: Cycles in the Case of the Insane', *British Journal of Psychiatry*, vol. 134, 1979, pp. 321–34.

28. A.S. Chamberlain, 'Early Mental Hospitals in Spain', *American Journal of Psychiatry*, vol. 123, 1966, pp. 143–49; R.D. Rumbaut, 'The Hospital at Zaragoza', *Bulletin of the Menninger Clinic*, vol. 39, 1975, pp. 268–73.

29. P. Anderson, *Lineages of the Absolutist State*, London, 1974, p. 64.

30. Further details of psychiatric facilities in pre-Renaissance Europe are given in the works cited by Rosen and Midelfort.

31. P. Doob, *Nebuchadnezzar's Children: Conventions of Madness in Middle English Literature*, New Haven, 1974; J. Neaman, *Suggestion of the Devil: The Origins of Madness*, New York, 1975.

32. W.H. Parry-Jones, *The Trade in Lunacy: A Study of Private Madhouses in the Eighteenth and Nineteenth Centuries*, London, 1972, p. 8.

33. Cited in Hunter and MacAlpine, *op. cit.* pp. 28, 35.

34. Stanley W. Jackson, 'Unusual Mental States in Medieval Europe. 1. Medical Syndromes of Mental Disorder. 400–1100 A. D.', *Journal of the History of Medicine*, vol. 27, 1972, pp. 262–97.

35. Menninger, Mayman and Pruyser, *op. cit.* p. 306.
36. V. Skultans, *Madness and Morals: Ideas on Insanity in the Nineteenth Century*, London, 1975, pp. 12–21, 98–100, 102–04, 107–13.
37. Cited in Hunter and MacAlpine, *op. cit.* p. 3. The treatment is portrayed also in a fifteenth-century picture of 'a frenzied person' in a religious psychiatric colony at Geel, Belgium: See Grace Golden, 'A Painting in Geel', *Journal of the History of Medicine*, vol. 26, 1971, pp. 400–12.
38. Rosen, *op. cit.* p. 132; Hunter and MacAlpine, *op. cit.* pp. 187, 254–55.
39. Aubrey Lewis, 'Melancholia: A Historical Review', in his *The State of Psychiatry*, London, 1967, p. 77.
40. See Stanley W. Jackson, *loc.cit.* for an account of this sophisticated and influential writer.
41. G. Rosen, 'The Philosophy of Ideology and the Emergence of Modern Medicine in France', *Bulletin of the History of Medicine*, vol. 20, 1946, pp. 328–39.
42. M. Hay, *Understanding Madness: Some Approaches to Mental Illness circa 1650–1800*, unpublished D Phil, University of York, 1979.
43. Rothman, *op. cit.* p. xviii.
44. Rosen's discussion (*Madness and Society*, pp. 158–64) parallels that of Foucault here, there with more coherence.
45. Hunter and MacAlpine, *op. cit.* pp. 402–10, 463–64, 538–42.
46. I. Wallerstein, *The Modern World System*, New York, 1974.
47. Tuke's observations on the utility of work are cited in Foucault, *op. cit.* pp. 247–48. In this regard, as in others, the example of the York Retreat as 'the ideal towards which institutions of every type must strive' was signalled in the questionnaire sent to asylum authorities by the Parliamentary Select Committee of 1827, which included five queries 'on occupation' ranging from manual labour to scientific and literary studies, drawing and gardening (Kathleen Jones, *Law, Lunacy and Conscience, 1744–1845*, London, 1955, pp. 139–40). Pinel's insistence on useful 'mechanical employment', in crafts and 'the soothing and delightful pursuits of agriculture and horticulture', (*A Treatise on Insanity*, English translation, 1806; reprinted New York, 1962, pp. 216–18), forms an important section of his theory. Dr Michael Fears has drawn my attention to the installation of weaving looms at the Yorkshire West Riding County Asylum, the first mental hospital in Britain to incorporate industrial therapy in its regimen, and the comment of its superintendent: 'If the patients are in good health, and in a proper state to work, they are allowed no beer, and every little indulgence is withheld, so long as they are idle. They soon find out that employment tends to their comfort' (W.C. Ellis, *A Treatise on Insanity*, London, 1838, p. 311).
48. See the extracts from Conolly's *An Inquiry concerning the Indications of Insanity*, London, 1830, in Hunter and MacAlpine, *op. cit.* pp. 805–09, and from his *The Treatment of the Insane without Mechanical Restraints*, London, 1856, in Skultans, *op. cit.* pp. 146–53, and Hunter and MacAlpine, pp. 1030–38.

49. Richard Hunter and Ida MacAlpine, *Psychiatry for the Poor: 1851 Colney Hatch Friern Barnet 1973*, London, 1974, p. 56.
50. Rothman, *op. cit.* pp. 265–87; Norman Dain, *Concepts of Insanity in the United States, 1789–1865*, Brunswick, N.J., 1964, pp. 79, 100–01; Gerald N. Grob, *Mental Institutions in America: Social Policy to 1873*, New York, 1973, pp. 178–256: 'prior to 1850 the gap between theory and practice of moral treatment was relatively narrow' (Grob, p. 176).
51. Dain, *op. cit.* pp. 104–08, 110–11; Albert Deutsch, 'The First US Census of the Insane (1840) and Its Use in Pro-Slavery Propaganda', *Bulletin of the History of Medicine*, vol. 15, 1944, pp. 469–82; Skultans, *op. cit.* pp. 23–25, 251–58.
52. *The Archaeology of Knowledge*, pp. 16, 47.
53. Illich, *op. cit.* pp. 116–21, 165–69.
54. *The Birth of the Clinic*, p. xix.
55. R. Carew, *The Survey of Cornwall, 1602*; in F.E. Halliday (ed.), *Richard Carew of Antony*, London, 1953, pp. 193–94. The practice is tentatively ascribed by Carew to a certain 'master of Bedlam' who cured his patients by keeping them bound in pools. Other forms of purification through water are discussed in Basil Clarke, *Mental Disorder in Earlier Britain*, Cardiff, 1975, pp. 127–133.
56. *op. cit.* pp. 240–42, 264–65. The original text speaks of 'les inconvenients sans nombre attachés à cette pratique' (*Traité Médico-philosophique sur l'Aliénation Mentale*, Paris, 1809, p. 324). Pinel's whole tendency is towards scepticism over any exterior medicaments distinct from the general asylum regimen.
57. *Traité*, pp. 205, 251. These repressive passages are censored from the contemporary English translation.
58. *A Treatise on Insanity*, p. 216.
59. *loc. cit.* pp. 217–18.
60. In an earlier passage (p. 198) he has said that Freud 'restored, in medical thought, the possibility of a dialogue with unreason'; but the later text incriminates Freud in giving 'a quasi-divine status' to the medical personage (even though Freud believed in non-medical analysts) and in transforming the powers of the asylum 'into an absolute observation, a pure and circumspect Silence, a Judge who punishes and rewards in a judgement that does not even condescend to language' (*loc. cit.*).
61. From J. Wing (ed.), *Schizophrenia from Within*, National Schizophrenia Fellowship, Surbiton, 1975, p. 56.
62. Segregation of residents according to social class as well as by sex and by practicability was an explicit feature of nineteenth-century asylum practice in both the public and private domains. See, for the USA, Grob, *op. cit.* pp. 221–56; the eminent psychiatric author Isaac Ray believed that the 'poor and laboring' classes needed only country walks and favourable employment, while those from 'educated and affluent backgrounds' could only 'be satisfied with long and repeated interviews with the superintendent'. In Britain, a similar situation held sway; even R. Gardiner Hill's small Lincoln Asylum, a

triumph for total non-restraint and the use of industrial occupation without compulsion, separated its patients 'according to payments made', into three Degrees of Rank, with varying amenities (Skultans, *op. cit.* p. 143).

63. Rothman, *op. cit.* pp. 265–87.

6. Psychiatry and Politics in Thomas Szasz pages 131–159

1. See e.g. Eric Berne, *Games People Play*, London, 1970, and the 'agonistic model' described in R. Harré and P. Secord, *The Explanation of Social Behaviour*, London, 1972, pp. 193–99.
2. *The Myth of Mental Illness*, New York, 1961, p. 305.
3. *ibid.* pp. 282–83.
4. See *ibid.* pp. 91–96 for a good discussion of organic theories of mental illness in the United States and Europe.
5. *ibid.* pp. 89–91, 267–71.
6. *ibid.* p. 194.
7. *ibid.* pp. 293, 310. See also his 'Freud as a Leader' *Antioch Review*, vol. 23, 1963, pp. 133–44, for a withering parallelism between institutional psychoanalysis and the business corporation.
8. *op. cit.* p. 108.
9. In the 1972 edition of *The Myth of Mental Illness*, Szasz withdraws the qualified judgement he made in the original text, on the role of psychiatrists in state mental hospitals, and replaces it by a caustic condemnation. Cf. p. 293 of the original and p. 266 of the revised edition.
10. *The Manufacture of Madness*, New York, 1970, pp. xxiii–xxv, 100–01 and *passim*. *Ideology and Insanity*, New York, 1970, pp. 243 *et seq.*
11. *The Manufacture of Madness*, pp. 23–24; and see pages above.
12. *The Myth of Mental Illness*, pp. 70–71.
13. *The Manufacture of Madness*, pp. 229.
14. *The Myth of Mental Illness*, p. 131; *Law, Liberty and Psychiatry*, New York, 1963, p. 27.
15. *The Manufacture of Madness*, pp. xxiii, 215.
16. The thoughts in the present section are largely indebted to discussion with Martin Gittelman, whose paper 'Sectorization: The Quiet Revolution in European Mental Health Care', presented at the 1971 Annual Meeting of the American Orthopsychiatric Association, makes a number of trenchant observations on the organisation and financing of community psychiatric services.
17. Szasz has contributed an excellent theoretical critique of the concept of schizophrenia (in 'The Problem of Psychiatric Nosology', *American Journal of Psychiatry*, vol. 114, 1957, pp. 405–13), but on logical grounds rather than from any material drawn from his own observation of patients; see also his comments on schizophrenia in *Law, Liberty and Psychiatry*, pp. 34–35.
18. 'The Concept of Transference', *International Journal of Psychoanalysis*, vol. 44, 1963, pp. 432–43.

19. Interview in Maggie Scarf, 'Normality is a Square Circle or a Four-sided Triangle', *New York Times Magazine*, 3 October 1971.

20. From a reminiscence of Larry Sloman, volunteered to me in the summer of 1971.

21. Phil Brown (ed.), *Radical Psychology*, New York, 1973, pp. xxi, 4.

22. The acquisitive evolutionary individualism of Herbert Spencer, for whom 'An argument fatal to the communist theory is suggested by the fact that a desire for property' – synonymous with 'the instinct of accumulation' – 'is one of the elements of our nature' (*Social Statics*, New York, 1954 reprint, pp. 119–20), had an extraordinary influence in intellectual and public circles in the United States. Richard Hofstadter's chapter on 'The Vogue of Spencer', in *Social Darwinism in American Thought* (1955 edition, pp. 31–50), provides a good discussion of Spencer's following among sociologists, philosophers, publicists and business leaders (Andrew Carnegie being the most devout of the last). The shortage of explicit references to Spencer among modern American conservatives testifies to the permanency of his ideas rather than to their disappearance: as Hofstadter puts it: 'If Spencer's abiding impact on American thought seems so impalpable to later generations, it is perhaps because it has been so thoroughly absorbed' (*op. cit.* p. 50).

23. Cited in J.D.Y. Peel, *Herbert Spencer: The Evolution of a Sociologist*, London, 1971, p. 58.

24. *The Man versus the State*, London, 1940 edition, pp. 10–17.

25. Peel, *op. cit.* pp. 17, 232–33.

26. Hofstadter, *op. cit.* pp. 54, 51.

27. *ibid.* pp. 195, 64.

28. *op.cit.* pp. 189–92.

29. *The Myth of Mental Illness*, pp. 308–10.

30. 'In the Church of America, Psychiatrists are Priests', *Hospital Physician*, October 1971.

31. *The Man versus the State*, p. 23.

32. *The Myth of Mental Illness*, p. 303.

33. *Social Statics*, p. 294.

34. Szasz, *op. cit.* pp. 13–14, 184–87, 303.

35. *Social Statics*, pp. 288–89. Spencer deleted 'the low-spirited' from later editions, perhaps following his own experience of psychological depressions; by an interesting coincidence, no ideologue of Social Darwinism has ever placed herself or himself in one of the doomed, inferior categories of humankind.

36. Spencer, *op. cit.* p. 201.

37. 'The Ethics of Suicide', in *The Theology of Medicine*, Oxford, 1977, pp. 68–85; 'The Ethics of Addition', in *ibid.* pp. 29–48.

38. 'The Ethics of Addiction', *loc. cit.* p. 38.

39. Hofstadter, *op. cit.* p. 41.

40. *The Myth of Mental Illness*, p. 192.

41. 'The Ethics of Addiction', p. 43.

42. *Facts and Comments*, London, 1907, p. 140.
43. *Social Statics*, p. 390.
44. *The Myth of Mental Illness*, p. 54.
45. *The Manufacture of Madness*, p. 220.
46. *Detroit Free Press*, 20 May 1970, excerpted in *The Abolitionist*, vol. I, no. 1, summer 1971, the organ of the American Association for the Abolition of Involuntary Mental Hospitalization established by Szasz himself.
47. *Facts and Comments*, pp. 65–66.
48. *Facts and Comments*, p. 152; Sir Edwin Chadwick, the pioneer of many investigations and reforms in urban life, is named as 'the leader of the movement'.
49. *Essays, Scientific, Political and Speculative*, New York, vol. 3, 1896, pp. 241, 248.
50. *Facts and Comments*, pp. 152–57.
51. *Social Statics*, p. 344 and *passim* in the chapter on 'Sanitary Supervision'.
52. *Social Statics*, p. 336.
53. *The Manufacture of Madness*, p. 281.
54. *Social Statics*, p. 352: 'It is highly probable that in the hands of a private company the resulting manure would not only pay the cost of collection but would yield a considerable profit.'
55. *The Manufacture of Madness*, pp. 210, 241.
56. *Social Statics*, p. 291.
57. *The Manufacture of Madness*, p. 220.
58. *The Man versus The State*, pp. 38, 41.
59. *'An "Unscrewtape" Letter: A Reply to Fred Sander'*, *American Journal of Psychiatry*, vol. 125, 1969, p. 1433.
60. 'Voluntary Mental Hospitalization: An Unacknowledged Practice of Medical Fraud', *New England Journal of Medicine*, vol. 287, 1972, pp. 277–78.
61. *Ideology and Insanity*, p. 243.
62. See e.g. *Psychiatry Justice*, New York, 1965; chapters 1, 4, 7, 8 and 12 of *Ideology and Insanity*; T.S. Szasz and G.J. Alexander, 'Law, Property and Psychiatry', *American Journal of Orthopsychiatry*, vol. 42, 1972, pp. 610–26.
63. 'Prison-Ethics', pp. 152–91 of *Essays, Scientific, Political and Speculative*. Spencer was concerned to argue (as Szasz is not) that the administration of penal justice on the absolute moral principles of equity would actually result in a greater practical reformation of the criminals than did the amoral expediencies (and cruelties) of the ongoing prison regime.
64. 'Justice in the Therapeutic State', *Indiana Legal Forum*, vol. 3, 1969, pp. 31, 27.
65. 'The Ethics of Addiction', p. 44.
66. From Green's essay, 'Liberal Legislation and the Freedom of Contract', cited in Steven Lukes, *Individualism*, Oxford, 1973, p. 130.
67. For a noteworthy (but partial) discussion of 'positive freedom', Isaiah Berlin's 'Two Concepts of Liberty', reprinted in *Four Essays on Liberty*, Oxford, 1969, pp. 118–72.

68. Lukes, *op. cit.* p. 66.
69. See the chapter on 'The Sociology of the Therapeutic Situation', pp. 52–72 of *The Myth of Mental Illness.*
70. Lukes, *op. cit.* p. 62 and *passim* in the chapter 'Privacy', pp. 59–66.
71. *The Myth of Mental Illness*, p. 55. He makes it clear that he is using 'capitalist' here as a synonym for 'individual-contractual': e.g. 'The Greek physician practised… in a capitalist society, selling his skills to the rich' (*loc. cit.*).
72. Friedrich Engels, *The Principles of Communism*, Appendix to Karl Marx and Friedrich Engels, *Manifesto of the Communist Party*, Moscow, 1971, pp. 74–75.
73. *Manifesto of the Communist Party, loc. cit.* pp. 34–35.
74. *Law, Liberty and Psychiatry*, p. 80.
75. See e.g. *The Manufacture of Madness*, pp. 49–50.
76. 'Justice in the Therapeutic State', *loc. cit.* p. 25.
77. See J.P. Bunker, 'Surgical Manpower: A Comparison of Operations and Surgeons in the United States and England and Wales', *New England Journal of Medicine*, vol. 282, 1970, pp. 135–44.
    I have looked at the therapeutic costs of the contract model both in surgery and psychotherapy in 'Medical Individualism', *Hastings Center Studies*, vol. 2, 1974, no. 3, pp. 69–80.

Part Two: Psychiatry and Liberation

7. Mental Health Movements and Issues: A Survey and Prospect pages 163–223

1. A.B. Hollingshead and F.C. Redlich, *Social Class and Mental Illness*, New York, 1958. This extraordinarily important work, documenting the various modes within psychiatry in which (as the authors note) 'the goddess of injustice may be blind, but she smells differences, and particularly class differences', has never to my knowledge been cited by any of the major 'radical' authors of psychiatry and anti-psychiatry.
2. The data which follow are reported from F. Redlich and S.R. Kellert, 'Trends in American Mental Health', *American Journal of Psychiatry,* vol. 135, 1978, pp. 22–28: this is, as the authors warn, a preliminary and provisional report at a stage when the study was still being completed.
3. As Redlich and Kellert point out, the nursing home, especially for the aged, mentally disturbed patient, had become the biggest source of expenditure in the mental-health field in the United States by 1975, accounting for 29 per cent of disbursements, funded by the general welfare and health system (Medicare) instead of through mental-health allocations. For a study of the policy of massive mental-patient discharges following budget cuts in New York State, see E.M. Markson and J.H. Cumming, 'The Post-Transfer Fate of 2,174 Relocated Mental Patients', *The Gerontologist*, vol. 2,

1975, pp. 104–08; for the effects of the run-down in California, where the state mental-hospital population was trimmed from over 35,000 in 1962 to less than 10,000 in 1972, see U. Aviram and S.P. Segal, The Exclusion of the Mentally Ill: Reflection on an Old Problem in a New Context', *Archives of General Psychiatry*, vol. 29, 1973, pp. 126–31; for the State of Hawaii, see S.A. Kirk and M.E. Thierrien, 'Community Mental Health Myths and the Fate of Former Hospitalised Patients', *Psychiatry*, vol. 38, 1975, pp. 209–17.

4. These last two citations are from follow-up reports on mental patients receiving community care in New York and California respectively, quoted in R.O. Rieder 'Hospitals Patients, and Politics', *Schizophrenia Bulletin*, no. 11, Winter 1974, pp. 9–15. Dr Rieder is responding to a partisan of the total dismantling of mental hospitals, Dr Werner Mendel, whose 'Leprs, Madmen – Who's Next?' forms pages 5–8 of the same issue.
5. J. Kovel, 'Therapy in Late Capitalism', *Telos*, no. 30, Winter 1976–77, pp. 73–92.
6. Their evaluation of the different propensities of the social classes to become mentally ill in the first place – and, in particular, their maxim that 'the lower social class, the greater proportion of patients in the population', is much more doubtful; see the review article by S.M. Miller and E.G. Mishler, 'Social Class, Mental Illness and American Psychiatry', *Millbank Memorial Fund Quarterly*, vol. 37, 1959, pp. 174–99. However, Miller and Mishler have no reservations in endorsing the book's revelations of class bias in treatment.
7. Between 1970 and 1975 the number of psychiatrists working full-time in the CMHCs declined from just under seven per cent to an average of 4.3, in a period when the total staff in the centres trebled. Qualified psychologists and social workers increased, but the biggest expansion was in uncertificated community residents performing therapeutic roles in the centres. The failure of federal funding to deliver resources was in large measure responsible for the move towards cheaper staffing. See P.J. Fink and S.P. Weinstein, 'The De-Professionalization of Community Mental Health Centers', *American Journal of Psychiatry*, vol. 136, 1979, pp. 406–09.
8. For the nineteenth century, Andrew Scull's *Museums of Madness* (London, 1979, pp. 50–51, 204–08) presents an admirable portrayal of such establishments as Ticehurst Asylum, a 300-acre site equipped with 'an aviary, bowling green, pagoda, summer house, music room, reading room, and so forth' for its 60 to 80 upper-class patients, who were attended by three medical superintendents, seven lady superintendents and companions, four gentleman companions (of the same class as the clientele), and a large number of menial attendants (over 150 in 1879, including coachmen for the 15 carriages and 26 horses). A pack of hounds was available for those patients who wished to hunt. Ticehurst House, re-titled as a nursing home rather than as an asylum, performs the same function to this day (doubtless with fewer horses) for mental patients admitted on a voluntary or compulsory basis for wealthy backgrounds.

9. Besides threatening to withdraw financial aid from two community-based detoxification centres for habitual drunken offenders – which were becoming accepted as a viable local alternative to court sentencing – the Department of Health and Social Services has proposed to end grant-aid to hostels for alcoholism, providing over 700 places for homeless people, during 1980. There is little chance that the local authorities of the United Kingdom will take over financial responsibility for these services when they have been ordered by central government to reduce their expenditures; see the letter from Richard Smith of the Bow Mission in London's East End, *Daily Telegraph*, 20 August 1979.

10. 'Mental Hospitals Will Close in 15 Years', *Guardian*, 8 December 1971; 'Mental Hospitals to be Swept Away', *Daily Mail*, 8 December 1971; 'Hospitals for the Mentally Ill to be Scrapped', *Daily Telegraph*, 8 December 1971: all reporting the gist of *Hospital Services for the Mentally Ill*, London, Department of Health and Social Services, December 1971. Ten years previously, the then Conservative Minister of Health, Enoch Powell, had envisaged the forthcoming demolition – again over the next decade and a half – of the old county asylums – 'isolated, majestic, imperious, brooded over by the gigantic water-tower and chimney combined, rising unmistakeable out of the countryside'. The same perspective of community-care provision in small local residential units – a 'colossal' undertaking of replacement, as he admitted – was outlined in this, the celebrated 'water-tower speech'. See *Co-ordination or Chaos? The Run-down of the Psychiatric Hospitals*, MIND Report no. 13, London, 1974.

11. Andrew T. Scull, *Decarceration: Community Treatment and the Deviant – A Radical View*, Englewood Cliffs, NJ, 1977.

12. See the following publications of the National Schizophrenia Fellowship, as an example of the havoc wrought among victims of the commonest severe mental disability: C. Creer and J.K. Wing, *Schizophrenia at Home*, London, 1974; *Living with Schizophrenia; by the Relatives*, London, 1974; D. Priestley, *Tied Together with String: A Two-Year Study of Care for the Schizophrenic*, London 1979.

13. *Better Services for the Mentally Ill*, DHSS, London, 1975, pp. 16, 40, ii, 83. The mental-health presure group MIND claimed that 116 out of 170 local authorities provided no residential places for the elderly mentally infirm (*Guardian*, 13 January 1976).

14. See the sections on women's self-help movements in J. Leeson and J. Gray, *Women and Medicine*, London, 1978, pp. 150–51, 190–96.

15. The argument is given, in considerable detail, in G.W. Brown and T. Harris, *Social Origins of Depression*, London, 1978, following a careful analysis of the personal and social situations of three samples of women (one drawn from a psychiatric register and two from the community at large). Although the subjects in this study were female, the authors regard their account of differential vulnerabilities leading to depression as having less

to do with sexual politics than with the differing life-chances conferred on individuals by social class.

16. For the latter position, see the works of Ivan Illich: *Medical Nemesis*, London, 1975, and its expanded version *The Limits of Medicine*, London, 1977. Illich advocates a programme of de-medicalising society, rendering individuals free to confront pain, sickness and death out of their own autonomous skills and resources rather than those of pretended experts. J. Ehrenreich (ed.), *The Cultural Crisis of Modern Medicine*, New York, 1978, has many important comments on the nature of medical reformism: see, in particular, its 'Introduction', pp. 1–35, the paper by B. and J. Ehrenreich, 'Medicine and Social Control', pp. 39–79, and the paper by I.K. Zola, 'Medicine as an Institution of Social Control', pp. 80–100. Zola remarks justly that, within the terms of his indictment, those criticisms of medicine as a social-control agency which insist on 'confining their concern to the field of psychiatry… have been misplaced. For psychiatry has by no means distorted the mandate of medicine, but indeed, though perhaps at a pace faster than other medical specialities, is following instead some of the basic claims and directions of that profession' (p. 80).
17. See, for example, R. Totman, *Social Causes of Illness*, London 1979; C. Herzlich, *Health and Illness, A Social Psychological Analysis*, London, 1974; R. Dingwall, *Aspects of Illness*, London, 1976. The stance of these texts varies from Dingwall's total questioning of the priority of medical explanations over folk-cultures of illness to Totman's attempt to integrate somatic approaches to the individual's health with a wider sense of the social rules that govern crisis and stress leading to breakdown. But these authors concur in seeing illness generally, and not simply psychiatric illness, as formed in the matrix of social behaviours.
18. J.K. Wing, *Reasoning About Madness*, Oxford, pp. 199–200. Scull (1977) documents the huge investment of the industry in the promotion of these psychochemicals (pp. 79–81).
19. The figures for mental-hospital resident patients are given in the *Annuaire Statistique de la France* published each year by the Institut National de la Statistique et des Etudes Economiques. The volumes for 1951, 1959, 1965, 1970/71 and 1975 reveal a rise in this patient total from 59,503 in 1944 to 83,396 in 1950, 101,278 in 1956, 113,430 in 1962 and 122,429 in 1969, following which the decline begins. For discussion of the post-war administrative currents in French psychiatry, the works of Robert Castel are indispensable: see e.g. 'Vers les nouvelles frontières de la medicine mentale', *Revue Française de la Sociologie*, vol. 14, 1973, 111–35.
20. F. Basaglia (ed.), *L'Instituzione Negata* (a collective report on Gorizia), Turin, 1968; M. Elkaim (ed.), *Réseau Alternative à la Psychiatrie: Collectif International*, Paris, 1977, pp. 146–47, 154–55 (Basaglia on Gorizia), 161–74 (Tommasini) and 175–93 (Jervis); S. Schmid, *Freiheilt Heilt: Bericht über die demokratischen Psychiatrie in Italien*, Berlin, 1977.

21. A. Maynard, *Health Care in the European Community*, London, 1975, pp. 181–82.
22. T. de Zulueta, 'No Patients – Just Consumers', *Guardian*, 20 November 1979.
23. Maynard, *op. cit.* pp. 28, 33, 41, 44.
24. T. Held, *Psychiatrie Politique: L'Affaire de Heidelberg (SPK)*, Paris, 1972, p. 123.
25. The mean patient-stay was 263 days in 1965, 259 days in 1973. See E. Gonzalez Duro, *La Asistencia Psiquiatrico, Cuadernos para el Dialogo*, Numero Extraordinario 46, May 1975, pp. 47–50; B. Gonzalez, *La Profesion Psiquiatrica en España, Doctor*, Barcelona, no. 150, May 1979. On the immobile character and traditionalist-authoritarian origins of psychiatry in Spain, Gonzalez Duro's book *Psiquiatria y Sociedad Autoritaria: España 1939–1975*, Madrid, 1978, is revelatory.
26. P. Westcott, *British Medical Journal*, 1979, 1, p. 989; H. Rollin, *ibid.* p. 1775.
27. The case is a dense and careful one, given for Britain in Scull, 1979, pp. 18–48 and more generally in Scull, 1977, pp. 15–40, references in notes 11 and 8 above.
28. Scull, 1977, reference in note 11 above, pp. 135–51. The financial assumptions of Scull's argument are queried in R. Matthews, "'De-carceration" and the Fiscal Crisis', in B. Fine, *et al.* (eds.), *Capitalism and the Rule of Law: From Deviancy Theory to Marxism*, London, 1979, pp. 100–17. It is not obvious to Matthews that a switch to community care would save the state any money since this would require additional resources on top of the (largely) fixed costs of the institution. As against this view, see the remarks by a publicist for the 'community care' programme of Napsbury Hospital, Hertfordshire: 'as more and more patients are integrated in the community, Napsbury Hospital has been able to close two-thirds of its admission wards... This reduction in bed occupancy represents a saving of a quarter of a million pounds each year' (L. Ratna, 'Crisis Intervention in Psychiatry', *CHC News*, March 1979).
29. Cambridge, Mass., 1973; a subsequent partial re-working by J.R. Marshall and D.P. Funch ('Mental Illness and the Economy: A Critique and Partial Replication', *Journal of Health and Social Behavior*, vol. 20, 1979, pp. 282–89), using New York State mental-hospital admission statistics over 1916–55, broadly confirms Brenner's findings for the patients of working age. Below the age of 15 and above 65, fluctuations in admission relate less to economic conditions and more to the state of mental-hospital provision.
30. Jervis records that in Bologna and Reggio Emilia the effect of the national economic crisis of the early 70s was to halt all attempts at creating community facilities as an alternative to the mental hospital; the trade unions and the Communist Party became much more conservative in their demands and welfare spending became concentrated increasingly on the old institutions (Elkaim, *op. cit.* pp. 188–89).
31. D. Widgery, *Health in Danger*, London, 1979, pp. 51–52.

32. Without providing a satisfactory complement of doctors and nurses (and, ultimately, of patients) earmarked for them; see the 1977 report of the *Cour des Comptes* on the over-provision of mental-hospital beds in France, summarised in C. Brisset, 'Une France Suréquipée', the second part of a series of 'Faut-il raser les hôpitaux psychiatriques?', *Le Monde*, 3 September 1980.

33. Scull, 1977, pp. 129–30. Equally, in Britain during the course of the 1870s, the Poor Law Board fought a successful battle to prevent the provision of dispensaries for the poor who were not in the workhouses. In this campaign against outdoor relief in general medicine, it became the duty of the local Poor Law officer 'to see the patient before the doctor so that he could force the patient into an institution as a condition of receiving medical relief' (B. Abel-Smith, *The Hospitals*, London, 1964, pp. 85–89).

34. G.V. Rimlinger, *Welfare Policy and industrialization in Europe, America and Russia*, New York, 1971.

35. Such is the principal approach to ideological challenges to his own position offered in J.K. Wing's otherwise helpful *Reasoning About Madness.*

36. S.H. Foulkes, On Group Analysis', *International Journal of Psychoanalysis*, vol. 27, 1946, p. 51.

37. For a history of this movement, see D.H. Clark, *Administrative Therapy: The Role of the Doctor in the Therapeutic Community*, London, 1964; and the works of Maxwell Jones himself.

38. R.D. Laing, *The Facts of Life*, New York, 1976, p. 122. Further reference to Laing's work in rehabilitation at this stage is made in chapter 4.

39. K. Lewin, *Resolving Social Conflicts*, New York, 1948. See the critique by H.S. Kariel, 'Democracy Unlimited: Kurt Lewin's Field Theory', *American Journal of Sociology*, vol. 62, 1956, pp. 280–89.

40. E.g. A.H. Stanton and M. Schwartz, *The Mental Hospital*, New York, 1954; M. Greenblatt, R.H. York and E.L. Brown, *From Custodial to Therapeutic Patient Care in Mental Hospitals: Explorations in Social Treatment*, New York, 1955; W.A. Caudell, *The Psychiatric Hospital as a Small Society*, Cambridge, MA, 1958.

41. *Symposium on Preventive and Social Psychiatry, 15–17 April 1957*, Walter Reed Army Institute of Research, Washington, DC, 1958.

42. Maxwell Jones, 'The Therapeutic Community, Social Learning and Social Change', in R.D. Hinshelwood and N. Manning, (eds.), *Therapeutic Communities: Reflections and Progress*, London, 1979, pp. 2–3; and *Beyond the Therapeutic Community*, New Haven, 1968.

43. S. Whiteley, 'Progress and Reflection', in Hinshelwood and Manning, *op. cit.*, p. 21. A further discussion of the ethical and political background to therapeutic communities is to be found on E. Jansen (ed.) *The Therapeutic Community*, London, 1980, with a strong emphasis in Elly Jansen's work with the Richmond Fellowship.

44. R. Castel, *Génèse et ambiguités de la notion de secteur en psychiatrie*, *Sociologie du Travail*, vol. 17, 1975, pp. 57–77.

45. Castel, *loc cit.* pp. 67–71, and the same author's *Le Psychoanalysme*, Paris, 1973.

46. L. Schittar, *L'ideologia della comunita terapeutica*, followed by a team discussion of 27 November 1969, pp. 153–78 in Basaglia, *op. cit.*

47. G. Jervis, *Le mythe de l'antipsychiatrie*, Paris, 1977, pp. 29–30.

48. Powell's resignation on monetarist grounds in January 1958 along with Nigel Birch and their mentor as Chancellor, Peter Thorneycroft, is hailed by the Thatcherite wing of modern Toryism as the founding act of post-war economic rationality in Britain. See G. Hutchinson, *The Last Edwardian at No. 10: An Impression of Harold Macmillan*, London, 1980.

49. On California's particularly intense activity in the running down of mental hospitals (from 50,000 in-patients in 1955 to 7,000 by 1973) see Scull, 1977, pp. 69, 73, 157–59, reference in note 11 above. S.I. Hayakawa, Reagan's own nominee to the headship of San Francisco State University and subsequently California's rabid rightist Senator, became a supporter of Thomas Szasz's American Association for the Abolition of Involuntary Mental Hospitalization, giving the keynote address at its first annual meeting in October 1971 (*The Abolitionist*, vol. 1, no. 1, 1971, p. 1).

50. L. Mosher, 'Social Barriers to Innovation', paper presented to the conference on 'Madness and Social Policy' held in Palo Alto, California, 17–19 June 1977.

51. Whiteley, *loc. cit.* p. 22.

52. Siegfried Hausner, another SPK member, received a three-year sentence at the trial in December 1972: see SPK, *Aus der Krankeit eine Waffe zu machen*, Munich, 1972. I have used the French version, *Faire de la Maladie une Arme, Paris,* 1973, and the documents collected by Tilo Held, *Psychiatrie Politique: L'affaire de Heidelberg* (SPK), Paris, 1972. While the SPK's theoretical position ('Illness and capital are identical: the intensity and extent of illness multiply in proportion to the accumulation process of dead capital') was highly involved, its practice, consisting of a multiplicity of patient peer-groups alternating with one-to-one therapy sessions or 'individual agitations', seems to have been simply and sensibly conceived and was quite conformable with the traditions of the therapeutic community as developed in more liberal societies. In the conditions of the German Federal Republic in the early seventies, which were marked by the polarisation between an extra-parliamentary student left and the conservative public opinion orchestrated by the hysteria of the Springer Press, the SPK became first marginalised and then effectively criminalised.

53. Interview with Félix Guattari, *Le Monde, 20* December 1979. On methods of La Clinique de La Borde, see J.C. Polack and D. Sabourin, *La Borde ou le droit à la folie*, preface by F. Guattari and J. Oury, 1976, and S. Turkle, *Psychoanalytic Politics*, New York, 1978, pp. 155–57.

54. Whiteley, *loc. cit.* pp. 15, 16.

55. I am indebted for this summary to the first chapter of D.G. Race and D.M. Race, *The Cherries Group Home: A Beginning*, London, 1979, an illuminating research report on a residential project for mentally-handicapped adults.

56. The most startling example of the latter being the Conservative William van Straubenzee's onslaught on Smythe (made under Parliamentary privilege) as a 'full-time agitator' whose 'interests lie on the side of the Irish Republican Army': this apropos of some publicity given by MIND to allegations (some of them later acknowledged to be true) that ECT was administered without anaesthetic precautions by members of the staff of Broadmoor special hospital, situated in Mr van Straubenzee's constituency. See 'Troubled MIND is Hit by a New Rumpus', *Sunday Times*, 25 May 1980.
57. Volume 1 of *A Human Condition*, sub-titled *The Mental Health Act from 1959 to 1975: Observations, Analysis and Proposals for Reform*, was published by MIND in 1975, and its sequel of the same title, Volume 2: *The Law Relating to Mentally Abnormal Offenders* in 1977.
58. Details of the project and its director are given in B.J. Ennis, *Prisoners of Psychiatry* (introduced by T.S. Szasz, M.D.), New York, 1972, and B.J. Ennis and L. Siegel, *The Rights of Mental Patients*, New York, 1973.
59. Thirty-seven court decisions within State or Federal jurisdiction are listed in Ennis and Siegel (*op. cit.* pp. 300–05), several of them in response to class actions filed as part of litigation projects such as theirs. Other important rulings have followed; e.g. the Supreme Court edict (*Donaldson vs. Connor*, 1975) to the effect that the state cannot confine a non-dangerous mental patient who is capable of surviving independently (*Psychiatric News*, 16 July 1975); and the judgement of October 1979, by a Federal District Court in Massachusetts, granting the right of committed mental patients to refuse anti-psychotic medication (see P.S. Appelbaum and T.G. Gutheil, 'The Boston State Hospital Case: The Constitution and "the Right to Rot"' *American Journal of Psychiatry*, vol. 137, 1980, pp. 720–23.)
60. Ennis, *op. cit.* pp. 244–53. Seldom has the link between the Powell-Joseph scheme of de-hospitalisation (in Britain) and the Reaganites' own plans for California been shown more clearly.
61. Gostin interviewed by M. Dean, 'Caring in the Courts', *Guardian*, 9 April 1980. Lucy Warner, contributing a note 'USA: Mental Patients' Rights' in *New Society*, 19 June 1980, reports a growing use of criminal law against patients since involuntary committment and compulsory treatment were curtailed: 'In California, arrests and convictions of the mentally ill have increased dramatically… While most charges are minor, bail is routinely denied.'
62. 'New Group Launched to Help Handicapped', *The Times*, 12 June 1981.
63. The Annual Reviews of MIND (National Association for Mental Health) provide a conspectus of the wide range of national and regional activities conducted by the organisation, as does MIND OUT, the bi-monthly produced by it.
64. In *The Second Sin*, London, 1974, p. 79; and *passim* in other works.
65. M. Lader, *Psychiatry on Trial*, Harmondsworth, 1977, p. 12.
66. C. Richards, 'The Crisis of Mental Illness in the Home', *New Society*, 10 April 1980.

67. For a history of this medical hegemony in British asylums, see A.T. Scull, 'From Madness to Mental Illness: Medical Men as Moral Entrepreneurs', *Archives Européenes de Sociologie*, vol. 16, 1975, pp. 218–61; for France, R. Castel, *L'Ordre psychiatrique: l'âge d'or de l'aliénisme*, Paris, 1976, pp. 60–127, 140–218. An important discussion of the role of medical authority in relation to 'para-medical' workers in British psychiatry is provided by N. Goldie, 'The Division of Labour among the Mental Health Professions: A Negotiated or An Imposed Order?', in M. Stacey, C. Heath and R. Dingwall (eds.), *Health and the Division of Labour*, London, 1977, pp. 141–62.

68. See *Handicapés Méchants*, the journal produced in Paris by the CLH, and *L'Exclu*, the organ of the Mouvement dê Defénse des Handicapés, for reports of these demonstrations and meetings.

69. 'Since we have received quite a few "refugees" from psychiatric clinics, we feel that our methods can equal many of the other ones. As per usual there has been little response [from a talk given to medical staff], for doctors are so SURE that their methods are superior': *Depressives Associated* (bimonthly newsletter), no. 9, April-May 1979.

70. For an account of the over-burdening of one such network, see M. Barnett, *People Not Psychiatry*, London, 1973.

71. From B. Boynton and S. Young, 'Red Therapy', *Humpty Dumpty: Radical Psychology Magazine*, no. 8, no date.

72. See, for instance, the three 'People's Psychiatry Sheets', dealing with general psychiatric emergencies, common drug emergencies, and suicide attempts, given in J. Agel (ed.), *Rough Times*, New York, 1973, pp. 151–66, reprinted from the 'alternative therapy' journal, *The Radical Therapist*.

73. I am aware that the Co-Counselling movement, with other forms of peer-counselling, forms a strong exception to this trend; but it constitutes, in the main, a formalised buddy-system for the normal, rather than a distinct therapy for problems of a psychiatric specificity.

74. Whose founding programme of late 1971 is reprinted in Agel, *op. cit.* pp. 60–63 as well as in P. Brown (ed.), *Radical Psychology*, London, 1973, pp. 521–25.

75. For an account of the founding of NAPA, and its successful campaign to limit the use of ECT by physicians in California, see L.R. Frank (ed.) *The History of Shock Treatment*, London, 1978, pp. ix–x, 146–52.

76. In Agel, *op. cit.* p. 63: Brown, *op. cit.* p. 524.

77. For a history of crisis clinics in the United States, and a comparative study of such centres in Europe, see J.E. Cooper, *Crisis Admission Units and Emergency Psychiatric Services*, WHO Regional Office for Europe, Public Health in Europe no. 11, Copenhagen, 1979. The bibliography is good.

78. Cooper, *op. cit.* p. 91.

79. J-L. Poisson, 'La Situation en France', in M. Elkaim, *op. cit.* p. 274; for the GIA movement, see also the review *Gardes-fous*, no. 1, February-March 1974, with documents (pp. 15–19) from GIA of the 17th arrondissement.

80. First published in its complete version in *Gardes-fous*, no. 8, Winter 1976, following a conference of the GIA's with other dissident mental-health

groups; and reprinted in Elkaim, *op. cit.*, pp. 258–61 and in N. Boulanger and J.F. Chaix, *Travail, Famille, Patrie*, Paris, 1977, pp. 223–28.

81. Reported briefly in *Le Monde*, 22 September 1977 in its account of the third (Trieste) meeting of the Réseau International d'Alternative à la Psychiatrie, which gathered a number of patient groups and radicalised professionals from several countries.
82. Elkaim, *op. cit.* pp. 253–56.
83. The MPUs Declaration of Intent, a set of 25 demands, is available in mimeographed form, and is printed in translation in *Gardes-fous*, special international issue, April 1975, pp. 39–41 along with some background briefing. A useful interview with several MPU activists in Hackney is given in *Humpty Dumpty*, nos. 6–7, no date but probably 1975, pp. 6–10.
84. See Elkaim, *op. cit.* pp. 261–64 for the aims of the Brussels GIA in this direction; and the *Humpty Dumpty* interview with the Mental Patients' Union members for a short account of the two residential households organised by them in London in this period.
85. A useful short treatment of these problems in a historical context is in M. Carpenter, *All for One: Campaigns and Pioneers in the Making of COHSE*, London, 1980 (a series of sketches in the development of the Confederation of Health Service Employees from its origins in such predecessors as the National Asylum Workers' Union, the Mental Hospital and Institutional Workers' Union and the Poor Law Workers' Trade Union).
86. See P. Good, 'Something Should Be Done', *Freedom*, vol. 40, no. 21, 17 November 1979, vol. 40, no. 21, for an account of this campaign, defeated after some particularly treacherous and discreditable management tactics, and culminating in the sacking of the leading militants.
87. See the interview by Terry Kelly of Derbyshire COHSE in *Militant*, 9 May 1980.
88. Scull, 1977, pp. 73, 75, reference in note 11 above.
89. D.H. Bennett, *The Changing Pattern in Mental Health Care in Trieste*, WHO Regional Office for Europe, Copenhagen, 1979, p. 2.
90. The special international issue of *Gardes-fous* (April 1975, pp. 27–36) has an interview with a psychiatrist-member of Basaglia's team covering the problems of de-hierarchising a health service from above, with special attention to trade-union divisions.
91. Gostin, 1977, pp. 49–51, reference in note 57 above.
92. In both cases, COHSE staffed the units and eventually the Rainhill branch of NUPE followed suit; Gostin, *op. cit.* p. 141 and L. Knights, 'Secure Units: Fact or Fiction?', *Mind Out*, no. 33, March-April 1979.
93. When, at a rally of one British revolutionary-left group in 1976, I argued the above position, I was met with a riposte accusing me of opposing 'the way COHSE members have refused to handle excessively violent patients'. An article in the health-workers' bulletin of the group took the view that 'we should support these members… They are taking this action to *defend their conditions of work*.' *I.S. Health Fraction Bulletin*, no date but probably May 1976, 'Mental Illness – What is the Revolutionary Position?'.

95. Interview in *Morning Star*, 20 August 1980. The hospital had experienced the killing of a psychiatric nurse by a patient – who was not, however, held there under any of the compulsory sections of the Mental Health Act against which the staff were operating their admissions ban.

95. P. Hunter, *Schizophrenia and Community Psychiatric Nursing*, Surbiton, 1978, pp. 61, 70, 71, 85. This extremely valuable pamphlet, published by the National Schizophrenia Fellowship, concludes with some suggestions on how mental-nursing visitors – some of whom have acquired a repertoire of counselling skills on their own – might be sensitised to a more social approach through a systematic training.

96. J-L. Poisson (Elkaim, *op. cit.*, p. 270) cites five examples 'out of a hundred which could be mentioned.'

97. Turkle, *op. cit.* pp. 157–59. Some patient groups, such as the GIA have of course refused any common membership with treatment staff, however enlightened.

98. I have been able to consult only a booklet produced by the Valencian section, *Per Una Nova Psiquiatria* (Valencia, 1978), which surveys the problems of a local traditional asylum and admits to some powerlessness in the face of backward welfare structure of the province.

99. P. Schrag and D. Divoky, *The Myth of the Hyperactive Child*, New York, 1975; P. Conrad, *Identifying Hyperactive Children: The Medicalization of Deviant Behaviour*, Lexington, 1976; S. Box, 'Hyperactivity: The Scandalous Silence', *New Society*, 1 December 1977, and correspondence in the 8 and 15 December 1977 and 5 January 1978 issues.

100. Box's article in *New Society* (note 99 above), critical of the very concept of hyperactivity, was assailed in subsequent letters to the journal by N. Tinbergen, the emeritus zoology professor from Oxford, and by D. Bryce-Smith, the professor of organic chemistry at Reading University, for its alleged tendency to minimise what both scholars regarded as a very real link between behavioural abnormality in children and impure food (Tinbergen) or lead ingestion (Bryce-Smith). On the hazards of lead intoxication in exposing children to hazards of poor learning and bad behaviour, see the excellent study by H.L. Needleman, C. Gunnoe, A. Leviton, R. Reed, H. Peresie, C. Maher and P. Barrett, 'Deficits in Psychologic and Classroom Performance by Children with Elevated Dentine Lead Levels', *New England Journal of Medicine*, vol. 300, 1979, pp. 689–94. While there was a relevantly infrequent rating of the children on a question about 'hyperactivity', there is some relation between its incidence and the children's dentine-lead burden. Other negative ratings (by teachers), on such factors as 'distractibility', were even more definitely dose-related to lead ingestion in the child.

101. P. Chesler, *Women and Madness*, London, 1974, p. 309, summarising a lengthy argument in earlier sections.

102. See the many articles by Walter Gove and his collaborators, e.g. W.R. Gove and J. Tudor, 'Adult Sex Roles and Mental Illness', *American Journal* *of Sociology*, vol. 77, 1973, pp. 812–35. These have been criticised, however on several grounds, such as their excluding from consideration the more male-related diagnostic categories (personality disorders, alcoholism). It has been argued, as an alternative account of the sex-relatedness of psychiatric illness, that women are more prone than men to depressive disorders, and conversely men more inclined to personality disorders of an anti-social description (D.P. Dohrenwend and B.S. Dohrenwend, 'Sex Differences in Psychiatric Disorder', *American Journal of Sociology*, vol. 81, 1976, pp. 1447–54). But one recent study has compared married women and men for the incidence of depressive illness in two types of marital relationship, one where the wife has a job and the other where her sole work-function consists of household labour; it is only in the latter case that wives had a higher frequency of depressive symptoms than husbands (S. Rosenfield, 'Sex Differences in Depression: Do Women Always Have Higher Rates?', *Journal of Health and Social Behavior*, vol. 21, 1980, pp. 33–42). The sample is small, but the result of the study indicates how misleading it can be to make sweeping generalisations about the sexual politics of psychiatric illness.

103. Chesler, *op. cit.* p. 108.
104. E.g. Leeson and Gray, *op. cit.* p. 161–63.
105. One careful study of different samples of university students seeking psychiatric or counselling assistance with emotional problems revealed a greater propensity for women to seek help even when the intensity of their distress (as measured, admittedly with some coarseness, by questionnaire) was held constant in the comparison. But the attribute 'having a father with postgraduate education' also yielded great help-seeking from these youngsters – an indicator at least as ambiguous as that of the gender of the help-seeker: J.R. Greenley and D. Mechanic, 'Patterns of Seeking Care for Psychological Problems', D. Mechanic *et al.*, *The Growth of Bureaucratic Medicine*, New York, 1976, pp. 177–96.
106. D. Mebane-Francescato and S. Jones, 'Radical Psychiatry in Italy: "Love is Not Enough"', in Agel, *op. cit.* p. 47.
107. M. Seem and J. Parkin, '"Santé Mentale" et Technologie de normalisation', in Elkaim *op. cit.* pp. 430–31.
108. Re-translated from the French text given in *Gardes-fous*, special international issue, April' 1975, pp. 55 (for the SPK) and 38 (for the MPU).
109. D. Cooper, *The Language of Madness*, London, 1978, p. 145.
110. For this last point, and for some of the discussion in the previous paragraph, I am indebted to Ursula Huws.
111. See, for example, *Schizophrenia from Within*, an anthology of autobiographical reports by patients, edited by John Wing for the NSF in 1975.
112. P. Hain and S. Hebditch, *Radicals and Socialism*, Nottingham, 1978, pp. 9–10.
113. D.B. Weiner, 'The Apprenticeship of Philippe Pinél: A New Document, "Observations of Citizen Pussin on the Insane"', *American Journal of Psychiatry*, vol. 136, 1979, pp. 1128–34. Gladys Swain (in *Le Sujet de la Folie:*

Naissance de la Psychiatrie, Toulouse, 1977) has sagely analysed the legend of Pinel as doctor-liberator.

114. See R.N. Baldwin (ed.), *Kropotkin's Revolutionary Pamphlets*, New York, 1970, pp. 219–35.

115. P. Kropotkin, *Mutual Aid: A Factor of Evolution*, London, 1908, pp. 194–95.

116. P. Kropotkin, *The Conquest of Bread*, London, 1906, pp. 179–85.

117. Kropotkin, 1908, *op. cit.* p. 282.

118. I have drawn on the papers, by several knowledgeable authors, in J.K. Wing and R. Olsen (eds.), *Community Care for the Mentally Disabled*, Oxford, 1979, as well as Wing's paper 'Innovations in Social Psychiatry', *Psychological Medicine*, vol. 10, 1980, pp. 219–30. Joseph Berke's *Butterfly Man: Madness, Degradation and Redemption* (London, 1977) is also useful.

119. Race and Race, *op. cit.* (reference in note no. 55 above). There is a film available for public showing about The Cherries project; it includes the wedding of 'Cathy' and 'Richard'.

120. P. Ryan, 'Residential Care for the Mentally Disabled' and J. Leach, 'Providing for the Destitute' in Wing and Olsen, *op. cit.* pp. 60–89 and 90–105. For Italy some bare details of the 116 small patient communities that replaced the asylum at Parma are given in Tommasini's 1977 interview (Elkaim, *op. cit.* pp. 169–70), without evaluation.

121. National Schizophrenia Fellowship, *Home Sweet Nothing*, Surbiton, 1979.

122. Kropotkin, 1908, *op. cit.* pp. 227, 228.

123. *Better Services for the Mentally Ill*, pp. 14, ii.

124. *Priorities for Health and Social Services in England*, Department of Health and Social Security, London, 1976, p. 57.

125. In one study of the outcome of spending decisions on 'joint funding' projects in a sample of 14 Area Health Authorities, very little expenditure was found to be taking place on community-based housing for mental illness: D. Wilson, 'Joint Financing: Where Does All The Money Go?', *Health and Social Service Journal*, 28 April 1978.

126. E. Roosens, *Mental Patients in Town Life: Geel – Europe's First Therapeutic Community*, Beverly Hills, Calif., 1979. Other studies, cited by Roosens, have appeared in Flemish and French.

127. *loc. cit.* p. 234.

128. Roosens, *op. cit.* p. 76.

Index